MW00835545

The Successful Completion of Your DNP Project

HOW TO ORDER THIS BOOK

BY PHONE: 866-401-4337 or 717-290-1660, 8AM–5PM Eastern Time

BY FAX: 717-509-6100

BY MAIL: Order Department
DEStech Publications, Inc.
439 North Duke Street
Lancaster, PA 17602, U.S.A.

BY CREDIT CARD: VISA, MasterCard, American Express, Discover, PayPal

BY WWW SITE: http://www.destechpub.com

The Successful Completion of Your DNP Project

A Practical Guide with Exemplars

Edited by

Mary A. Bemker, PhD, PsyS, MSN, LPCC, CNE, RN
Core Faculty, College of Nursing, Walden University

Christine M. Ralyea, DNP, MS-NP, MBA, NE-BC, CNL, OCN, CCRN-Alumnus
Chief Nursing Officer, Prisma Health-Baptist and Baptist Parkridge
Queens University Adjunct Faculty
University of South Carolina Adjunct Faculty

Barb Schreiner, PhD, RN, CDCES, BC-ADM
Education Specialist and Independent Consultant

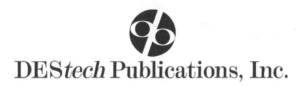

DEStech Publications, Inc.

The Successful Completion of Your DNP Project

DEStech Publications, Inc.
439 North Duke Street
Lancaster, Pennsylvania 17602 U.S.A.

Copyright © 2022 by DEStech Publications, Inc.
All rights reserved

No part of this publication may be reproduced, stored in a
retrieval system, or transmitted, in any form or by any means,
electronic, mechanical, photocopying, recording, or otherwise,
without the prior written permission of the publisher.

Printed in the United States of America
10 9 8 7 6 5 4 3 2 1

Main entry under title:
    The Successful Completion of Your DNP Project: A Practical
    Guide with Exemplars

A DEStech Publications book
Bibliography: p.
Includes index p. 367

Library of Congress Control Number: 2021938161
ISBN No. 978-1-60595-569-8

Table of Contents

PART 2: EDUCATION EXEMPLARS

Chapter 6. Exemplar for Educational Practice: A Collegial Mentoring Program **127**
LAURA M. SCHWARZ

PART 3: CLINICAL EXEMPLARS

Chapter 7. Increase Advance Directives Knowledge Among African Americans in the Faith-Based Organization **149**
KOTAYA GRIFFITH

Chapter 8. Exploring the Effectiveness of Sepsis Protocol in the Emergency Department: A Quality Improvement Project **163**
JAYANTHI HENRY

Foreword

It is my distinct pleasure to introduce you to *The Successful Completion of your DNP Project: A Practical Guide with Exemplars*. Over the last decade, the number of Doctor of Nursing Practice (DNP) programs, student enrollments, and graduates from DNP programs has increased substantially across the United States. Today's healthcare environment is highly complex, and nurses with a professional doctorate must be able to readily translate evidence into practice to improve outcomes. The practical value of this book is that it will better prepare DNP students to complete meaningful final projects and disseminate their findings to other healthcare professionals. Additionally, students will become more marketable after having completed projects that are designed to translate evidence and improve clinical outcomes.

Since the inception of the DNP program in 2004, I have taught several DNP classes, worked with DNP students in planning their projects, and have served on several DNP committees. I was fortunate to be a part of the development of some of early DNP programs and the development of guidelines for DNP projects. In my experience as an educator, one of the most stressful parts of any DNP program, other than statistics of course, is the DNP project—from topic selection to dissemination. However, nursing programs continue to improve the final project experience and are exploring new ways of meeting requirements for this project. This book embodies these improvements by providing a clear framework for developing final projects, along with exemplars of actual student projects to provide a point of reference for DNP students.

The editors of this book are all highly accomplished professionals who have generated new nursing knowledge in their careers and have translated existing evidence into practice. They have all mentored students in doctoral education programs, and they are exemplary professionals who strive to provide the best possible education to their students. This book draws on their combined experiences to provide a valuable roadmap explaining how to successfully complete the DNP project from start to finish. This book is extremely relevant to all DNP students, because their peers provide examples of projects they have completed and assist them in mitigating the challenges in the journey to ensure high quality projects and dissemination of outcomes. Additionally, when graduates of DNP programs are applying for jobs, they can use their projects as an example of work they completed to improve clinical outcomes, develop policy, enhance nursing education, and advance nursing practice.

Every DNP student should read *The Successful Completion of Your DNP Project: A Practical Guide with Exemplars* to learn from their peers' experiences and become better prepared to enter the DNP project journey. The requirements for the DNP project vary from school to school. However, this book provides a standard approach for success in any DNP program. If students take the time to read this book, they will be fully prepared to focus on and complete the DNP project in a reasonable timeframe. This book is exactly what DNP students need to be successful in their respective programs and to conduct projects that will demonstrate their abilities to translate evidence into practice.

GEORGE A. ZANGARO, PHD, RN, FAAN
The American Association of the Colleges of Nursing

Preface

The Successful Completion of Your DNP Project: A Practical Guide with Exemplars is written as both a reference and practical guide for DNP students. It offers an overview of the Doctor of Nursing Practice (DNP) project and has the depth needed to be a reference source for students and practitioners alike. With changes in curriculum and nomenclature, this text offers a clear differentiation between the DNP, Ph.D., EdD, and other terminal degrees related to advanced practice nursing. This book shares important information about why selecting the DNP as a terminal degree is practical and how this degree differs from other terminal degrees offered to nurses. If one is interested in research, the student would be guided early to seek out a degree that is culminated into a dissertation. However, if one is interested in taking current research, applying it to practice, seeking successful outcomes and generating big data, then the DNP degree is right for that student.

This text offers a clear understanding of the DNP degree as it builds upon evidence-based practice (EBP), and the eight essentials (CCNE) or five standards (NLN) that serve as the underpinning of their particular program's accreditation. Regardless of the specific accreditation obtained at their institute of study, the DNP degree supports the nurse's ability to take EBP from the review of the literature and apply it in practice to advance care delivery, healthcare systems, nursing education, policy development, or nursing practice.

Within this text, content is shared on how to successfully complete a DNP project start to finish. With the use of project exemplars in leadership, education, clinical, and policy development, efforts are inclusive of how to overcome barriers with a review of the literature, narrowing the topic, getting through the institutional review board, data analysis, developing and working from an outline for a project, and dissemination of findings. Exemplars are included by recent DNP graduates from across the nation to provide an array of examples of accomplished DNP projects. These exemplars also demonstrate how to complete a DNP process successfully (both in the school and within the clinical setting). Dissemination of the DNP project process and findings by recent graduates also affords the DNP graduate and practitioner a new array of insights focusing on multiple areas of nursing (education, leadership and clinical practice). Specific criteria as to how one can discover opportunities for dissemination are included. Practical insights as to successful application and delivery of findings are also noted in this text.

From an earlier version of this text, questions were received from students regarding the selection of a mentor or advisor for their DNP project. Students also wanted to know how to develop a strong collaborative relationship with the mentor. Specific tips were requested for polishing or completing their DNP project. Based on these common questions, a survey was completed, and some suggestions were provided with answers to these very questions and more.

Topics often do not fit exclusively within one area of a textbook. Because of this, many common threads are noted throughout the book. The history of the DNP degree is intertwined with policy and the DNP curriculum. Therefore, content related to these topics is addressed in more than one area of the book. In addition, references to exemplars for understanding through the specific application is highlighted. By using these strategies, readers of this text will have the advantage of an integrated, as well as a specialized examination of key areas, linked to the DNP project.

Words of Wisdom from students who have successfully navigated the DNP project provide a glimpse of their struggles and how they overcame these barriers. Thus, the reader has guidance from those who have completed the process and reflected on what would have made their journey easier. Additionally, Chapter 19 was added to explain the collaboration between the mentor and student. Both perspectives are shared to guide the students to success and could also be used by a new DNP prepared nurse moving into their advanced role.

This book will offer DNP students and those considering this terminal degree practical guides for making the best choice for the DNP degree and success with their DNP project, including selecting their topic and committee, through completion with dissemination of their hard work. Each of the three editors and these authors are dedicated to advance the profession, elevate the practice of nursing, and make a difference. This book will afford others to learn and stimulate the commitment to excellence.

MARY BEMKER
CHRISTINE RALYEA
BARB SCHREINER

Contributors

Obed Asif, DNP, RN

Shawana Burnette, DNP, RNC-OB, NEA-BC, CLNC
Nurse Manager
Atrium Health- Carolinas Medical Center

Gerlyn Campbell, DNP, APRN, PMHNP. RN

Fred Cantor, DNP, RN

Colleen Crosby, DNP, MS, RN, NE-BC
Clinical Director of Nursing
Norther GI Endoscopy

Selena A. Gilles, DNP, ANP-BC, CNEcl, CCRN

Nicholas M. Green, DNP, RN
Alumnus CCRN
Curry College School of Nursing

Kotaya Griffith, DNP, MSN, APRN, AGNP-C, CNL
Atrium Health—Senior Care
East Carolina University Faculty

Staci J. Harrison, DNP, RN
Director of Adult Care Services
Regional Patient Care Services
Southern California
Kaiser Foundation Hospitals

Theresa Katerina Haley, DNP, MSN-ED, MSN-FNP, NP-C

Jayanthi Henry, DNP, RN-BC, CIC
Nursing Professor

Lina Najib Kawar, PhD, RN, CNS
Nurse Scientist
Translational Research; Regional Nursing Research Program
Southern California Patient Care Services
Kaiser Permanente

Patrick S. LaRose, DNP, MSN/Ed, RN
Associate Professor, Doctor of Nursing Practice Degree Program
Chamberlain University College of. Nursing

Nancyruth Leibold, EdD, RN, MSN, PHN, CNE, AHN-BC
Southwest Minnesota State University
Department of Nursing

Jennie Pattison, DNP, RN, CNE
Assistant Professor
Chamberlain College of Nursing

Veronica Rankin, DNP, RN-BC, NP-C, CNL, NE-BC
Magnet Program Director/Clinical Nurse Leader Program Administrator
Atrium Health—Carolinas Medical Center
Queens University Adjunct Faculty

Laura Schwarz, DNP, RN, PHN CNE, AHN-BC
Professor, Nursing
Minnesota State University, Mankato

Audrey A. Sutton-Taylor, DNP, RN
Nurse Educator
Brooke Army Medical Center

Jill S. Walsh, DNP, RN, CEN, NEA-BC, RN
Dean, Doctor of Nursing Practice Degree Program
Chamberlain University College of Nursing

Part 1: Introduction to DNP Completion

CHAPTER 1

What Is a DNP?

NANCYRUTH LEIBOLD, EDD, RN, MSN, PHN, CNE, AHN-BC

The development of the Doctor of Nursing Practice (DNP) as a terminal degree is fairly recent and dynamic. The DNP emphasizes advanced clinical nursing practice (AACN, 2006a; ANA, 2011) in a variety of settings, across the lifespan, and in a variety of roles. The initial clinical doctorate in nursing was the Nursing Doctorate (ND) (AACN, 1996). Later, this evolved into a practice doctorate and transformed into the DNP. The DNP degree addresses the changing health care climate and needs of society, especially related to advanced clinical leadership, a focus on patient-centered care, and improving health care systems to improve patient safety. The transformation of the practice doctorate in nursing parallels a swift growth in the number of DNP programs available. Due to health care reform and recommendations by the Institute of Medicine (2003a), nurses are being prepared to lead in complex health care systems to improve patient outcomes. Some have raised concerns about the roles of the DNP, such as the faculty role (Kelly, 2010). The faculty role was not one of the original roles for the DNP. However, the intent of the Doctor of Philosophy (PhD) was directed toward the research role, so many PhD programs do not provide nurse educator courses. Therefore, graduates of both programs wishing to pursue the faculty role may take additional nurse educator courses as needed (AACN, 2006). This chapter will address what the DNP is and what it is not. Also included is a background discussion of the DNP topic, including a historical perspective of doctoral degrees in nursing, the types of doctorate degrees for nurses, and history of events leading up to the DNP. Exemplars of final DNP student projects, which relate to the AACN (2006) DNP essentials, are included in this text. Additionally, DNP roles, practice settings, DNP outcomes, and future work are given.

THE DNP VERSUS PHD?

There are two types of nursing doctorates: the research concentrated doctorate and the practice focused doctorate. The core of the research doctorate is original research, whereas a practice doctorate prepares the nurse for an advanced level of evidence-based practice, quality improvement, and leadership in a practice setting. The EdD is the research doctorate focused on preparing the nurse for an academic role. There are some DNP programs that include nurse educator content (NLN, 2013). The research doctorates include EdD, PhD, DNSc, DSN, and the DNS, whereas the clinical doctorate is the ND and the practice doctorates are the DrNP and DNP. It is important to determine the focus a nurse wants to pursue to know if the research doctorate or the practice doctorate is the best individual choice. The following sections in the chapter describe the degrees, focus, and role options.

TYPES OF DOCTORATE DEGREES FOR NURSES

There are several doctorate degrees for nurses (see Table 1.1). The evolution of these degrees is important to understand in the context of how the DNP came about. Nursing education has an active role in the development and advancement of the discipline of nursing.

Educational Doctorate

The Educational Doctorate (EdD) has a variety of majors, such as a major in Educational Leadership, Nursing Education, or Education of Health Care Professionals. The first doctorate in nursing, an EdD in

TABLE 1.1. Doctoral Education for Nurses.

EdD	Educational Doctorate
PhD	Doctor of Philosophy in Nursing
DNSc	Doctor of Nursing Science
DSN	Doctor of Science of Nursing
DNS	Doctor of Nursing Science
ND	Nursing Doctorate
DNP	Doctor of Nursing Practice

Nursing Education, started in 1933 at the Teacher's College, Columbia University (Dreher, 2010; Fitzpatrick, 2008). The EdD is a terminal degree. The EdD varies from a practice degree to a research degree, depending on the program and institution. The EdD dissertation may be teaching practice oriented or for original research to discover new knowledge. Graduates of the EdD are prepared for the faculty role and focus on teaching practice and research to advance the science of education.

The EdD has a research dissertation with an educational focus. Today, there are several EdD programs for nurse educators. For example, at the University of Alabama, the EdD in Instructional Leadership for Nurse Educators focuses on preparation of graduates in designing instructional programs, using technology, educational evaluation, and research related to nursing education (Graves *et al.*, 2013; University of Alabama, 2019). The EdD role is specific to teaching at a university and conducting educational research.

Doctor in Philosophy in Nursing

The Doctor in Philosophy in Nursing (PhD), a terminal degree, is research oriented and prepares graduates with the knowledge to discover new knowledge (AACN, 2010). In the 1930s, the first PhD program in nursing started at New York University (Fitzpatrick, 2008) at the Teachers College of Columbia University (Rice, 2016). It was originally an EdD program but became a PhD in nursing program in 1934 (Fitzpatrick, 2008). The PhD in nursing did not become a commonly existing degree until after the development of the practice doctorate (Frances Payne Bolton School of Nursing, 2013). Fitzpatrick (2008) explains that rapid growth of PhD programs in nursing occurred between 1975 and 1990. The PhD in Nursing degree project is a research dissertation focused on a nursing topic. The nurse who desires to do nursing research should strongly consider the PhD in Nursing.

Doctor of Nursing Science

The Doctor of Nursing Science (DNSc) degree was an early approach to develop a clinical nursing doctorate (Dreher, 2010). It was first started at Boston University in 1960 and later dispersed to University of California at San Francisco (UCSF), Rush, Columbia, Yale, and Widener (Dreher, 2010). Many DNSc programs have faded from operation, and nurses interested in research should consider the PhD. The

University of Medical Sciences Arizona (2018) is the only institution that continues to offer the DNSc degree. The program focuses on preparing graduates with research skills and the ability to provide expert patient care, including knowledge in "scholarship, clinical leadership, and organizational skills," (University of Medical Sciences Arizona, 2018, para. 2). DNSc programs required an original research dissertation (AACN, 2019). The DNSc was more of a research doctorate than a clinical doctorate.

Doctor of Science of Nursing

The next approach to address the need for a clinical doctorate in nursing was the Doctor of Science of Nursing (DSN). This terminal degree was first at the University of Alabama in Birmingham in 1975. This degree was later at East Tennessee State, University of Texas Health Sciences-Houston, and West Virginia (Dreher, 2010). The DSN was similar to PhD programs and more of a research degree than a clinical degree. According to the University of Alabama (2013) School of Nursing website, all graduates of the DSN program may convert their degree to a PhD. Still, the nursing discipline searched for a clinically focused nursing doctorate.

Doctor of Nursing Science

The third wave of clinical doctorate programs in nursing was the Doctor of Nursing Science (DNS). This degree was also a terminal degree and was first at Indiana University in 1976. According to Fitzpatrick (2008), the DNS programs were very similar to the PhD programs. The DNS degree is still currently offered at Louisiana State University Health New Orleans (2019), Kennesaw State University (2019), and the Sage Graduate Schools (2019). Louisiana State University refers to the DNS as a professional degree with a focus on research (Louisiana State University Health New Orleans 2019). According to the AACN (2001) position statement for indicators of quality in research-focused doctoral programs in nursing, the same quality indicators are used for the PhD or DNS degree.

Nursing Doctorate

The first nursing doctorate (ND) was pioneered by the Frances Payne

Bolton School of Nursing at Case Western Reserve University in 1979 (AACN, 2004; Frances Payne Bolton School of Nursing, 2013). The ND focused on clinical practice instead of research (Bellack, 2002). The degree model was similar to the medical degree (MD) with a requirement of a baccalaureate degree to enter a ND program and then a four-year doctoral level nursing program that produced graduates for entry-level practice in nursing. However, for nurses wanting a practice doctorate and advanced practice specialization, the early ND did not meet both goals (AACN, 2004) because the preparation was in general nursing. Other schools that offered the ND were Rush University, The University of Colorado, and the University of South Carolina (O'Sullivan *et al.*, 2005). Later, Case Western Reserve University added an advanced practice nursing aspect to the ND and subsequently revised the ND offering to a DNP program (Tibbitts, 2005). O'Sullivan *et al.* (2005) report the schools that offered the ND accepted the AACN recommendation to end the ND and modify the offering to a DNP program.

The Doctor of Nursing Practice (DrNP)

Drexel University began offering the DrNP degree, which is a clinical research program (Dreher, Donnelly, and Naremore, 2006). It incorporates practice and research similar to a doctorate in public health (DrPH). Dreher, Donnelly, and Naremore (2006) report that the Drexel University faculty was aware of the developments with the DNP, however, they choose the DrNP degree that focuses on practice and research. Therefore, the main difference between the DrNP and the DNP is the DrNP focused on clinical research and practice, whereas the DNP focuses on leadership practice and use of research evidence in practice. Later, Drexel changed to the current DNP offering (Drexel, 2018).

The Doctorate in Nursing Practice

The doctorate in nursing practice degree prepares the nurse with advanced skills in clinical nursing practice and leadership to practice in the dynamic health care world. The intent of the DNP degree is to prepare the nurse with advanced leadership skills and to practice at the highest level of nursing practice. The DNP focuses on the translation of research into practice settings, known as evidence-based practice. DNP educational programs should prepare nurses in at least one area of advanced clinical nursing expertise, or an organizational focus, or both

(AACN, 2006b). The DNP is a terminal degree. The DNP is a Scholar-Practitioner who has the skills to combine ethical practice, application of research evidence, theory, and experiential knowledge.

In 2004, the AACN voted to approve the DNP as entry level into advanced practice nursing (instead of the MSN), effective 2015. The position statement suggests using the phrase practice doctorate, instead of clinical doctorate in nursing. Key differences in the DNP should focus on less theory and meta-theory, less research methods, and a final project instead of dissertation approach. The position statement notes that the term dissertation may have various meanings. More of a focus should be on practice experience, practice improvement, practice interventions and evaluations, health policy, and leadership (AACN, 2004). The DNP was forecasted to replace the master's degree in nursing (AACN, 2006a) but this is not yet fully realized. Some master's degree in nursing programs have closed and the number of BSN to DNP programs is on the rise (Killien *et al.*, 2017).

The first DNP program was at the University of Kentucky (Killien *et al.*, 2017). The DNP has experienced dramatic growth in a short time. In 2014 the AACN reported 241 DNP programs in the United States and an additional 59 programs in the planning phase. Doctor of Nursing Practice programs outnumber research-focused Doctor of Nursing programs in the United States (AACN, 2014). In 2018, the AACN reported 336 DNP programs with 121 new DNP programs in planning. AACN (2018) also reported the current number of students in DNP programs during 2016–17 amplified from 25,289 to 29,093. Growth in DNP programs continue to increase in the U.S.

The DNP Final Student Project

The DNP program culminates in the final student project to demonstrate the competencies of the education with their educational experience (Kirkpatrick and Weaver, 2013). For the purposes of this chapter, the reference to the final project is as the DNP student project. Each university has a requirement for the DNP student project, based on program outcomes. Many programs require a topic for the DNP student project that is clinically based. In Chapter 6, Dr. Laura M. Schwartz, DNP, RN, CNE, AHN-BC, describes her experiences with selecting a DNP study project and explains how she chose a final topic of mentoring in nursing. Essentially, theory courses and clinical courses prepare the DNP learner for the student project, prior to graduation for practice in healthcare.

A FOUNDATION OF THE DNP: EVIDENCE-BASED PRACTICE

A major aspect of DNP programs is advanced training and skill development in evidence-based practice. Instead of practicing "because we have always done it this way," evidence-based practice (EBP) is the act of using research evidence, values and beliefs, and experiential knowledge to guide nursing practice. The purpose of EBP is a scholarly and systematic problem-solving process for the delivery of quality healthcare for the patient/family/community (American Nurses Association, 2017). There are many EBP models for use by nurses. Six commonly used EBP models are The Iowa Model: Evidence-Based Practice to Promote Excellence in Health Care©, Advancing Research and Clinical Practice Through Close Collaboration Model, Johns Hopkins Nursing Evidence-Based Practice Model, Rosswurm and Larrabee Model, and Promoting Action on Research Implementation in Health Services (PARIHS) Framework, and the Clinical Scholar Model (Boswell and Cannon, 2020).

An outstanding example in this book of developing EBP is shared in Chapter 8 by Dr. Jayanthi Henry, DNP, MSNCH, MSNIPC, GNEd, RN-BC, which includes a description of an evidence-based sepsis program in the emergency department. Knowledge and skill acquisition of advanced EBP and the ability to lead others with EBP is the foundation of the DNP program.

A narrative, the story of flowers/plants, to illustrate why evidence-based practice is necessary is told by Leibold (2019). During an orientation on the evening shift, the preceptor told the orientee nurse that at 9 pm, all flowers/plants are removed from the patient rooms and placed in a storage room. When asked why, the preceptor explained that the flowers/plants robbed the oxygen from the nighttime air the patient's breathed. The orientee responded that in biology class, she learned the flowers/plants provide more oxygen to a hospital room than they use. The preceptor said it is "how we do it here." This true story is an example of why EBP is important (Leibold, 2019). The skill of being able to lead others in the use of EBP is the crux of the DNP degree program.

ACCREDITING BODIES FOR DNP PROGRAMS

Three organizations accredit DNP programs in the U.S.: The

Commission on Collegiate Nursing Education (CCNE) (AACN, 2006a), the National League for Nursing (NLN) Commission for Nursing Education Accreditation (CNEA) (NLN, 2016), and the Accreditation Commission for Education in Nursing (ACEN) (ACEN, 2017a). The accreditation process is similar, but each organization has their own set of standards, criteria, and process. Since the accreditation standards can impact the program outcomes and DNP student project, the differences in accreditation by CCNE, CNEA, and ACEN are explained in this chapter. Some knowledge of the accrediting body standards may provide insight about the expectations in the DNP program.

CCNE Essentials

The CCNE Essentials support a student project. Eight areas essential for DNP education programs to include are (AACN, 2006a, 8–16):

1. Scientific underpinnings for practice.
2. Organization and system leadership/management, quality improvement and system thinking.
3. Clinical leadership and analytical methods for evidence-based practice.
4. Information systems/technology and patient care technology for the improvement and transformation of health care.
5. Health care policy for advocacy in health care.
6. Interprofessional collaboration for improving patient and population health outcomes.
7. Clinical prevention and population health for improving the nation's health.
8. Advanced nursing Practice.

In the following chapter sections, project examples illuminate the essentials and give examples from final DNP student projects (see Table 2.2). Keep in mind that DNP student projects vary from one institution to another, but often demonstrate competency in multiple essentials. Doctorate students should obtain the instructions for their school and be familiar with the expectations in the school document/instructions. Therefore, recognize that DNP student projects demonstrate multiple essentials, however the examples illustrate each essential (see Table 1.2).

TABLE 1.2. DNP Final Student Projects and Essentials.

CCNE Essential	Example of Project and Author to Illustrate Essential
I. Scientific Underpinnings for Practice	Implemented EMR to improve patient health care in rural setting. (Smith, 2013).
II. Organizational and Systems Leadership for Quality Improvement and Systems Thinking	Initiated an on-going quality improvement program on value-based purchasing in health care organization (Heard, 2012).
III. Clinical Leadership and Analytical Methods for Evidence-Based Practice	Developed an evidence-based guideline for school nurses to use in determining exclusion from school for head lice (Myer, 2012).
IV. Information Systems/Technology and the Transformation of Health Care	Led a quality improvement project to use smartphones by nurses in acute care (Whitlow, 2013).
V. Health Care Policy for Advocacy in Health Care	Studied community service organizations position on sharing a client record (Friberg, 2010).
VI. Interprofessional Collaboration for Improving Patient and Population Health Outcomes	Developed and implemented a performance improvement project to track patients with spinal cord stimulator implants to track outcomes (Rajala, 2013).
VII. Clinical Prevention and Population Health for Improving the Nation's Health	Designed and led intervention to prevent prediabetes from becoming diabetes in adult population (Bolinger, 2012).
VIII. Advanced Nursing Practice	Clinical scholarship project to introduce rural NPs to the use of telehealth video (Langley, 2012).

Scientific Underpinnings for Practice

The AACN essentials (2006) support the DNP student project. Essential I is "Scientific Underpinnings for Practice" (AACN, 2006, 8). DNP learners' study and incorporate a wide variety of scientific theories, such as biology, organizational theories, psychology, and genomics to guide practice and benefit patient outcomes (AACN, 2006). A student project on the topic of the process and implementation of electronic medical records (EMRs) in a rural health care setting by Smith (2013) is an applied example of the AACN DNP essentials. The scientific foundation used for the project was Keshavjee's EMR framework. Three major concepts incorporated in the framework are people, process, and technology. Keshavjee's EMR framework has three phases, the pre-implementation, implementation, and post-implementation phase. The application of change theory in the health care organization was present. For example, in Keshavjee's pre-implementation phase, hospital and clinic staff were actively involved and received training for use of the new software program. The project was evidence-based because the project included a review of evidence on barriers to EMR implementation and improved clinical outcomes with EMR implementation and application throughout the project. Collaboration between the disciplines and departments was present in all phases of the implementation project. The EMR included complete and accurate information in a format easy to access, and Smith (2013) reported that this improved the rural population health outcomes. One specific example given by Smith (2013) was a small group of diabetic patients that had improvement from pre-to-post EMR implementation in terms of glucose control. The application of Keshavjee's EMR framework to address a clinical problem is a strong aspect of this project.

DNPs, Leadership and Performance Improvement

Graduates of DNP programs are well versed in exploring practice questions from a performance improvement standpoint. The AACN Essential II: "Organizational and Systems Leadership for Quality Improvement and Systems Thinking" is a critical skill to improve patient outcomes (AACN, 2006, 10) such as decreasing medical errors. DNPs are practice scholars who have the expertise to ask clinical questions and use quality improvement models and information technology to improve patient outcomes (Nickitas, 2011). A specific example is the DNP student project by Heard (2012) on the topic of initiating value-based purchasing to set the organization up for an ongoing quality improvement project. The purpose of the student project was to provide education and consultation for organizational nurse executives about Hospital Consumer Assessment of Healthcare Providers and Systems (HCAHPS) and Value Based Purchasing (VBP). Robbs' framework for value-based purchasing consultation guided the project. The focus is on Essential II: Organizational and Systems Leadership for Quality Improvement and Systems Thinking and Essential V: Health Care Policy for Advocacy in Healthcare (Heard, 2012).

Clinical Leadership and Analytical Methods for Evidence-Based Practice

In the third AACN (2006) essential, "Clinical Leadership and Analytical Methods for Evidence-Based Practice," the DNP scholar identifies a problem and applies nursing practice scholarship to address the problem. Myer (2012) developed an evidence-based guideline for school exclusion related to head lice. Since school exclusion polices influence a student's attendance, it is best to base decisions on accurate information and evidence. To develop the exclusion guideline, Myer used current clinical guidelines, a review of the literature, grading of the literature, and a Delphi process to seek expert opinions. After the Delphi process, a guideline for exclusion from school for head lice was developed (Myer, 2012). This project is an example of using evidence to develop health policies.

Technology for the Improvement and Transformation of Health Care

Essential IV is "Information Systems/Technology and the Transformation of Health Care" (AACN, 2006, 12). DNPs use technology and informatics to organize and maintain health care information and measure effectiveness of technology related to patient care. Whitlow (2013) completed a quality improvement project in which nurses used smartphones at the bedside to increase communication times between nurses and physicians in the acute care setting. The project design was pretest/post-test. The use of smartphones decreased patient interruptions, decreased wait times between nurse and physician communication, and increased the time nurses spent with patients. Whitlow concluded the smartphone technology improve nurse-physician communication response time related to patient management and granted nurses more time with patients.

Health Care Policy

The DNP essential V is "Health Care Policy for Advocacy in Health Care" (AACN, 2006, 13) and focuses on policies that can improve health care practices or facilitate provider services. A DNP student project by Friberg (2010) identified interest from community service organizations about the use of a shared client record in the elderly population. Aday's framework for health policy evaluation and open systems theory guided the project, which focused on functional assessments in the community. All participating community organizations ($n = 15$) reported interest in a shared client record. Friberg (2010) concluded the use of shared functional assessment data would increase the effectiveness of patient care services provided. The shared client record has health care policy implications.

Interprofessional Collaboration to Improve Patient and Health Care Outcomes

"Interprofessional Collaboration for Improving Patient and Population Health Outcomes" is the AACN (2006, 14) DNP essential VI. A multidisciplinary team followed patients with spinal cord stimulator implants (SCSI) to track improvement of patient's outcomes, specifically implant longevity and efficacy (Rajala, 2013). The student DNP led final project focused on performance improvement. Rajala (2013) created a database for information related to the SCSI, such as device information and patient outcomes gathered from medical records and a questionnaire. The team completed an analysis of the data to study areas for improvement and having met the desired outcome. Rajala (2013) led a multidisciplinary approach to address patient needs related to improving outcomes, such as SCSI reprogramming to provide better pain management.

Clinical Prevention and Population Health

The ACCN (2006, 15) DNP essential VII, "Clinical Prevention and Population Health for Improving the Nation's Health," targets promoting health and reducing risks for health concerns in the US population. The evaluation of a practice changes to prevent diabetes by identification and treatment of prediabetes is the topic for a DNP student project by Bolinger (2012). Adults 25 to 70 years of age in Wirt County with prediabetes were the population of focus in the project. Rogers Diffusion of Innovations Theory provided the theoretical framework for the education session with staff and EMR reminders for health care. Evidence from the literature was the basis for the intervention plan and took place in a health care facility that had three sites. Interprofessional collaboration took place between facility administration, medicine, nursing, project champions at each site, a clinical nurse midwife, laboratory services, and a pharmaceutical company. All key stakeholders received education about the EMR reminders. The EMR reminders serve as use of technology to improve health care, AACN essential VII. Data collection and analysis for outcomes took place. The project objectives were met or partially met. Bolinger (2012) reports screening, education, and actions to prevent diabetes. This DNP project is a clear example of the application and leadership of EBP.

Advanced Nursing Practice

Essential VIII addresses "Advanced Nursing Practice." DNP graduates have preparation in a clinical area and advanced role (AACN, 2006), such as nurse practitioner, nurse midwife, nurse anesthetist, and clinical nurse specialist. Langley (2012) recognized the clinical problem of elderly receiving timely and economical healthcare from nurse practitioners in rural Mississippi to address in her DNP student project. This is an example of an advanced nursing practice project to improve healthcare to a population. Clinical scholarship in the project involved the application of a new technology (clinical video telehealth) in a clinical practice situation by nurse practitioners (NP). Lee and Kotler's social marketing framework guided the project. Langley (2012) used a focus group survey technique to gather data from twelve NP in Mississippi. Langley (2012).reported success with using social marketing to educate NP about clinical video telehealth use.

NLN CNEA Accreditation and Standards

The CNEA accreditation standards were approved in 2016 by NLN CNEA. The CNEA was established in 2013 to foster quality and excellence in nursing education (NLN CNEA, 2016). CNEA does support nurse education content in DNP programs (NLN, 2013). The five accreditation standards for NLN CNEA DNP programs are (NLN CNEA, 2016, 2) (see Table 1.3 for descriptions):

1. Culture of Excellence—Program Outcomes;
2. Culture of Integrity and Accountability—Mission, Governance, and Resources;
3. Culture of Excellence and Caring—Faculty;
4. Culture of Excellence and Caring—Students; and
5. Culture of Learning and Diversity—Curriculum and Evaluation Processes

NLN has four core values (NLN CNEA, 2016) that are rich and clear within the NLN CNEA standards. A culture of caring, diversity, in-

TABLE 1.3. NLN CNEA Standards and Descriptions.

Standards	Descriptions
I. Culture of Excellence—Program Outcomes	Clear program outcomes; related to goals, faculty achievement, curriculum, student learning
II. Culture of Integrity and Accountability—Mission, Governance, and Resources;	Related to goal setting, decision-making, consistency between the institution and nursing mission, goals, outcomes, and values
III. Culture of Excellence and Caring— Faculty;	Related to faculty competence, diversity, lifelong professional development
IV. Culture of Excellence and Caring— Students;	Related to learning environment and caring support for students
V. Culture of Learning and Diversity—Curriculum and Evaluation Processes	The curriculum is current, evidence-based, and reflects societal needs

(NLN CNEA 2016)

tegrity, and excellence are in harmony with the program accreditation process (see Table 1.4 for descriptions).

ACEN Accreditation of DNP Programs

The third organization that accredits DNP programs is the Accreditation Commission for Education in Nursing (ACEN). The ACEN seeks to support nursing education, practice, and the public with accreditation

TABLE 1.4. NLN Core Values.

Values	Descriptors related to Accreditation Process
Culture of Caring	Advocacy and collaboration with stakeholders
Culture of Diversity	All levels of nursing education and types of programs, curricula, faculty, students
Culture of Integrity	Open communication, ethical decisions, timely responsiveness
Culture of Excellence	Continuous quality improvement, student-centered learning environments

(NLN CNEA 2016)

of programs (ACEN, 2017a). The Standards at the doctorate program level are referred to as Clinical Doctorate/DNP Specialist Certificate by ACEN (2017a). ACEN defines the DNP Specialist Certificate as:

> *A selected series of courses that are a subset of courses within a clinical doctorate program specific to one (1) area of practice (e.g., certificates in nursing administration, certificates in nursing education, certificate as a family nurse practitioner) which are taken after an individual is already credentialed with a doctorate degree in nursing in a different specialty (ACEN, 2017b, 4).*

They do accredit DNP programs with a specialization in educational leadership, such as the American Sentinel University (2018). ACEN's six accreditation standards for the clinical doctorate programs are (ACEN, 2018) (see Table 1.5 for descriptions):

1. Mission and Administrative Capacity
2. Faculty and Staff
3. Students
4. Curriculum
5. Resources
6. Outcomes

TABLE 1.5. ACEN Standards and Descriptions.

Standards	Descriptors
1. Mission and Administrative Capacity	Governing organization mission and nursing mission in sync; clear end of program outcomes
2. Faculty and Staff	Faculty that are qualified and credentialed; qualified staff to support the program
3. Students	Student resources support learning; student records comply with federal law
4. Curriculum	The curriculum supports the end of program learning outcomes
5. Resources	The fiscal, physical, and learning resources support the end of program learning outcomes
6. Outcomes	End of program learning outcomes are met and validated through program assessment/evaluation

(NLN CNEA 2017)

The standards have some overall similarities (missions, faculty competence, resources, etc.) among all three accrediting bodies, yet unique specifics in the details.

HISTORY OF THE DNP (OR THE PROLOGUE TO THE DNP)

Origin of the DNP

In 2001, the AACN had serious deliberations about the Doctor of Nursing practice degree. The development of the DNP has been through a stimulating path to where it is today. This section includes a prologue story to the revolutionary development of the DNP to add background and context.

Driving Forces for Development of the DNP

The Institute of Medicine (IOM) (1999) Report, *To Err is Human: Building a Safer Health System*, is a significant driving force in the development of the DNP degree because it called attention to patient safety and medical errors. This report opened the eyes of many nurse leaders that it was time for a progressive and innovative approach. Up to 98,000 people die each year in the United States from medical errors (IOM, 1999). The report included that health systems (including hospitals) need to add systems in place to reduce medical errors. The recommended systems would require advanced clinical education for leaders and the DNP was a solution to provide education for leaders to develop the skills to put the necessary systems in operation in health systems.

The IOM (2001) Report, *Crossing the Quality Chiasm*, calls for re-thinking and restructuring of healthcare to improve the safety, effectiveness, efficiency, and timeliness of patient care. In addition, the report also recommends patient centered care practice. The provision of equitable care was also a key point addressed and included quality care that did not vary due to age, gender, ethnicity, socioeconomic status, or geographical location (IOM, 2001). The degree prepares a nurse to improve healthcare delivery systems, and to improve the quality of patient care and reduce medical errors (Chism, 2009).

A task force by the AACN to revise the *Quality Indicators for Doctoral Education* found that the indicators applied to PhD or DNS degrees (AACN, 2001). This spurred further discussion of the practice doctorate in nursing. Also, in 2001, a *Practice Doctorate Task Force* was formed by the National Organization of Nurse Practitioner Faculties (NONPF) to examine the issues of a clinical doctorate (NONPF, 2002).

The IOM (2003a) report, *Health Professions Education: A Bridge to Quality* focused on the education needed to improve patient safety. The report stated that healthcare providers are not educated in methods to reduce medical errors. The report presented five core areas for health care professionals and students to develop and maintain proficiency. The five areas include the provision of patient centered care, interdisciplinary team approach, evidence-based practice, quality improvement, and information technology (IOM, 2003a). These five areas are all included in the AACN (2006a) eight essentials for DNP education.

The IOM (2003b) Report, *Keeping Patients Safe: Transforming the Work Environment of Nurses*, recommended clinical nursing leadership roles in the executive aspect of healthcare agencies. The report stresses solutions to reducing medical errors by improving the work environment of nurses. Specifically, the report addresses work design, management practices, workforce skills and education, and the cultures of organizations. Specific issues, such as mandatory overtime, work hours, and nurse to patient ratios are discussed (IOM, 2003b). Again, DNP education is a tool to increase the skills that nurse executives need to address these issues. These events led up to the decision of the DNP being a practice or clinical doctorate with a major focus on evidence-based practice, quality improvement, and systems leadership.

In 2004, the AACN voted to require the DNP as the entry level for advanced practice nurses by 2015 (AACN, 2006a). Advanced practice nurses include nurse anesthetist, nurse midwives, nurse practitioners, and clinical nurse specialists. In the next sections, descriptions of the advanced practice nurses are given.

Nurse Practitioner

The role of the nurse practitioner (NP) is to provide advanced nursing practice within their clinical specialty. The NP can obtain health histories, complete physical examinations, diagnose, prescribe treatments, and evaluate for responses. NPs also provide patient and family education. NPs specialize in an area, for example, family NP, acute care NP, mental health NP, geriatric NP, neonatal NP, pediatric NP, women's health NP, and their practice is limited to that area (AANP, 2013).

The National Organization of Nurse Practitioner Faculties (NONPF, 2002) has led the discussion regarding the NP and DNP entry issue, starting in 2001 with a task force to address the topic. The 2002 Clinical Doctorate Initiative document states that the NONPF supports clinical nursing doctorate education. The document stressed multiple entry and exit levels for a clinical doctorate (NONPF, 2002). The White Paper: The Doctor of Nursing Practice Nurse Practitioner Clinical Scholar by NONPF (2016) states that increasing the number of doctorally prepared NPs is essential to transforming the healthcare system. In the same White Paper, the NONPF (2016) notes their continued recommendation that the DNP is the entry level for NP practice. A concern stressed by the AANP (2016) is the DNP prepared NP clinical scholar needs clear descriptions and development.

Nurse Anesthesia

The role of the nurse anesthetist includes individualized care for patients, pre-operatively, intra-operatively, and post-operatively to provide safe, quality anesthesia (AANA, 2018). The nurse anesthetist provides pre-operative patient and family education about the perioperative experience and anesthesia process (AANA, 2018). In addition, the nurse anesthetist prepares the equipment and anesthesia for use, administers the anesthesia, and evaluates for desired effect or complications of anesthesia. Airway management is provided along with assessment and provision of any emergency care needed during the perioperative time. Intravenous (IV) sites are started and IV fluids are infused by the nurse anesthetist.

The American Association of Nurse Anesthetist's (AANA) (2009) position statement on doctoral education supports doctoral education as mandatory entry level into practice for nurse anesthetists by 2025. It does not specify the doctorate to be a DNP (Hawkins and Nezat, 2009). The AANA states that the doctorate is consistent with advancing knowledge to suit the complex healthcare systems of today.

Several schools have nurse anesthetist/DNP programs in operation. Rush University (2019) is set up for nurses to earn a DNP with the specialty of nurse anesthesia. Other universities offering nurse anesthesia DNP programs are University of Minnesota School of Nursing (2019), Duke University School of Nursing (2019), and University of Maryland School of Nursing (2019).

Certified Midwifery

The role of the certified nurse midwife is to provide primary care services for women throughout the lifespan (ACNM, 2016). The practice role focuses on assessments, diagnostics, therapeutics, evaluation, and health promotion. Specific services include family planning, gynecology cares, preconception care, pregnancy care, child birthing, postpartum care, and newborn care in the first 28 days of (ACNM, 2011).

Since nurse midwives are advanced practice nurses, the requirement of the DNP for entry into advanced practice nursing has an impact (Avery and Howe, 2007). The American College of Nurse-Midwives (ACNM, 2012) responded with a position statement titled *Mandatory Degree Requirements for Entry into Midwifery Practice*. The statement does not support the requirement of a doctorate for nurse midwives to enter practice (ACNM, 2012). However, ACNM does include in the position statement that graduate nurse education for nurse midwives is valued. In addition, the position statement stipulates that certified nurse-midwives (CNMs) and certified midwives (CMs) educated before 2010 should keep their licensure to practice and not be required to complete graduate education.

Clinical Nurse Specialist

The role of the clinical nurse specialist (CNS) is to provide advanced nursing practice to improve the health of patients, families, groups, and communities in a specialized area such as a population (pediatrics, woman's health) or practice area (burn trauma, coronary care) (NACNS, 2019). The CNS serves as an expert resource for staff, have advanced assessment skills, can diagnose, and treat within their specialized area. In addition, the CNS is a change agent in the healthcare organization and works to improve healthcare delivery systems.

The NACNS (2015) endorses the DNP as the entry into practice for the CNS. In their White Paper, NACNS (2015) explains the change from their position of neutrality to endorsing the DNP degree due to complex needs of patients, healthcare transformation, and recommendations by various reports and agencies about the future of healthcare. The NACNS (2016) recognizes the PhD in Nursing as the highest form of nursing research degree, but states that the CNS is a closer link to the DNP due to the nature of the CNS practice.

Leading Change and Advancing Health

The IOM published *The Future of Nursing: Leading Change, Ad-*

vancing Health in 2011. Four key messages were of focus in the report that considers practice barriers with the intent to move nursing ahead for the future.

The four key messages:

• Nurses should practice based on their education.
• Nurses should obtain higher degrees in an improved educational system.
• Nurses should collaborate with other healthcare professionals.
• The workforce should have a better information infrastructure.

The first key point is that nurses should be able to practice based on their education, rather than state laws setting where they practice nursing. The report gives the example of a nurse practitioner who can prescribe medications in one state, but not in another (IOM, 2011). Therefore, even though the nurse practitioner has received education to prescribe medications, they are not allowed to do so in the state of practice.

The second key point is that nurses should have higher education levels through an improved education system (IOM, 2011). Nurses should be able to obtain higher levels of education (for example, a nurse should be able to earn a graduate degree in nursing).

The third key point is nurses should partner with all healthcare providers in leading the way for improved healthcare (IOM, 2010). Nurses should lead and receive credit for their contributions. Interprofessional collaboration is one of the AACN (2006a) essentials for DNP programs.

The fourth key point is that the information infrastructure needs improvement to create an environment for workforce planning and policy development (Institute of Medicine, 2010). This includes a better way to collect data and analyze data regarding workforce information and demographics. This is another good fit for the DNP curriculum. The AACN (2006a) essentials include informational technology, health policy, and organizational leadership, which support this key point of the IOM report.

Quality and Safety Education for Nurses

Quality and safety education for nurses (QSEN) criteria were developed for quality and safety education for advanced nursing practice (Cronenwett *et al.*, 2009). The advisory board included the incorporation of the Institute of Medicine competencies, QSEN faculty, members from professional organizations with a stake in advanced nursing practice, and a National Advisory Board to develop quality and safety competencies for graduate programs and the development of advanced practice nurses (AACN, 2012a; Cronenwett *et al.,* 2009). The six criteria developed include quality improvement, safety, teamwork and collaboration, patient centered care, evidence-based practice, and informatics. Educational units incorporate the six criteria the related knowledge, skills, and attitudes (KSAs) DNP programs.

DNP ROLE EMPHASIS IN DIRECT ADVANCED CLINICAL HEALTHCARE

DNP prepared advanced practice nurses are practice leaders. There are diverse advanced practice roles for nurses with DNP degrees, such as nurse practitioners, nurse midwives, nurse anesthetists, and clinical nurse specialists. Their skills go beyond clinical expertise and include advanced skills in organizational leadership and management, advanced communication, interprofessional collaboration skills, and systems thinking (AACN, 2006a; Sonson, 2013). The roles in the future for the DNP are plentiful. The University of Washington School of Nursing (2018) website lists many options for the DNP, such as gerontology nurse practitioner, nurse-midwifery, pediatric clinical nurse specialist, and population health nursing.

Clark and Allison-Jones (2011) used a qualitative design to study roles of DNP graduates. A snowball sampling that resulted in 25 DNP graduates participated in the study. The participants reported a change in their practice after the DNP program that included a consistent theme of their enhanced ability to practice evidence-based practice. Also reported was the ability to collaborate and communicate with professionals from other disciplines also increased. Most participants reported they had a clinical role, such as a CNS. Specific aspects of the clinical roles were reported as clinical leadership, using evidence-based practice, teaching clinical, being a change agent, and advanced practice clinician (Clark and Allison-Jones, 2011). DNP graduates reported that goals for DNPs should include, "system change, participating in policy development, teaching, research, and publication" (Clark and Allison-Jones, 2011, 74). DNP graduates in Clark and Allison-Jones' (2011) qualitative study about DNP graduate roles include expansion of the DNP to an independent practitioner.

An issue related to the roles of advanced practice nursing and the DNP is the requirement for entry into advanced practice nursing voted in effect by AACN (2004). This change affects nurse practitioners, nurse midwives, nurse anesthetists, and clinical nurse specialists (Avery and Howe, 2007). For example, will existing advanced practice nurses be allowed to continue their practice if they do not have a doctorate? Will reimbursement changes exclude master prepared advanced practice nurses? The American Nurses Association (ANA) (2011) position statement states the ANA supports masters or doctoral level entry into advanced nursing practice. An explanation of the advanced practice roles and the specialty association's position on entry into advance nursing practice follows.

The Health Systems and Clinical Leadership/Administration Role

The nurse administrator role is a complex one that requires a broad skill set. According to Marquis and Huston (2017), the functions of the manager include planning, organizing, staffing, directing, and controlling. Within each of the five functions, there are many skills, such as fiscal responsibility and patient care delivery. The DNP offers the graduate many skills that are suited to the business model role due to the AACN essentials (Swanson and Stanton, 2013). Swanson and Stanton (2013) completed a DNP student project that used an online survey method to study the use of the DNP in an organizational business model. The authors report that most chief nursing officers reported that the DNP preparation fits the role of the nurse executive (Swanson and Stanton, 2013).

The Faculty Role

Diverse nursing faculty education preparation provides a balanced and rounded approach to preparing nurses. That is, a variety of faculty grounding and credentials are best suited to work together to provide the best education for preparing nurses. Since nurse graduates are educated in practice and research, DNP graduates in the faculty role may share their gift of expertise in clinical practice to help prepare nurses for practice (AACN, 2006a).

A few DNP programs offer an educator track, however not all DNP programs include courses in the educator role. One criticism of the DNP in the faculty role is that the DNP programs do not include courses that prepare the graduate for the faculty role. However, many PhD programs do not offer courses in the educator role to prepare graduates for the faculty role (AACN, 2009; AACN, 2012b). The National League for Nursing (NLN) (2007) position supports including education courses in the DNP curriculum. The AACN position is that a primary purpose of the DNP program is not to prepare graduates as educators and that additional coursework is available for those who wish educational preparation. For example, at Creighton University School of Nursing (2019), the DNP tracks are Advanced Practice Registered Nurse (APRN) and Nurse Leader Track. Just as PhD programs, some DNP programs may offer educator role preparation, while others may not (AACN, 2004). In cases where a university does not offer education courses as part of the DNP degree, the graduate may take additional courses in teaching effectiveness, educational assessment, and evaluation.

DNP PRACTICE SETTINGS

DNP practice settings include a large variety of locales that are dependent on the specialty track of the DNP. Nurse practitioners' practice in a variety of settings, from acute care to primary care, and specialty settings (AANP, 2013). Nurse anesthetists' practice in operating rooms, ambulatory surgical centers, psychiatric departments, emergency departments (EDs), pain management centers, the United States Military, and intensive care units. Dental practices and plastic surgery centers are also employing nurse anesthetists (AANA, 2014). Nurse midwives' practice in a variety of settings, such as hospitals, birthing centers, ambulatory care centers, health departments, private practice, and health maintenance organizations (HMOs) (ACNM, 2011). Clinical nurse specialists' practice in clinics, hospitals, public health departments, and the community (NACNS, 2014).

DNP Outcomes

Since the DNP is a relatively new degree program, there is limited outcome data available. In 1999, the University of Kentucky conducted a market analysis survey (AACN, 2004). The participants included 111 acute care, long-term, and public health executives in Kentucky that completed the survey (29% response rate). Most participants responded that they would hire DNP graduates. The participants identified positions that they would hire DNPs for as Vice President for Clinical Services, Program Director, Vice President for Patient Care, Chief Executive Officer, Quality Improvement Director, Director of Clinical Services, Faculty Member, Direct Care Clinician, and Clinical Information Technology Specialist (AACN, 2004).

A study of the doctorate in nursing practice by DeMarco, Pulcini, and Haggerty (2009) examined the perceptions of registered nurses (RNs) in Massachusetts. A convenience sample of 376 RNs participated in an online survey of 17 items about DNP structure, process, and program outcomes. Findings were mixed, but the DNP is slightly preferred to the PhD by the participants. Another interesting finding is that older nurses reported stronger support for the DNP. DeMarco, Pulcini, and Haggerty (2009) offered a reason for these as older nurses have witnessed much change in healthcare and see the value of the DNP to lead in healthcare systems. The authors report the data was gathered in 2006 and that viewpoints may change over time.

Completion of a DNP program evaluation plan and analysis of the transition was undertaken by The University of Washington (Kaplan and Brown, 2009). Post program employer evaluations are collected of the outcomes of DNPs in the healthcare organization. Data collection includes faculty and student interviews. Seven tools were developed to assist in gathering data.

Broome, Riner, and Allam (2013) studied publication practices of DNP graduates with a published article with one or more authors with a DNP from 2005 to 2012. The authors found 175 articles for study inclusion. One finding noted is that DNP graduates are contributing to the knowledge of nursing. The most common articles related to the evaluation of an intervention with nurses or patients. Most publications relate to practice topics. Many publications were interprofessional publications and the authors relate this to the AACN (2006a) essential for interprofessional collaboration. The first author was most commonly a DNP. Broome, Riner, and Allam (2013) attach this to the leadership role of DNPs. One AACN essential that lacked in the articles was translational science underpinnings. Broome, Riner, and Allam (2013) suggest the strengthening of this area in programs. This is an area for evaluation by faculty in DNP programs. In addition to journal publications, books, conference presentations, and webinars are ways to reach professionals with information about improving clinical practice.

Nichols, O'Connor, and Dunn (2014) studied the use of DNPs in healthcare organizations. A convenience sample of 17 chief nursing officers (CNOs) in Michigan responded to the survey. Most participants reported their organizations did not employ DNPs. However, a majority of CNOs reported they would hire a DNP in their organization. The most beneficial roles to the organization were the nurse practitioner and nurse executive DNP. Seventy-one percent of CNOs responded that nurses have organizational incentives to earn a DNP (Nichols, O'Connor, and Dunn, 2014). The DNP degree is encouraged by healthcare organizations, although they are not completely being used in the workplace. Utilization of the DNP in healthcare organizations is encouraged.

Nurses with DNPs have had an impact on the contributions in healthcare, thus far. The impact of 1,308 DNPs were studied by Minnick, Kleinpell, and Allison (2018) using a descriptive survey design. DNP participants reported 98% employment. Full-time, part-time, and full-time employment with additional part-time work was reported. Hospital settings (45.3%), nursing education (17.5%), and ambulatory care (22.4%) were the most often settings employed. Fifty-nine percent of participants reported the DNP was not required nor preferred by their employer. Forty-one percent of the participants reported a scholarly publication. Over 70% of participants reported their DNP program promoted their ability to use quality improvement, EBP, and leadership (Minnick, Kleinpell, and Allison, 2018). Further study of the DNP impact is warranted.

AACN (2017) reports there are DNP programs in all 50 United States. A count of DNP graduates in 2016 was 4,855 and in 2017 was 6,090. The number of DNP students in 2016 was 25, 289, and increased to 29,093 in 2017 (AACN, 2017).

THE FUTURE FOR THE DNP DEGREE

The DNP student project has a vast value, as it actualizes a substantial document that demonstrates acquired proficiency of the degree outcomes. As stated earlier, each university has a DNP student final project that is specific to the program outcomes. System thinking and clinical projects that require critical thinking and problem-solving abilities are often the impetus for the DNP student project.

Patient safety and improved patient, family, and society health outcomes are the focus of the DNP student project. Core areas include patient centered care, interdisciplinary team approach, evidence-based practice, quality improvement, and information technology. These five areas identified in the IOM (2003a) report, *Health Professions Education: A Bridge to Quality center on patient safety. In Keeping Patients Safe: Transforming the Work Environment of Nurses*, another IOM (2003b) report the work environment is the locus for improvement as this impacts the patient's safety. These reports served as driving forces for the AACN (2006) Essentials for DNP education and eventually for the focus of the DNP student project.

Areas for improvement related to DNP education and practice are evident. As reported by Broome, Riner, and Allam (2013) there is a need for increased focus in the application of theoretical frameworks in advanced nursing practice. DNP programs may evaluate the inclusion and application of theoretical frameworks and revise the curriculum as needed to allow for a stronger focus on theory application. Evidence of substantive DNP graduates' publication practices relates to the educational essential of interprofessional collaboration (Broome, Riner, and Allam, 2013). Since future dissemination of DNP work has the potential to advance nursing by sharing ideas and projects that may improve patient/family outcomes, DNP programs may add even more emphasis about publishing, presenting, and networking with colleagues to share knowledge.

Future dissemination of DNP work is of utmost importance because the DNP expertise lies in promoting patient safety and improving patient, family, and society health outcomes. Promulgation of this urgent and vital work is paramount toward advancing the nursing profession. DNP student projects submitted to dissertation and thesis databases reach a sizable audience, and so this activity is encouraged. Avenues for dissemination of DNP endeavors include conference presentations, poster sharing, journal publications, books, and webinars.

The clarity and rigor are areas identified that needs further addressing in the future. Root *et al.* (2018) voice concerns about the wide variety of rigor in the DNP programs. A qualitative content analysis of DNP students' perceptions to explore, analyze, and describe issues was conducted by Volkert and Johnston (2018). Students shared concerns about the lack of clarity regarding the translation of research into practice settings. Student concerns with academic settings included difficulties of non-DNP faculty and advisors. A predominant concern was non-DNP faculty as the lead for DNP projects. A need for standardized DNP project expectations were found (Volkert and Johnston, 2018), which provides clear focus for needs to address in the future.

The future for the DNP degree, including the final student project is positive, and yet unknown in terms of the impact that DNPs in practice will have on the healthcare system. The final student project demonstrates competency in critical thinking and problem solving as applied to clinical practice and/or practice issues. There is further need for evidence collection and analysis on the use of DNPs in their various roles and settings. Grey (2013) published an article discussing the next steps for the DNP. Grey notes the consensus areas surrounding the DNP to be that there is much interest in the DNP degree, and that the DNP includes health policy, and population health. Controversies described by Grey include the differences in clinical experiences, clinical hours, and the DNP student project. Evaluation and data collection of DNP programs and DNP graduates will provide information for analysis of these concerns. From the number of nurses with DNPs by year to the impact that this has had on the use of evidence-based practice, quality improvement, and systems leadership—there are many opportunities for valuable research data to study the products. Evidence to illustrate the significance the DNP degree has made for advanced practice nurses is justified.

Since DNP education is still in the early years of existence, early reports such as program evaluation and published research are providing guidance to shape and refine DNP programs. Yet more research about the DNP role, performance, and DNP program evaluations are necessary to cultivate the quality of DNP education. Evidence from further research and program evaluation data, along with the healthcare needs of society will guide the enhancement of DNP education.

REFERENCES

Accreditation Commission for Education in Nursing (ACEN). (2017a). ACEN Accreditation Manual-2017 Standards and Criteria. Retrieved from https://www.acenursing.org/resources-acen-accreditation-manual/

ACEN. (2017b). ACEN Accreditation Manual Glossary. Retrieved from http://www.acenursing.net/manuals/Glossary.pdf

American Association of College of Nursing (AACN). (1996). 1995–1996 Enrollment and graduations in baccalaureate and graduate programs in nursing. Washington, DC: AACN.

AACN. (2001). Indicators of quality in research-focused doctoral programs in nursing. Retrieved from http://www.aacn.nche.edu/publications/position/quality-indicators

AACN. (2004). AACN position statement on the practice doctorate in nursing. Retrieved from http://www.aacn.nche.edu/publications/position/DNPpositionstatement.pdf

AACN. (2006a). The essentials of doctoral education for advanced nursing practice. Retrieved from https://www.aacn.nche.edu/publications/position/DNPEssentials.pdf

AACN. (2006b). Roadmap task force report. Retrieved from http://www.aacn.nche.edu/dnp/roadmapreport.pdf

AACN. (2009). About the DNP: Frequently asked questions. Retrieved from http://www.aacn.nche.edu/dnp/about

AACN. (2010). The research-focused doctoral program in nursing. Pathways to excellence. Retrieved from https://www.aacn.nche.edu/education-resources/PhDTaskForceReport.pdf

AACN. (2012a). Graduate-level QSEN competencies: Knowledge, skills, and attributes. Retrieved from: http://www.aacn.nche.edu/faculty/qsen/competencies.pdf

AACN. (2012b). Leading initiatives. Retrieved from http://www.aacn.nche.edu/dnp/faqs

AACN. (2014). DNP fact sheet. Retrieved from http://www.aacn.nche.edu/media-relations/fact-sheets/dnp

AACN. (2017). DNP fact sheet. Retrieved from https://www.aacnnursing.org/News-Information/Fact-Sheets/DNP-Fact-Sheet

AACN. (2019). DNP education. Retrieved from https://www.aacnnursing.org/Nursing-Education-Programs/DNP-Education

American Association of Nurse Anesthetists (AANA). (2009). Doctor of nurse anesthesia practice (DNAP). Retrieved from http://www.dnap.com/

AANA. (2018). Professional practice. Retrieved from https://www.aana.com/practice

American Association of Nurse Practitioners (AANP). (2013). Your partner in health: The nurse practitioner. Retrieved from http://www.aanp.org/images/documents/about-nps/npbrochure.pdf

American College of Nurse-Midwives. (ACNM) (2011). Definition of nurse midwifery and scope of practice of certified nurse midwives and certified midwives. Retrieved from http://www.midwife.org/ACNM/files/ACNMLibraryData/UPLOADFILENAME/000000000266/Definition%20of%20Midwifery%20and%20Scope%20of%20Practice%20of%20CNMs%20and%20CMs%20Dec%202011.pdf

American College of Nurse-Midwives. (ACNM) (2016). Essentials facts about nurse midwives. Retrieved from http://www.midwife.org/Essential-Facts-about-Midwives

ACNM. (2012). Position statement: Mandatory degree requirements for entry into midwifery practice. Retrieved from http://www.midwife.org/ACNM/files/ACNMLibraryData/UPLOADFILENAME/000000000076/Mandatory%20Degree%20Requirements%20Position%20Statement%20June%202012.pdf

American Nurses Association (ANA). (2011). The doctor of nursing practice: Advancing the nursing profession. ANA position statement. Retrieved from http://gm6.nursingworld.org/MainMenuCategories/Policy-Advocacy/Positions-and-Resolutions/ANAPositionStatements/Position-Statements-Alphabetically/The-Doctor-of-Nursing-Practice-Advancing-the-Nursing-Profession.html

American Nurses Association. (2017). Research tools. Retrieved from https://www.nursingworld.org/practice-policy/innovation-evidence/improving-your-practice/research-toolkit/

American Sentinel University. (2018). Online DNP Program in Educational Leadership. Retrieved from https://www.americansentinel.edu/degrees-programs/nursing/online-doctoral-degree-programs/dnp-educational-leadership/

Avery, M. and Howe, C. (2007). The DNP and entry into midwifery practice: An analysis: Doctor of Nursing Practice. *Journal of Midwifery & Women's Health, 52*(1), 14–22.

Bellack, J. P. (2002). A matter of degree. *Journal of Nursing Education, 41*(5), 191.

Bolinger, M. C. (2012). *Evaluation of a practice change to improve screening, identification, and management of patients with prediabetes.* (Order No. 3538247, West Virginia University). *ProQuest Dissertations and Theses, 86.*

Boswell, C. and Cannon, S. (2020). Introduction to nursing research. (5th ed.). Burlington, MA: Jones & Bartlett Learning.

Broome, M. E, Riner, M. E. and Allam, E. S. (2013). Scholarly publication practices of doctor of nursing practice-prepared nurses. *Journal of Nursing Education, 52*(8), 429–434. doi:http://dx.doi.org/10.3928/01484834-20130718-02

Chism, L. A. (2009). Understanding the DNP. Retrieved from http://nurse-practitioners.advanceweb.com/Editorial/Content/Editorial.aspx?CC=191812

Clark, R. and Allison-Jones, L. (2011). The Doctor of Nursing Practice Graduate in Practice. *Clinical Scholars Review, 4*(2), 71–77.

Creighton University. (2019). Doctor of Nursing Practice. Retrieved from https://nursing.creighton.edu/program/doctor-nursing-practice-dnp

Cronenwett, L., Dracup, K., Grey, M., McCauley, L., Meleis, A. and Salmon, M. (2011). The Doctor of Nursing Practice: A national workforce perspective. *Nursing Outlook, 59,* 9–17. doi: doi:10.1016/j.outlook.2010.11.003

Cronenwett, L., Sherwood, G., Pohl, J., Barnsteiner, J., Moore, S., Sullivan, D., Ward, D., Warren, J. (2009). Quality and safety education for advanced nursing practice. *Nursing Outlook 57*(6), 338–348.

Dreher, H. M. (2010). The historical and political path of doctoral nursing education to the doctor of nursing practice degree. In. H. M. Dreher and M. E. Glasgow (Eds.), *Role development for doctoral advanced nursing practice.* (pp. 7–43). New York, NY: Springer Publishing Company.

Dreher, H.M., Donnelly, G. and Naremore, R., (2006). Reflections on the DNP and an alternate practice doctorate model: The Drexel DrNP. *Online Journal of Issues in Nursing.* Vol. 11 No. 1. doi: 10.3912/OJIN.Vol11No01PPT01

Drexel University. (2018). Doctor of nursing practice: DNP. Retrieved from http://www.drexel.com/online-degrees/nursing-degrees/dnp/index.aspx

Duke University. (2019). Nurse anesthesia and DNP. Retrieved from https://nursing.duke.edu/academic-programs/dnp-program-nursing/nurse-anesthesia-dnp

Fitzpatrick, J. J. (2008). History of graduate nursing education. In J. J. Fitzpatrick and M. Wallace (Eds.), *Doctor of nursing practice and clinical nurse leader: Essentials of program development and implementation for clinical practice* (pp. 1–12). New York, NY: Springer Publishing Company.

Frances Payne Bolton School of Nursing. (2013). History of the DNP at FPB. Retrieved from http://fpb.case.edu/DNP/history.shtm

Friberg, E. E. (2010). *Community service organizations use of functional assessment to enhance the delivery and coordination of regional long-term care services.* (Order No. 3437480, University of Virginia). ProQuest Dissertations and Theses, 192.

Gatti-Petito, J., Lakatos, B. E., Bradley, H. B., Cook, L., Haight, I. E. and Karl, C. A. (2013). Clinical scholarship and adult learning theory: A role for the DNP in nursing education. *Nursing Education Perspectives, 34*(4), 273-276.

Graves, B. A., Tomlinson, S., Handley, M., Oliver, J. S., Carter-Templeton, H., Gaskins, S. and . . . Wood, F. (2013). The Emerging Doctor of Education (EdD) in Instructional Leadership for Nurse Educators. *International Journal of Nursing Education Scholarship, 10*(1), doi:10.1515/ijnes-2012-0024

Grey, M. (2013). The doctor of nursing practice: Defining the next steps. *Journal of Nursing Education, 52*(8), 462-465. doi:http://dx.doi.org/10.3928/01484834-20130719-02

Hawkins, R. and Nezat, G. (2009). Doctoral education: Which degree to pursue? *AANA Journal, 77*(2), 92-96. Retrieved from https://www.aana.com/docs/default-source/aana-journal-web-documents-1/educnews_0409_p92-96.pdf?sfvrsn=e24c5ab1_6

Heard, J. D. (2012). *Value based purchasing: Positioning a healthcare organization for the future.* (Order No. 3534854, The University of Southern Mississippi). *ProQuest Dissertations and Theses,* 51.

Institute of Medicine. (1999). To Err is human: Building a safer health system. Washington, DC: National Academy Press. Retrieved from http://www.iom.edu/Reports/1999/To-Err-is-Human-Building-A-Safer-Health-System.aspx

Institute of Medicine. (2001). Crossing the quality chasm. Washington, DC: National Academy Press. Retrieved from http://www.iom.edu/Reports/2001/Crossing-the-Quality-Chasm-A-New-Health-System-for-the-21st-Century.aspx

Institute of Medicine. (2003a). Health professions education: A bridge to quality. Washington, DC: The National Academies Press. Retrieved from http://www.iom.edu/Reports/2003/Health-Professions-Education-A-Bridge-to-Quality.aspx

Institute of Medicine. (2003b). Keeping patients safe: Transforming the work environment of nurses. Washington, DC: The National Academies Press. Retrieved from http://www.iom.edu/Reports/2003/Keeping-Patients-Safe-Transforming-the-Work-Environment-of-Nurses.aspx

Institute of Medicine. (2011). The Future of Nursing: Leading Change, Advancing Health. Washington, DC: National Academies Press; Retrieved from http://www.thefutureofnursing.org/sites/default/files/Future%20of%20Nursing%20Report_0.pdf

Iowa Model Collaborative. (2017). Iowa model of evidence-based practice: Revisions and validation. *Worldviews on Evidence-Based Nursing, 14*(3), 175–182. doi:10.1111/wvn.12223

Kaplan, L. and Brown, M. (2009). Doctor of nursing practice program evaluation and beyond: Capturing the profession's transition to the DNP. *Nursing Education Perspectives, 30*(6), 362–6.

Kelly, K. (2010). Is the DNP the answer to the nursing faculty shortage? Not likely! *Nursing Forum, 45*(4), 266-270. doi:10.1111/j.1744-6198.2010.00197.x

Kennesaw University. (2019). Nursing Science, DNS. Retrieved from https://graduate.kennesaw.edu/admissions/apply/program-information/dns.php

Killien, M., Thompson, H., Kieckhefer, G., Bekemeier, B., Kozuki, Y. and Perry, C. K. (2017). Re-envisioning a DNP program for quality and sustainability. *Journal of Professional Nursing, 33*(3), 194–203. doi:10.1016/j.profnurs.2016.09.006

Kirkpatrick, J. M. and Weaver, T. (2013). The doctor of nursing practice capstone project: Consensus or confusion? *Journal of Nursing Education, 52*(8), 435–41. doi:http://dx.doi.org/10.3928/01484834-20130722-01

Kutash, M. (2015). *The relationship between nurses' emotional intelligence and patient outcomes* (Order No. 3718094). Available from ProQuest Dissertations & Theses Global. (1707900396).

Langley, T. L. (2012). *Impact of social marketing on nurse practitioners' acceptance of clinical video telehealth for elderly patients in rural Mississippi.* (Order No. 3534857, The University of Southern Mississippi). *ProQuest Dissertations and Theses,* 65.

Leibold, N. (2019). *The praxis of critical thinking in nursing.* St. Paul, MN: Nanza Publications

Louisiana State University Health New Orleans. (2019). Doctor of nursing science. Retrieved from https://nursing.lsuhsc.edu/DNS/

Marquis, B.L. and Huston, C.J. (2017). *Leadership roles and management functions in nursing: Theory and application, 9th edition.* Philadelphia: Lippincott, Williams & Wilkins.

Meleis, A. and Dracup, K. (2005). The case against the DNP: History, timing, substance, and marginalization. *Online Journal of Issues in Nursing, 10*(3), 3. Retrieved from https://www.researchgate.net/publication/7541772_The_case_against_the_DNP_History_timing_substance_marginalization

Minnick, A. F., Kleinpell, R. and Allison, T. L. (2018). DNPs' labor participation, activities, and reports of degree contributions. *Nursing Outlook*, doi:10.1016/j.outlook.2018.10.008

Myer, M. L. (2012). *Using a consensus process to develop an evidence-based practice guideline for school exclusion for head lice (pediculosis capitis).* (Order No. 3507134, University of South Carolina). ProQuest Dissertations and Theses, 267.

National Association of Clinical Nurse Specialists (NACNS). (2019). What is a CNS? Retrieved from https://nacns.org/about-us/what-is-a-cns/

NACNS. (2015). Position statement on the nursing practice doctorate. Retrieved from https://nacns.org/advocacy-policy/position-statements/position-statement-on-the-doctor-of-nursing-practice/

NACNS. (2016). PhD position statement. Retrieved from https://nacns.org/advocacy-policy/position-statements/phd-position-statement/

National League for Nursing (NLN). (2007). Doctor of Nursing Practice. Retrieved from http://www.nln.org/aboutnln/reflection_dialogue/refl_dial_1.htm

National League for Nursing. (2013). A Vision for Doctoral Preparation for Nurse Educators: A Living Document from the National League for Nursing. Retrieved from http://www.nln.org/docs/default-source/about/nln-vision-series-%28position-statements%29/nlnvision_6.pdf?sfvrsn=4

National League for Nursing and Commission for Nursing Accreditation. (2016). Accreditation standards for nursing education programs. Retrieved from http://www.nln.org/docs/default-source/accreditation-services/cnea-standards-final-february-201613f2bf5c78366c709642ff00005f0421.pdf?sfvrsn=12

National Organization of Nurse Practitioner Faculties (NONPF). (2002). Strategic initiative. Retrieved from http://www.nonpf.org/?page=83

NONPF. (2016). The White Paper: The Doctor of Nursing Practice Nurse Practitioner Clinical Scholar. Retrieved from https://cdn.ymaws.com/www.nonpf.org/resource/resmgr/docs/ClinicalScholarFINAL2016.pdf

Nickitas, D. M. (2011). The clinical doctor of nursing (DNP): What's the value?. Connecticut Nursing News, 84(3), 11.

O'Sullivan, A., Carter, M., Marion, L., Pohl, J., Werner, K., (September 30, 2005). Moving forward together: The practice doctorate in nursing. *OJIN: The Online Journal of Issues in Nursing. 10*(3), Manuscript 4. doi: 10.3912/OJIN.Vol10No03Man04

Pieper, B. and Colwell, J. (2012). Doctoral education for WOC nurses considering advanced practice nursing. *Journal of Wound, Ostomy & Continence Nursing. 39*(3, 249–255.

Rajala, I. (2013). *Development and implementation of a quality improvement initiative: Systematic follow-up of patients who have spinal cord stimulator implants.* (Order No. 3590159, University of Nevada, Las Vegas). *ProQuest Dissertations and Theses, 82.*

Rice, D. (2016). The research doctorate in nursing: The PhD. *Oncology Nursing Forum, 43*(2), 146-148. doi:10.1188/16.ONF.146-148

Rhodes, M. K. (2011). Using effects-based reasoning to examine the DNP as the single entry degree for advanced practice nursing. *Online Journal of Issues in Nursing, 16*(3), 20–8.

Root, L., Nuñez, D. E., Velasquez, D., Malloch, K. and Porter-O'Grady, T. (2018). Advancing the rigor of DNP projects for practice excellence. *Nurse Leader, 16*(4), 261–265. doi:10.1016/j.mnl.2018.05.013

Rush University. (2019). Nurse anesthesia (CRNA) DNP program information. Retrieved from https://www.rushu.rush.edu/college-nursing/programs-admissions/nurse-anesthesia-dnp-crna-program

Sage Graduate Schools. (2019). DNS at the School of Health Sciences. Retrieved from https://www.sage.edu/academics/programs-degrees/health-sciences/nursing-education-and-leadership/

Smith, M. A. (2013). *Implementation of electronic medical records in a rural healthcare setting.* (Order No. 3590903, State University of New York at Binghamton). *ProQuest Dissertations and Theses*, 91.

Sonson, S. L. (2013). DNP-prepared APRNs: Leading the Magnet® charge. *Nursing Management, 44*(7), 49–52. doi: 10.1097/01.NUMA.0000431425.39076.81

Swanson, M. L. and Stanton, M. P. (2013). Chief nursing officers' perceptions of the Doctorate of Nursing Practice Degree. *Nursing Forum, 48*(1), 35–44. doi:10.1111/nuf.12003

Tibbitts, T. (2005). A matter of degree: AACN adopts the doctor of nursing practice. *The Frances Payne Bolton Case Western Reserve University Alumni Magazine.* Retrieved from http://fpb.cwru.edu/Alumni/magazines/Fall05/Fall2005-6.pdf

University of Alabama School of Nursing (2013). DSN to PhD conversion. Retrieved from http://www.uab.edu/nursing/home/dsn-to-phd-conversion

University of Alabama. (2019). Overview—EdD in Instructional Leadership, concentration in Nurse Education. Retrieved from https://bamabydistance.ua.edu/degrees/edd-in-instructional-leadership-nurse-education/index.php

University of Maryland School of Nursing. (2019). Nurse anesthesia-doctor of nursing practice. Retrieved from https://www.nursing.umaryland.edu/academics/doctoral/dnp/nurse-anesthesia/

University of Medical Sciences Arizona. (2018). Doctor of nursing science. Retrieved from http://www.umsaz.org/dnp.html

University of Minnesota School of Nursing. (2019). Doctor of nursing practice and nurse anesthesia. Retrieved from https://www.nursing.umn.edu/degrees-programs/doctor-nursing-practice/post-baccalaureate/nurse-anesthesia

University of Washington School of Nursing. (2018). Degree programs and tracks: A community of scholars. Retrieved from https://nursing.uw.edu/programs/degree-programs-tracks/

Volkert, D. and Johnston, H. (2018). Unique issues of DNP students: A content analysis. *Nursing Education Perspectives*, 39(5), 280–284. doi:10.1097/01.NEP.0000000000000379

Whitlow, M. L. (2013). *Bringing technology to the bedside: Using smartphones to improve interprofessional communication.* (Order No. 3574432, University of Virginia). *ProQuest Dissertations and Theses*, 121.

Planning and Conducting the DNP Project: A Toolkit for Success

BARB SCHREINER, PhD, APRN, CDE, BC-ADM

INTRODUCTION

Chapter 2 explores the differences among typical culminating scholarly works, the masters' thesis, the doctoral dissertation, and the DNP project. The American Association of Colleges of Nursing's *The Essentials of Doctoral Education for Advanced Nursing Practice* (AACN, 2006) provides a guiding framework for a discussion of applicable directions for the DNP project. Examples of published projects are offered, leading into a practical guide for planning, delivering, and evaluating the practice-change or quality improvement initiative.

DNP PROJECT, DISSERTATION, AND MASTER'S THESIS

A thesis, dissertation, and DNP project are similar in that they all demonstrate mastery of the core essentials required from the graduate nursing student's program of study. These milestones represent the culmination of an academic program that moves the student forward in her or his knowledge toward a specific outcome. Each of these scholarly forms of assessment demonstrates the student's advanced level of understanding, addresses an issue related to the specific course of study and provides specific evidence to inform clinical practice. Each form of assessment is assigned to a particular type of course of study.

Because the focus of each type of degree (PhD, DNP and MSN) differs with regard to concentration and academic mastery, achievement is verified through a detailed process designed to highlight the outcomes assigned to that particular academic program. The dissertation and thesis formats have been used in the academic environment for

35

many years. There is a general, legacy understanding as to what each of these milestones require for completion. With the DNP being the newest academic degree, there are often differing opinions as to what defines or constitutes an appropriate DNP project. Both DNP programs and students are in flux about the elements of a quality DNP project. For instance, what does a DNP project do for the field of nursing, for the student's environment, or for the student's career path? How does one go about designing and implementing a DNP project?

Theses and dissertations are formal documents traditionally used to support a student's standing for a graduate degree. A master's thesis is an original piece of scholarship that focuses on an area of interest within a student's chosen field of study. A master's thesis is typically shorter and narrower in focus than a dissertation, and the form of inquiry may only focus on assessing previous research findings. A master's thesis is designed to respond to a problem or debate noted in the literature or is a piece of inquiry that brings forth new evidence within the topic of concentration.

A dissertation, on the other hand, is an original piece of research that focuses in detail on a specific topic or sub-topic in the student's chosen field of investigation (Merriam-Webster, 2014). Typically comprised of five parts, a dissertation provides evidence that supports a conclusion through identification of an area of study, literature review, research methodology, findings and discussion. This method of inquiry is used to develop theory or test theory as a means toward best practices.

Finally, the DNP project is based on transformative methodology that addresses quality improvement within nursing or healthcare. Application of research to practice is a key component of the DNP project, and practice can be focused on a nursing or healthcare problem, organization, or policy. The DNP project reflects the student's command of knowledge and expertise at applying such proficiency to contemporary real-world problems. One aim of the DNP project is to propose or test sustainable changes that positively impact nursing (AACN, 2006). Conducted as an individual or collaborative venture, the DNP project must meet an identified need, utilize an evidence-based interventions and acceptable nursing actions, has defined, actionable metrics, produce outcomes that can be evaluated with structured analytics and demonstrate sustainability (Ahmed, 2013; NONPF, 2012). Throughout the project, DNP students demonstrate their ability to evaluate and apply current practice approaches. This in turn provides the foundation for creating clinical strategies that improve nursing outcomes (Brown and

Crabtree, 2013). Table 2.1 demonstrates the rich variety and distinctions among the thesis, dissertation and DNP project.

Expansion of a Thesis into a DNP Project

A DNP project can expand a master's thesis by directing the thesis findings to current application. As previously noted, the master's thesis can define a problem currently noted in nursing or healthcare. Review of current literature, analysis of previous research and research in a sub-section of an area of interest provide a solid foundation for a DNP Project. For instance, the Master's thesis may explore the risk factors leading to food insecurities in older Americans, while the DNP project would provide a depth and analysis of the literature, perhaps including interviews, and would design and implement evidence-based interventions to address the health concern.

Expanding a Master's thesis, the DNP student can ask how the information in the Master's thesis impacts nursing. The answer to this question will provide the direction for the DNP project. For example, a nurse might have investigated the literature that evaluated school-based clinics to improve overall health of elementary school children as a thesis. The nurse could then utilize the findings from that work to decide as to what might be needed in schools to support health among children and adolescents. A DNP project to impact such an area within nursing and healthcare could evolve into a sustainable solution. The initial area of interest remains the same. However, the DNP student takes the initial findings and transforms that information into an intervention that impacts quality of care.

This intervention might take the form of establishing a health clinic in a school, providing a needed service within the already established health clinics, or offering educational materials to students via a kiosk at the health clinic. The direction the nurse chooses to expand upon the thesis will depend upon the findings and the nurse's area of interest. Additional literature and research may need to be considered before the overall project is finalized; however, a large part of the foundation needed for a DNP project will have been accomplished through the work conducted at a master's level.

Act Locally, Think Globally

By addressing local problems, a DNP nurse may, in turn, impact

TABLE 2.1. Sample Dissertation Thesis and DNP Project Topics: A Comparison.

Type	Title	Description
Dissertation	Adolescent Substance Abuse: A Research Investigation of Risk Factors in Vulnerable Populations	A qualitative investigation that allows thematic representation of risk factors linked to substance use among adolescents to emerge. This research study provides a theoretical model that can be applied to practice.
Thesis	Assessment of Intervention Practices with Substance Abuse in Adolescents	A thesis that investigates and evaluates therapeutic practices for intervention with substance use disorders in adolescents. This comprehensive exploration of treatment models and outcomes is a thorough representation of the literature present at the time of publication.
DNP Project	Educational Intervention with High Risk Youth	A therapeutic, nursing intervention was developed that can be used in both the school and community setting. Based on current literature and research, this 14-week intervention was developed, implemented and evaluated to serve the needs of high-risk youth in a school system in the Southeastern Portion of the United States.
Dissertation	An Assessment of Holistic Practices to Palliative Care	A multivariate analysis of 15 holistic was conducted in relation to palliative care units in inpatient and outpatient setting throughout the United States. Finding link type and combinations to specific outcomes determined to be essential to palliative care within multiple settings.
Thesis	A Review of Literature Addressing the Use of Holistic Practices in Palliative Care	A literature survey was conducted among nursing, holistic care, and behavioral sciences to ascertain the types and ways holistic practices are used in palliative care. An argument for increasing the use of holistic practices was presented and supported as part of this thesis.
DNP Project	Use of Holistic Interventions to Improve Palliative Care Practices	Using findings from current literature and research, a holistic approach to palliative care was developed using an integrative approach to holism and nursing care. This approach was incorporated into the strategic program initiative for a palliative care unit in the Midwest. Note: After the results were seen at this institution, the system adopted this approach for all their hospitals within their healthcare system.

(continued)

TABLE 2.1 (continued). Sample Dissertation Thesis and DNP Project Topics: A Comparison.

Type	Title	Description
Dissertation	Lateral Violence: An Assessment of Variables that Impact Nursing Practice	A mixed method investigation utilizing grounded theory and survey assessment was conducted to obtain information related to lateral violence in nursing. Information related to personal experience and variables believed to support lateral violence were assessed. The population surveyed included nurses working in rural, suburban, and urban settings. Three percent of the participants were randomly selected to participate in the grounded study portion of the investigation.
Thesis	Assessment of Lateral Violence Among Nurses in a Hospital Setting	An investigation of beliefs about lateral violence was conducted in a rural hospital and medical center to determine if there were any differences in experiences and beliefs about lateral violence and nursing. A survey was conducted via an online system to obtain nurses' opinions and experiences related to lateral violence in these two settings.
DNP Project	Lateral Violence, Safety and Best Practices: An Educational Intervention Program for Hospital Administrators	A two-day workshop was developed and presented to hospital administrators in the Northeast portion of the United States. Based on current findings, a program to make hospital administrators aware of the problem of lateral violence, safeguards that can be put into place and potential intervention strategies when lateral violence occurs was offered. This workshop was open to senior managers, CEOs, CNOs, and other leadership with an interest in this topic.

national and international concerns. The reverse is also true. Whenever a DNP project is developed at the local level, consideration as to what national and international trends and findings need to be included. The Institute of Medicine, QSEN, Center for Disease Control, UNICEF, the American Nurses Association are good examples of resources to ascertain trending within healthcare and the nursing profession. Consider what other national and international resources can you determine that might impact your area of interest for a DNP project.

When programs are developed, it is important that they are sustainable. Utilizing information from national and global organizations offers the DNP student and practitioner a lens into current and future issues in healthcare. Best practices mandate that we address current issues and that we look toward future needs. Having insights into what is needed locally and what is occurring on a larger scale, provides a foundation for the DNP student or DNP-prepared nurse to consider next steps and possible funding sources for the current or future projects.

As the Affordable Care Act emerged on the healthcare scene, prevention became a primary area of interest (Shearer, 2014). DNPs can have a strong presence in both prevention and intervention practices. Being aware of healthcare issues and trends allows the DNP to predict what programs and other clinical practices will be needed to meet the demands within his or her current practice and community. It is important that the DNP take the lead in addressing application of research to practice in a meaningful way. This practice can be developed during the DNP course of study, and it can be reflected in the DNP project chosen.

HOW TO CHOOSE A DNP PROJECT: AN OVERVIEW

Whatever a student selects, it is important that he or she has a passion for the topic. The student will be living with the subject matter for many months, and if there is not a compelling interest from the start, it will be easy for the student to be less than enthusiastic the longer the project progresses.

Once one or more areas have been chosen, a review of the research and current literature related to the topic is needed. Looking at what has been written about specific areas within the nursing focus of interest, the DNP student needs to consider what has and has not been successfully accomplished related to the topics under review. At this stage, it is important to consider problems that are emerging and research that may be used to address such problems.

For instance, if the DNP student is interested in diesel emissions and the potential link to healthcare issues noted in rural communities, it would be important to review what is known about diesel emissions and health concerns. The student would also need to review the unique characteristics found in rural communities that are related to the impact of diesel emissions. The next step might be to explore what research suggests as proactive choices in dealing with the problem. The DNP student would then investigate what had been done in similar circumstances. This exploration will provide an outline of possible interventions and perhaps trigger creative or innovative solutions. To expand the perspective, the student should also consider what some national organizations, like the CDC, have said about the problem. Based upon these findings, the DNP student then can decide if this is an area that needs further intervention, and if so, what that intervention might be.

Next the DNP student must consider if he or she will have the means to develop an intervention that flows from the area of interest. Special consideration needs to be placed on identifying key stakeholders and their support for a possible intervention. The student should also be ready to address pushback from possible sources or stakeholders. Access to the population or individuals necessary for the intervention to take place, and resources need to generate the intervention are also major concerns when selecting a project. This might be a good point in which to do a SWOT Analysis of strengths, weaknesses, opportunities and threats linked to the problem and possible intervention (Berry, 2014).

Sometimes students conducting DNP projects and dissertations have hit snags because of timing. The student may need to consider whether the intervention must be carried out at a time of the year. For example, if simulation and nursing student skill levels are the focus of the DNP project, then the intervention needs to occur during the time a nursing program is in session. This one piece might make the difference in which site is chosen, specific population within the area of interest utilized and even the preceptor selected who will be supporting the DNP student. Considering your project, what issues might need to be addressed up front so that similar timing issues do not occur as the project emerges?

It is imperative that the DNP student focus on what needs are noted within nursing and healthcare, and special attention needs to be assigned to the direction that will be taken within the practice change process. This may be difficult for a student in a BSN to DNP program. In that case, it will be important that a foundational piece be included that reflects the skills developed through a Master's thesis or something similar. By providing this foundation, the BSN to DNP student will have time to grasp the necessary information needed to discern how to choose a problem for investigation, have the research that will offer an understanding of the scope and potential interventions for the DNP Project and provide time needed to acclimate to the scope and role assigned to the DNP practitioner. The understanding of what it means to be a DNP practitioner is especially important when conceptualizing the DNP project, as the project is how the student is able to demonstrate knowledge and skills needed to demonstrate mastery of AACN's *The Essentials of Doctoral Education for Advanced Nursing Practice* (AACN 2006).

Revisiting the Essentials

The doctoral essentials were established to direct advanced practice nursing. Broad in scope, the essentials provide guidance as to the scope and role of practice. For consideration, three of the essentials will be addressed in further detail.

Essential II: Organizational and Systems Leadership for Quality Improvement and Systems Thinking (AACN, 2006). These essential addresses the organizational and systems leadership evidenced within the scope of DNP practice. In addition to directing attention to the needs of individuals, the DNP practitioner needs to be prepared to work with specific groups of stakeholders within the healthcare systems. These systems can be as small as a panel of patients or as large as sets of populations. DNP prepared nurses need to be equipped to conceive new healthcare delivery models that are based on current research and are viable within current and future healthcare environments. Such delivery models must consider organizational, economic and other impacting dynamics to eliminate health disparities and to promote optimal care that supports safety and excellence in practice.

Working alone or in partnership with other health professionals, the DNP practitioner has the vantage of an academic preparation that supports developing and evaluating delivery approaches within the DNP's area of expertise. These approaches must be broad enough in scope to meet current and future demands of specific populations, while continuing to promote healthcare and patient safety. Accountability is a major part of this process, and DNP prepared nurses must be willing to apply scientific findings and ethical mandates to interventions specific to the identified problem or need that is emergent within their scope of practice. While research and statistics are not the primary focus of a DNP preparation, they become tools to help the DNP assess and evaluate sustainable interventions. (AACN, 2006).

An example of what this AACN Essential might look like in practice is as follows:

> *Patients at a medical center where a DNP works are continuing to contract MRSA on the specialty units in large numbers. While MRSA has been contained on the medical surgical floors, there are an exceedingly large number of patients contracting MRSA on the specialty units. The DNP was assigned to review this problem.*

The first thing the DNP might do is examine the literature for the latest information regarding MRSA and how it is being tracked nationally. For example, knowing about new MRSA strains would prove useful. This information would be combined with chart reviews and determination of any significant commonalities other than location of patients that did and did not contract MRSA on the specialty units. Perhaps ancillary services or rotation of staff between units is the key. Working with the nurse epidemiologist and the quality care team, the DNP can collaborate with other healthcare professionals to find the problem source. He or she can interview and observe practices of healthcare professionals within the specific units where MRSA is being contracted and lead the intervention to address any issues noted.

In a situation such as this, the best practices need to be validated on all units affected. An in-service education might be recommended to the nurse educator for the organization. The DNP could coordinate that effort. In addition, protocols for assessment of best practices by nurse managers, the nurse epidemiologist and others could be developed as a preventative practice. These measures could also be included in new employee orientation.

The point is that skills learned during the DNP project are translatable to the DNP's future work as a doctorally prepared nurse.

Health Care Policy for Advocacy in Health Care

The 2010 *Patient Protection and Affordable Care Act* (ANA, 2009) ᴶearly exemplifies the importance of advanced practice nurses and the influence on healthcare. The ANA position statement on Ethics and Human Rights (ANA, 2010) indicates that the profession of nursing has an obligation for the health and well-being of individuals and society. This fits well with the scope and role of practice for the DNP prepared nurse. DNP graduates are equipped to assume a leadership role within organizations and on a more global front as decisions pertaining to policy are addressed. This role of the DNP prepared nurse and political impact will be discussed in detail in Chapter 9; however, it is important to look at the overview of that essential in relation to DNP practice.

DNP Essential V (AACN, 2006) clearly states that DNP Programs are mandated to guide their students to be at the fore in all areas of advocacy. Therefore, it stands to reason that the DNP prepared nurse has the capability to design, implement and advocate for equity and social justice in health policy and within the political arena. The DNP role is well defined and fits well with this mandate. As leaders in clinical practice, the DNP graduate is in a key position to facilitate the integration of policy, research, and practice. The DNP is prepared to articulate and apply advocacy within professional organizations, the workplace, community organizations, and international platforms. Whatever the venue, it is important for the DNP prepared nurse to remain current on pertinent topics related to her or his area of expertise. Knowledge related to both nursing and current state of affairs is necessary for the DNP to have an impact on such issues.

Looking at education as one example, a DNP prepared nurse has multiple opportunities to impact healthcare and advocacy. A DNP prepared nurse could:

- Teach a course related to leadership and social advocacy within a nursing program.
- Chair a committee that explores pertinent issues in healthcare and patient support in the workplace.
- Design and implement relevant educational programs considering social, cultural, gender, and ethnic needs.
- Design and facilitate educational groups with a health focus within the school setting.
- Write a column at the current workplace or for a community newspaper.
- Develop a blog addressing specific health issues related to patient needs and advocacy.

- Serve as a presenter at professional conferences on topics related to healthcare and nursing advocacy.
- Offer to speak at community events—such as community health fairs and PTA meetings.
- Write letters to the editor on timely health topics.
- Offer evaluations of health policy and advocacy information found on the internet and social media to patients and through public venues.
- Serve on the speaker bureau of a professional nursing organization.

Clinical Prevention and Population Health for Improving the Nation's Health

DNP Essential VII (AACN, 2006) clearly focuses on health promotion and disease prevention to improve the overall health of our nation. The DNP analyzes of scientific data from environmental, epidemiological, and other sources to inform effective preventive interventions for individuals and groups. The Essential reinforces a holistic approach of assessment and implementation which accounts for the unique qualities and strengths of a population.

In addition, this Essential, paramount to achieving the national goal of improving the health status of the United States, could apply to other nations similarly. Unhealthy lifestyle choices account for a majority of preventable mortalities, yet this focus is under-represented when looking at healthcare interventions (United Nations, 2013; U.S. Department of Health and Human Services, 2010). The DNP graduate can utilize information related to social determinants of health, public health, sociocultural factors, and environmental conditions to craft health prevention and promotion strategies. The DNP is in a position to participate in and lead projects promoting the Institute for Healthcare Improvements' Triple Aim for populations: improving the patient experience of care, improving the health of populations, and reducing the cost of health care (Whittington *et al.*, 2015).

The following example helps the DNP student look at this Essential from a community perspective. A DNP prepared nurse has multiple opportunities to impact healthcare and advocacy. A DNP prepared nurse could:

- Analyze data as a means to define emerging problems and develop prevention interventions

- Conduct community assessments to determine prevention and early intervention needs
- Apply current research to specific population program development for cardiovascular disease.
- Utilize data from national organizations to predict prevention education within a city or town.
- Develop educational programs that support local prevention services based on national initiatives.
- Develop, implement and evaluate prevention and early intervention services in a school-based health program.
- Teach community programs specific to developmental needs of various populations.
- Coordinate and develop an intervention program with other health professionals geared toward nutritional health.

The DNP student should review the AACN Essentials and consider how the proposed DNP project might link to one or more Essentials. Table 2.2 provides ideas for projects and their connections to an Essential.

TABLE 2.2. Sample DNP Projects Addressing Select AACN Doctoral Essentials.

Essentials	Possible DNP Projects
Essential II: Organizational and Systems Leadership for Quality Improvement and Systems Thinking	• Possible DNP projects • Addressing incivility • Nurse practitioner scope of practice • Interprofessional practice • Inter-facility communication • Nurse-driven protocols • Leadership styles
Essential V: Health Care Policy for Advocacy in Health Care	• Barriers to care • Health literacy • Social determinants of health • Improving utilization of services • International collaborations
Essential VII: Clinical Prevention and Population Health for Improving the Nation's Health	• Reducing hospital readmissions • Clinical practice guidelines • Risk screening • Role of technology • Provider stress

THE DNP PROJECT

DNP projects are written as a testament to the student's knowledge that was learned and can be applied to practice. The DNP Project must reflect the course of study taken, and the project's focus needs to be an area that will support nursing and healthcare. Examples vary depending upon the focus and interest of the DNP student. The following are a few examples of what can be found in the literature regarding the DNP Project.

McCoy (2018) addressed the shortage of clinical sites for undergraduate nursing students by creating an education program for faculty. Faculty experienced high fidelity simulation and its benefits. As a result, faculty were more likely to support and adopt simulation in the nursing curriculum

Collaboration between nurses and physical therapists was the major emphasis of another study (Bullock, 2018). The author found that physical therapists were not routinely monitoring pulse and blood pressure during and after therapy sessions. To address this patient safety issue, Bullock employed the Plan-Do-Study-Act (PDSA) rapid cycle of improvement to establish an communicate policy in an orthopedic clinic. As a result, therapists were more likely to stop sessions and refer patients for cardiac follow up care.

Roth (2018) addressed health literacy by using a machine learning database system to help patients understand their electronic medical records. Patients found the tool useful and easy to understand. The author speculated that such tools will improve health literacy and patient safety.

DNP projects run the gamut of issues related to education, collaboration, technology, and leadership. Reid (2018), for instance, instituted a 12-week education and support program to help nurse leaders uncover and enhance "the conditions that contribute to joy in the workplace." Following the program there was a noticeable 18% decrease in expected turnover.

Defining the Scope of the Project

Happy is the student who enters the DNP program with a project idea already in place. But more often than not, the student has a vague interest area but not a fully articulated project idea. One of the first steps is to decide the scope of the project. Are you interested in patient groups or populations? Are organizations, models of care, or quality improvement more interesting? Do you prefer systems, cost analyses, or community care? Regardless of the scope, there are several resources to help. Several DNP programs list student projects on the school's website. Table 2.3 provides a list of DNP programs with such lists. Several professional organizations also list DNP student projects including the National Organization of Nurse Practitioner faculty and the Doctor of Nursing Practice organization. If chronic illness care is of interest, the site www.improvingchroniccare.org may provide inspiration. If nursing care in healthcare facilities is the interest area, the case studies coming from the National Database of Nursing Quality Indicators are models for further DNP scholarly work or practice inquiries (Montalvo and Dunton, 2007; Dunton and Montalvo, 2009; Duncan, Montalvo, and Dunton, 2011).

In reviewing completed DNP projects, it is apparent that students have taken a variety of approaches. Projects cover clinical practice and interventions (including guidelines and protocols), products (including

TABLE 2.3. Academic Programs Listing DNP Projects.

Program	Website/URL
Boise State University	https://www.boisestate.edu/nursing-dnp/scholarly-projects/
Duke University School of Nursing	https://nursing.duke.edu/sites/default/files/publications_by_dnp_graduates_9-13-2018.pdf
Old Dominion University	https://www.odu.edu/nursing/graduate/dnp/advanced-practice/student-presentations#tab682122356095=2
Rutgers School of Nursing	http://nursing.rutgers.edu/students/DNPExecutive/files/CompletedCapstoneList.pdf
University of Iowa College of Nursing	http://www.nursing.uiowa.edu/academic-programs/dnp/leadersip-project-abstracts
University of Kentucky	https://uknowledge.uky.edu/dnp_etds/
University of Massachusetts Amherst	http://scholarworks.umass.edu/nursing_dnp_capstone/
University of Missouri Sinclair School of Nursing	https://nursing.missouri.edu/academic-programs/dnp/doctor-nursing-practice-program-projects/
University of San Francisco	https://repository.usfca.edu/dnp/
Vanderbilt University	https://nursing.vanderbilt.edu/dnp/scholarlyproject.php

patient-care technology aids, usability and human factors), programs (including feasibility, cost, and impact), and policies (including clinical, organizational, or educational) (Hickey and Brosnan, 2012). One area particularly amenable to DNP study is patient safety (Hughes, 2008; Newhouse, 2006). The National Organization of Nurse Practitioner Faculties (NONPF) (2007) has offered a sampling of DNP projects including: conducting quality improvement for care processes, developing and analyzing policy, designing and using decision-making tools, evaluating impact of technology use at the bedside, designing new care models, collaborating with legislators, and developing or evaluating community health programs.

According to Titler *et al.* (1994) and Titler *et al.* (2001), practice inquiries, or practice change projects may be derived from practice-focused triggers or knowledge-focused triggers. For example, the DNP student reviews risk management data and notices that the fall rates on a nursing unit have exceeded the average for the institution. This practice-focused trigger developed from quality data and clinical observations. The knowledge-focused trigger, on the other hand, derives from new standards, guidelines, or evidence from the literature. For example, the recent revisions to blood pressure (Whelton *et al.,* 2018) and lipid guidelines (Grundy *et al.,* 2018) would serve as knowledge-focused triggers.

Triggers may help the DNP student to isolate a project topic. Exploratory questions may also help. Magyary, Whitney, and Brown (2006) suggested a number of questions to help isolate the focus of a practice inquiry or practice change project (see Table 2.4).

Rather than an individual project, DNP practice inquiry projects often depend on the needs of the agency or organization. DNP students may need to "be open to formulate projects based on agency needs and view the project goal as learning the practice change process" (Brown and Crabtree, 2013, 334). In such cases, the student must be adept at identifying key stakeholders and project champions and be willing to explore existing quality initiatives.

Finally, Stevens and Ovretveit (2013) of the Improvement Science Research Network identified topics which will guide investigators to "determine effective strategies in quality improvement and patient safety" (Improvement Science Research Network, 2010). The priorities include coordination and transitions of care, high performing care processes, evidence-based quality improvement strategies, and human factors and cultures of quality.

TABLE 2.4. Probing Questions to Trigger DNP Project Ideas (Magyary, Whitney, and Brown, 2006).

- Who does/does not have access to nursing services and healthcare programs, and why?
- How are nursing services and programs being delivered in a timely and cost-effective way?
- What types of clinical, demographic, process, and outcome variable data need to be systematically collected and analyzed to monitor and evaluate clinical patterns over time and to monitor variance in healthcare services and outcomes that account for health disparity across subpopulations?
- How can clinical epidemiological benchmark comparison studies yield viable quality-improvement information?
- What system, structural, and technological changes are necessary to capture relevant and critical data?
- What types of evidence-based prevention and treatment nursing clinical guidelines are/are not implemented?
- What are the issues and barriers that prevent implementation of evidence-based nursing clinical guidelines?
- What are successful approaches for implementing and evaluating evidence-based nursing clinical guidelines to influence clinical processes and outcomes?
- Who is most/least likely to benefit from certain types of nursing services and programs (differential effects)?
- What types of moderating and mediating variables are linked to nursing intervention processes and outcomes?
- How are nursing interventions appropriately modified for subpopulations?
- How are evidence-based nursing clinical guidelines modified to be culturally relevant for diverse populations?
- How are individuals, families, and populations motivated to engage in intergenerational patterns of healthy lifestyles?
- What types of organizational structures, financial incentives, and healthcare policies positively or negatively impact how nursing practice and programs are delivered?
- What types of relational partnerships with patients, families, and communities are linked to health outcomes?

Narrowing the Topic to a Manageable Project

Often, identifying the problem and selecting an interest area will result in a project much too broad for a DNP final project. Narrowing the topic can be one of the most challenging steps in developing the project. Hulley and colleagues (Ogrinc *et al.,* 2012) suggested applying FINER to narrow the focus of research (or quality improvement) projects. FINER reminds the DNP students to develop projects which are feasible, interesting, novel, ethical, and relevant. Consider the topic, "the best way to provide diabetes education to a homeless population." Is this narrow enough for a DNP project? Does it meet the FINER assessment? How might the topic be further refined?

Several resources may help the student to further narrow a topic of interest. Mind mapping or the use of fishbone diagrams are two of several brainstorming tools. A variety of tools may be found at www. mindtools.com. How might the student isolate a reasonable, manageable project from the topic of diabetes education for the homeless? A simple place to begin is to answer these questions:

- Why is this a problem?
- Who is it a problem for?
- Who benefits from a solution?

While it may be enticing to begin with a solution in mind, try to avoid such an approach. Rather, thoroughly consider the problem and the possible causes by beginning with the problem, not the solution.

To further define the problem, Bonnel and Smith (2014) recommended using self-exploration. Why do you want to study this topic? What do you already know about the topic? How will your background support the project? What areas will you need to gain further knowledge or skill? When the project is completed, what expertise will you have gained?

When you apply these questions, you are assuring that your clinical interests and expertise are incorporated in the project. For the DNP student, the process of graduate study fine tunes your scholarly skills and intellectual curiosity. These skills allow you to "know how to frame compelling questions about clinical phenomena as experienced and observed in practice" (Magyary, Whitney, and Brown, 2006).

Revisiting the topic, the best way to provide diabetes education to a homeless population, what will help to narrow the focus? The Figure 2.1 illustrates how a mind map refines the topic. Notice how the original interest area (diabetes education for the homeless) now incorporates the DNP student's clinical experience (prescription filling behavior for low income/homeless patients). The solution (diabetes education) has been replaced with a more expansive analysis of the underlying problems.

Another approach is to compare the current state with the desired state. The questions in Table 2.5 address both risks and benefits of change.

Waldrop *et al.* (2014) described five criteria for developing and completing a meaningful DNP project using the phrase "EC as PIE": E =

Enhances; C = Culmination; P = Partnerships; I = Implements; E = Evaluates". Successful DNP projects are designed to enhance health outcomes or healthcare policy. At the culmination of the project, the resulting change should be pragmatic and practical as well as timely, reproducible, and sustainable. DNP projects use various approaches and strategies but should demonstrate partnerships through collaborative interdisciplinary teams. Further, the DNP student implements evidence-based practice and evaluates the outcomes of the practice or policy change. It might be argued that a sixth criteria, dissemination also be included in successful DNP projects. Sharing both the process and the outcomes of the project will help enhance and advance nursing care.

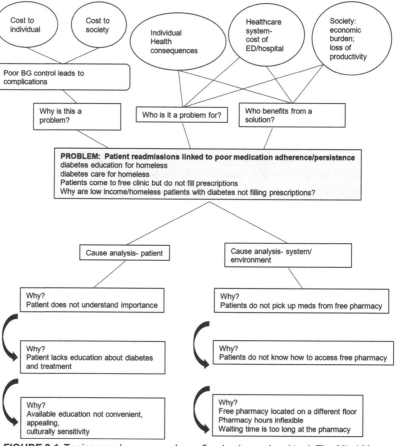

FIGURE 2.1. Topics may be narrowed or refined using a visual tool, The Mind Map.

TABLE 2.5. Narrowing the Focus: Comparing Current to Desired.

Topic/Interest Area	
Current Situation	**Desired Situation**
Why is this a problem?	Why is this a better state?
What is the evidence that this is a problem?	What is the evidence that this is a better state?
What is maintaining the current state (internal and external drivers and constraints)?	What would have to change to reach the desired state (internal and external drivers and constraints)?
What are the benefits in maintaining the current state?	What are the benefits of achieving the desired state?
What are the risks in changing the current state?	What are the risks in changing to the desired state?

Selecting a Theoretical Framework

Refining the project will also help the student to select a theoretical foundation. There are several constructs which may help the DNP student to isolate features of the project to study. For instance, Donabedian's (1966, 2005) structure-process-outcomes model suggests that quality is derived when three primary pathways are aligned. In his original work, Donabedian focused on the relationship between physician and patient and identified the setting of care or the structure of the organization includes the processes that support the delivery of quality care. This pathway includes the "the adequacy of facilities and equipment; the qualifications of medical staff and their organization; the administrative structure and operations of programs and institutions providing care; fiscal organization and the like." The process pathway, on the other hand, concerns whether care is delivered in accordance with current standards, or as Donabedian wrote, "whether medicine is properly practiced." Finally, Donabedian defined the outcome of medical care "in terms of recovery, restoration of function, and of survival" and noted that "outcomes, by and large, remain the ultimate validators of the effectiveness and quality of medical care." Donabedian's model has been expanded to encompass healthcare in general and for the DNP student, this model may adequately serve as an underlying theoretical construct.

Scholars have expanded on Donabedian's model. Talsma *et al.*

(2014), for instance, further operationalized the 'structure' component. The authors proposed a "Quality, Implementation, and Evaluation" (QIE) model to better understand the forces driving implementation of evidence-based practice. Talsma *et al.* identified several forces, including policy, patient preparedness, provider competency, and performance/accountability.

Others have expanded Donabedian's concept of outcomes. Aday *et al.* (2009) proposed that not only are quality and effectiveness important, but equity and access must be considered in an evaluation of quality. The works of Talsma *et al.*, Aday *et al.*, and others underscore the complexity of program evaluation. The DNP student must appreciate that multiple variables intersect to produce program outcomes and that an appropriate framework will guide the DNP project.

As practice inquiries or practice change initiatives, DNP projects should also have a theoretical underpinning addressing change. Kotter's 8 step model, Bridges' transition model, or Rogers' diffusion of innovation, are all models amenable to the change process defining DNP projects.

Articulating the Project Question

Using a tool such as PICOT or PICOT/S assists the DNP student in describing the focus or boundaries of the project. PICOT/S, the acronym for population, intervention, comparison, outcomes, timeframe and setting, was introduced by Richardson *et al.* (1995) and adapted by McDonald, Chang, and Schultz (2013) as a method of framing a researchable clinical question. Stillwell *et al.* (2010) proposed several templates to help formulate a PICOT-style question. While all the elements may not apply to every DNP project, the components may change a nebulous idea into a refined question of great merit. Take, for instance, the question posed earlier: Why are low income/homeless patients with diabetes not filling prescriptions? The DNP student decided to develop a multifaceted intervention incorporating systems change (pharmacy hours and role of pharmacist) and an educational approach (diabetes education curriculum change). The resulting PICOT/S was thus crafted: In low income/homeless patients with diabetes (P), how do systems and educational changes (I) compared to standard care (C) affect prescription filling behaviors (O) within 9 months (T) in a community clinic (S)?

DNP students sometimes struggle with fitting their projects into a PICOT framework. There may not be a comparison group, for example.

In these cases, the current state is the comparison. Here is an example: In a pediatric clinic (P), how would a triage system (I) work to decrease waiting time (O) within 6 months (T)? The comparator in this case is the current situation—no triage system.

Once the student has isolated a viable and interesting project, determined the underlying theoretical framework, and has developed a viable question, it is time to apply a project management approach. Preparing the project mimics the nursing process and thus the scientific method: assessing, planning, intervening, and evaluating.

TABLE 2.6. Narrowing the Focus: Comparing Current to Desired.

PDSA (Shewhart/Deming) Cycle (Best and Neuhauser, 2006)	1. Plan 2. Do 3. Study 4. Act
Six SIGMA (Black and Revere, 2006)	1. Define 2. Measure 3. Analyze 4. Improve 5. Control
CDC (U.S. Department of Health and Human Services, 2011)	1. Engage stakeholders 2. Describe the program 3. Focus the evaluation 4. Gather credible evidence 5. Justify conclusions 6. Ensure use of evaluation findings and share lessons learned
Human Performance Technology Model (Van Tiem, 2004)	1. Performance analysis (organization, environmental, gap) 2. Cause analysis 3. Intervention selection, design, and development 4. Intervention implementation and change 5. Evaluate (summative, formative, confirmative)
Evidence-based Practice Models (Lusardi, 2012)	1. Identify a clinical problem 2. Gather the best evidence 3. Critically appraise and evaluate strength of the retrieved evidence 4. Determine a potential practice change 5. Plan and implement a practice change 6. Evaluate practice change outcomes over time

Mitchell *et al.* (2010) reviewed 47 models for evidence-based practice and translational science, finding that the models provided four purposes: "(a) evidence-based practice and knowledge transformation processes; (b) strategic change to promote adoption of new knowledge; (c) knowledge exchange and synthesis for application and inquiry; and (d) designing and interpreting dissemination research" (3). In addition to the evidence-based practice models, there are several models or frameworks to assist the DNP student to organize and plan the project (Table 2.6). An organizing framework or model helps the project team to organize the workflow, delineate the processes, and logically sequence the steps toward completion.

EVALUATION MODELS

Evaluation models grew up in the business world with leaders such as Walter Shewhart, W. Edwards Deming, and others. The Plan-Do-Study-Act cycle, developed by Shewhart and later promoted by Deming, is a tool for continuous quality improvement (Best and Neuhauser, 2006). In the plan phase, a team asks key assessment questions. What could be improved? Why is improvement needed? What can be done? Who will do it? In the Do phase, the practice change is implemented, and outcomes tracked. In the Study phase, the team analyzes the outcomes and compares findings to desired results. Finally, the team must decide next steps: sustain change or enter the PDSA cycle once again. An example of the application of PDSA has been posted by the Institute for Healthcare Improvement (2014).

Six Sigma is another quality improvement methodology widely embraced by industry and business, and, within the past decade, by healthcare systems (Black and Revere, 2006; Liberatore, 2013). The Six Sigma process involves five steps: define, measure, analyze, improve, and control, often abbreviated DMAIC. In the define stage, the team identifies goals stakeholders for the project. The next stage, measure, involves collecting data about the current state or current process. Information from this stage drives the proposed solution or practice change. In the improve stage, the team implements the chosen intervention. It is during this stage that data is collected and analyzed to evaluate the outcomes. Finally, in the control stage, a change management process is implemented to sustain the gains and improvements.

Reports of nurses using Six Sigma methodology are beginning to populate the literature. For example, Donovan *et al.* (2016) successfully applied Six Sigma methodology to the problem of increasing rates of unit-acquired pressure ulcers in high-risk patient populations. Godley and Jenkins (2019) also used a Six Sigma approach to improve patient satisfaction by decreasing waiting time in a radiology department.

In addition to PDCA and Six Sigma, other evaluation models are applicable for DNP projects. The Centers for Disease Control and Prevention (CDC), for instance, advocates a Framework for Evaluation in Public Health (U.S. Department of Health and Human Services, 2011). In this six-step model, there is added emphasis on stakeholder identification and involvement for effective change within public health systems. The model is particularly designed for evaluating programs of care. Stakeholder engagement includes determining which individuals would enhance the credibility of the evaluation, who would actively implement the interventions, who would advocate for the evaluation findings, and who would champion continued funding for the program. In addition to describing the stakeholders, the program must be described in terms of needs, target audience, objectives, activities, deliverables, and outcomes. Visual tools such as logic models can help with this description (U.S. Department of Health and Human Services, 2011).

The next step in the Framework for Evaluation in Public Health is focusing the evaluation on the most critical questions, those that will achieve the greatest utility and are the most feasible. Focusing the evaluation addresses the purpose of the assessment, who wants or needs the results, what will be done with the findings, and what resources will be needed to conduct the evaluation. One or more methods are then used to collect the necessary data. Both the quantity and quality of the data are concerns at this stage. The evidence is then analyzed, and the results interpreted. The final step of the Framework, using and sharing the findings, underscores the philosophy that "the ultimate purpose of program evaluation is to use the information to improve programs." The Framework for Evaluation in Public Health is thus another model available to the DNP student.

The models described thus far share components of the scientific method with varying emphasis. The Human Performance Technology (HPT) Model particularly expands the assessment component (Van Tiem, 2004). HPT is an approach to identifying and solving performance gaps within organizations. In this model, the team would conduct several selected assessments: organizational or business analysis, workforce performance, gap analysis, environmental analysis, or cause analysis.

Based on the extensive assessment, the intervention is designed, implemented, and evaluated. The HPT Model has been used in healthcare quality projects. Lange and Coltham (2005) described the use of the HPT model in improving communication and services to member physicians within a healthcare system. Duman *et al.* (2011) applied the model to a hospital's problem with errors in the radiology department.

Finally, evidence-based practice models are popular in nursing-focused projects. Lusardi (2012) highlighted a number of models (Johns Hopkins Model, Rossworm and Larrabee Model, Stetler Model, and Iowa Model) and extracted the similarities. Nursing models tend to focus on the supporting evidence from both peer-reviewed sources and clinical experience. The models consistently address identifying the clinical problem, gathering and critically appraising scientific and experiential evidence following by defining the practice change. As in other models, the evidence-based practice models include planning, implementing, and evaluating the practice change. Levin *et al.* (2010) were one of the first to propose a merging of the evidence-based models with performance improvement (PI). In their Evidence-Based Practice Improvement model, the authors capitalize on the strong component of searching for and synthesizing existing evidence with the PI approach of testing change with repeated cycles of PDSA (Plan-Do-Dtudy-Act).

Tools for Analyzing the Current State

All models described above mention some form of needs assessment. Depending on the clinical or practice question, the assessment may focus on people, performance, processes, practices, products, or policies. Assessment tools and resources are listed in Table 2.7.

Identifying stakeholders is a critical element for any change project. Stakeholders have varying interest in the project. Some will be supportive and champion or sponsor the projects and its scope and processes. Others, however, are more interested in stopping or interfering with the project. Each type must be carefully engaged and have carefully tailored communication. A stakeholder analysis should include the elements noted in Table 2.8.

Yet another assessment to conduct at the start of a practice change project is a risk assessment. Consider what might hinder the successful completion of the project. Resources are often a pivotal element for the DNP student. Will there be enough time, funding, interest, and people to effectively conduct the project? Is the project feasible? Will there

TABLE 2.7. Forms of Analysis and Resources.

Analysis	Content	Sources
Organization	Improving Primary Care	http://www.improvingprimarycare.org/assessment/full
Organization	NCQA's Patient-Centered Medical Home (PCMH) Recognition Program	https://www.ncqa.org/programs/health-care-providers-practices/patient-centered-medical-home-pcmh/
Organization	Policies, procedures, structure, culture, context, finances, mission, philosophy	Cultural web: http://www.mindtools.com/pages/article/newSTR_90.htm Organizational assessment tools: https://www.centerfornonprofitexcellence.org/sites/default/files/OrganizationalAssessmentsToolsCCF.pdf
Business	Stakeholder analysis: power and interest grid; influence map	Power/interest grid: http://www.mindtools.com/pages/article/newPPM_07.htm Influence map: http://www.mindtools.com/pages/article/newPPM_83.htm
Process	Cause-effect diagrams, flowcharts, work-flow diagrams, process maps	http://www.thinkreliability.com/excel-tools.aspx https://www.health.state.mn.us/facilities/patientsafety/adverseevents/toolkit/ http://www.skymark.com/resources/tools/management_tools.asp
Performance	Knowledge, skills, motivation, capacity, confidence, management, training needs assessment, task analysis	Job performance, training needs, individual needs: http://www.nwlink.com/~donclark/analysis/analysis.html
Cause	Fishbone (cause and effect), flowcharts	http://asq.org/learn-about-quality/process-analysis-tools/overview/overview.html
Economic	Cost benefit; cost utility; cost-effectiveness	Cost analysis tool: https://www.mindtools.com/pages/article/newTED_08.htm
Risk	Risk impact; failure mode and effect analysis (FMEA)	Risk impact tool: https://www.smartsheet.com/all-risk-assessment-matrix-templates-you-need Techniques: https://projmgmtguru.blogspot.com/p/pm-tools.html

TABLE 2.8. Stakeholder Analysis.

Stakeholder Name:
Role in Organization:

Characteristics:
• Interest in project or outcomes
• Perspectives (known areas of concern or resistance)
• Motivators
  —Role in the project (change agent, champion)
  —Input to the project
  —Acquired benefit from the project
  —How and when to engage
  —How and when to update/keep informed
  —Influences
  —Influenced by
  —Aware
  —Understands
  —Accepts
  —Aligned
  —Committed

Adapted from: CDC 2010

be enough support from management or administration or the nursing program? Other questions address the nature of the project itself. Has there been enough assessment of the problem? Are complex solutions needed which are beyond the scope of a DNP project? Will correcting one problem create more issues? How realistic are the goals for a DNP project? DNP students (and advisors) truly want to make a difference. Yet projects must be realistic, address the right question, and allow the student to graduate in time.

Tools for Describing the Program or Project

Recall that the Framework for Evaluation in Public Health (U.S. Department of Health and Human Services, 2011) suggests using a logic model approach to visually describe healthcare programs. A logic model diagrams key components of a program permitting a visual and sequential view (see Figure 2.2). These components form a series of if-then relationships: "*if* resources are available to the program, *then* program activities can be implemented; *if* program activities are implemented successfully, *then* certain outputs and outcomes can be expected" (Innovation Network, Inc., 2010). Knowlton and Phillips (2013) added that if outcomes are achieved, what is the overall impact to the organization or system, to the stakeholders, to constituents, or the community?

Longest (2005) identified three purposes for logic models: strategizing, designing, and leading. The model serves as a roadmap and summary of the program. In its strategizing role, the model graphically depicts the path from resources to outcomes. As a design tool, the model summarizes the program's resources, processes, and activities (inputs), the program's deliverables or products (outputs), and desired short, medium, and long-term outcomes. As a tool for leadership, the logic model provides a roadmap for allocating program resources to logically achieve the results.

Further, logic models guide evaluation and may help the project team communicate the linkage between activities and outcomes. Finally, a logic model "builds common understanding and promotes buy-in among both internal and external stakeholders about what the program is, how it works, and what it is trying to achieve" (Innovation Network, Inc., 2010). Reports in the literature provide numerous examples of ways nurses have applied the logic model to clinical and organizational problems. Frye *et al.* (2018), for instance, effectively used the model to improve the effectiveness of a call program for patients discharged with congestive heart failure. In a different project, Herold *et al.* (2018)

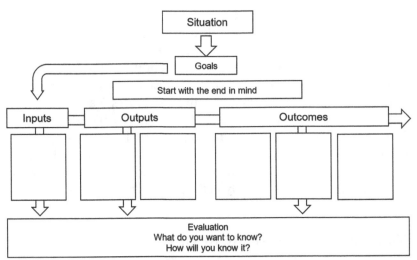

FIGURE 2.2. A logic model template demonstrates the flow of thinking from the problem to the evaluation of the solution.

TABLE 2.9. Resources for Developing Logic Models.

Resource	Materials	Source
University of Wisconsin-Extension, Cooperative Extension, Program Development and Evaluation	Training guide; templates; example; slides; bibliography	https://fyi.extension.wisc.edu/programdevelopment/logic-models/
W. K. Kellogg Foundation	Logic Model Development Guide and Evaluation Guide	https://www.wkkf.org/resource-directory/resource/2006/02/wk-kellogg-foundation-logic-model-development-guide
CDC, Division for heart disease and stroke prevention	Evaluation guide: Developing and using a logic model	https://www.cdc.gov/eval/logicmodels/
Betty C. Jung, RN, MPH, MCHES	A compendium of credible internet resources for evaluation	https://www.bettycjung.net/Evaluation.htm

systematically applied the logic model to integrate pediatric nurse practitioners into the medical child abuse team. For the DNP student, a logic model can assure that there is consistency and alignment across all elements in the program or project (Sun and Cheery, 2018).

Several resources to further explore the logic model as a tool for practice change projects are provided in Table 2.9.

Another tool, the CIPP (context-input-process-product) model, similar to the logic model, was described by Stufflebeam and Shinkfield (2007). The CIPP model addresses the context, input, processes, and product. The program is described in terms of the setting, the presenting problem and program goals (context), resources and characteristics of people in the program (input), activities (process) and anticipated outcomes (product). Hall, Daly, and Madigan (a DNP) (2010) used the CIPP model to develop a documentation tool for clinical nursing educators. Both the logic model and the CIPP model are effective tools for the DNP student to describe a program, link goals to actions and to evaluation, and to plan evaluation early in the project development.

ROLE OF THE LITERATURE REVIEW

Recall that while other evaluation models focused on assessment or

evaluation, the evidence-based evaluation models emphasize the importance of peer-reviewed and other evidence. The literature review serves
to benchmark current practice and helps the DNP student to identify
best practices and to consequently identify gaps in the current state. The
literature supports the rationale for a chosen intervention. However, the
evidence is not equally valid, reliable, credible, or generalizable. The
Agency for Healthcare Research and Quality (AHRQ, 2002) identified
domains and elements to use in reviewing individual articles. For example, AHRQ recommended, in critiquing observational studies, the
reviewer should consider the study question, the sample, the intervention, the outcome measurement, the analysis and results, as well as the
funding source. Melnyk and Fineout-Overholt (2011) advocated for a
rapid appraisal of randomized controlled trials through the use of three
questions:

- Are the findings valid? (i.e., as close to the truth as possible)
- Are the findings important? (i.e., what is the impact of the
  intervention [the size of the effect or the extent to which the
  intervention or treatment worked]?)
- Are the findings clinically relevant or applicable to the patients for
  whom I am caring?

Systems for grading the evidence are important as the student distin-
guishes quality sources of information. While there are many grading
systems, the US Preventive Services Task Force (USPSTF) Evidence
Grading System reflects recommendations for clinical practice (USP-
STF, 2012). The GRADE (Grading of Recommendations, Assessment,
Development, and Evaluation) appraisal system reported by Guyatt
and colleagues (2008) is a systematic approach to categorizing "quality of evidence and strength of recommendations" using a four-level
approach. Melnyk and Fineout-Overholt (2011) offered a seven- level
system based on research design while Evans (2003) ranked evidence-
based on effectiveness, appropriateness, and feasibility. Daly *et al.*
(2007), recognizing that most evidence hierarchies placed qualitative
studies low on the list, devised a system which placed well-crafted
generalizable studies high on the list of qualitative studies followed by
conceptual studies, descriptive studies and single case studies. When
building the literature review, the DNP student should filter published
studies through one or more of these evidence hierarchy systems.

Extracting credible, contemporary evidence and managing the pleth-
ora of citations can be a nightmare. The DNP scholar should decide

TABLE 2.10. Resources for Developing Logic Models.

	P	I	C	O	T	S
Search Terms	Low income/ homeless patients with diabetes	System and educational changes	Standard care	Prescription filling behaviors	Within 9 months	Community clinic
	Low income	Quality improvement		Prescriptions		Community clinic
	Homeless	Support		Prescription filling		Primary care
	Minority	Diabetes education		Medications		Outpatient clinic
	Diabetes	DSMT/E		Adherence		
	Diabetes mellitus			Persistence		
	Type 2 diabetes			ompliance		

TABLE 2.11. Record of Searches.

Clinical Question: Why are low income/homeless patients with diabetes not filling prescriptions?

PICOTS: In low income/homeless patients with diabetes (P), how do systems and educational changes (I), compared to standard care (C), affect prescription filling behaviors (O), within 9 months (T), in a community clinic (S)?

Date of Search	Source	Terms Used	Scope of Search	Number of Citations	Notes
9/1/19	PubMed	Diabetes AND prescription filling	All	39	Use MeSH (Medical Subject Headings) terms for diabetes and medication filling
9/1/19	PubMed	Diabetes mellitus AND medication Adherence	All	1118	Add "persistence"
9/1/19	PubMed	Diabetes mellitus AND medication Adherence AND persistence	All	39	Review references in Meece (2013) article
9/1/19	CINAHL	Diabetes AND medication AND adherence	Searched in abstracts imited to: English Full text Peer-reviewed Exclude Med-line records 2009–2014	36	Refine search for in-terventions to improve adherence/persistence

early in the project how to keep the accumulated information organized and easily retrievable. Three tools will help: creating a search strategy, documenting a record of searches, and using a reference matrix. Creating the search strategy relies heavily on the project question or PICOT/S. Table 2.10 demonstrates a search strategy for the medication adherence project mentioned earlier. Literature searches can be complex with many branches and side roads. A record of searches describes the steps taken in searching the literature and chronicles the decisions made in adjusting the search. It includes the search terms and phrases used (from the search strategy), inclusion and exclusion criteria, and databases searched. A sample record of searches for the clinical question posed early is provided in Table 2.11.

Once the articles or sources are selected, it is important to archive them in a retrievable database or a literature review matrix. This might be as simple as a spreadsheet or as sophisticated as reference management software such as EasyBib, Reference Manager, Endnote, Mendeley, RefWorks, or Zotero. The Cochrane Collaboration recommends a free software program, GRADEpro, developed by the GRADE Working Group. The program and supporting resources are available from https://gradepro.org/. A simple spreadsheet for organizing the literature review is provided in Table 2.12.

TABLE 2.12. Literature Review Matrix.

Source
Purpose/ study questions
Sample (Size, characteristics, inclusion, exclusion criteria, power)
Research design
Variables (dependent, independent)
Instruments
Methods
Results/ Outcomes
Discussion/ Conclusions
Evidence grading
Funding source
Notes

The components of the DNP project addressed thus far include selecting the question, narrowing the focus, conducting a stakeholder analysis, and reviewing the supporting literature. These elements inform the intervention and the evaluation. Once developed, the project is ready to be implemented and the tools of project management should be used.

PLANNING THE EVALUATION

Planning the evaluation of a project should occur early in the development and should closely link to the goals and interventions. In fact, Guerra-López and Thomas (2011) affirmed that "the key ingredient for successfully collecting relevant, reliable, valid, and complete data is alignment" across the components of the project. Using a logic model can visually depict this alignment. The evaluation plan must include key success indicators, data sources, and an analysis plan. Let us say that in the medication adherence project described earlier, the clinical issue is that patients do not fill or refill their prescriptions and their hospital readmissions are linked to these behaviors. The goal of the project is to decrease hospital readmissions which are linked to lack of medication adherence or persistence. The DNP student, with input from stakeholders, decides to implement two interventions. One will address a system problem and will change processes in the pharmacy to make refills easy and automatic. The other approach will address a knowledge deficit and will use phone texts to remind and educate patients about the need to continue prescribed medications. Table 2.13 is the evaluation plan for this project.

Notice that there are several types or levels of evaluation. Evaluation might address the ends (outcomes or products) or the means (processes). Guerra-López and Thomas (2011) noted that "performance indicators, also referred to as *measures* or *metrics*, are specific and concrete gauges of a result, process, or activity that allows us to make complex systems palpable and manageable." Sometimes the metrics are dictated by regulatory or quality entities. For example, the Centers for Medicare and Medicaid (CMS, 2019) and the Joint Commission (2014) have published measures for hospital quality. The National Quality Strategy (NQS) domains highlight priorities for healthcare quality improvement for the Department of Health and Human Services. The NQS domains are patient and family engagement, patient safety, care coordination,

TABLE 2.13. Evaluation Plan.

Project Question/Goal	• Hospital readmissions due to poor medication adherence will be decreased.	
Desired Outcome	• 80% or prescribed medications will be filled or refilled in the defined population.	
Intervention	• Pharmacy system change to easier and automatic process • Message texting within 2 weeks of needed refill	
Key Success Indicators	• Time between refills • Number of patients reached with message texting • Time between healthcare visit and initial filling of medication • Satisfaction of pharmacy staff • Patient satisfaction	
Data Collection Plan	**Pharmacy Records**	**Phone Records**
Data Source(s)	Satisfaction survey Hospital admission data	Satisfaction survey Hospital admission data
Responsible for collecting	Project associate in pharmacy	DNP student
Time needed to collect	Quarterly for 9 months	Monthly for 9 months
Analysis Plan		
Resources needed	Project database, statistical software, DNP Committee statistician, clinic IT support	
Responsible for analysis	DNP student	
Time needed to analyze	1–2 months	

population/public health, efficient use of healthcare resources, and clinical process/effectiveness. The CMS website provides a description of the clinical quality measures used in 2019 for targeted hospitals. The Joint Commission also posts standards and measures for healthcare services across the delivery continuum. These metrics advocated by the organizations may help the DNP in determining key measures for the project.

The National Voluntary Consensus Standards for Nursing-Sensitive Care is another resource for selecting appropriate metrics. The consensus standards identify patient outcomes directly influenced by nursing

TABLE 2.14. Kirkpatrick Evaluation Model Applied to Project Questions.

Level of Evaluation	Sample Project Questions	Sample Sources of Data
1. Reaction	• Did the environment support learning? • Did the learner like the teaching approaches? • Would the learner recommend the program to others?	• Participant satisfaction survey • End-of-class survey • Faculty survey
2. Learning	• What did the participant learn? How well did the participant learn? • What content was difficult? • What additional training is needed? • Which attitudes changed after the classes?	• Pre and post knowledge tests • Skills test • Standardized exams • Attitude assessments
3. Behavior	• How has a behavior or skill changed as a result of the training?	• Skills check list • Behavior diary • Supervisor evaluation • Peer review
4. Results	• What happened to the key organizational goal following training?	• Safety metrics (e.g. number of falls, number of medication errors) • Change in patient satisfaction scores • Change in attrition of staff • Change in clinical outcomes

care (National Quality Forum, 2004). Patient safety, patient education, and nurse staffing are examples of the standards which may apply to the DNP project. In addition to nursing or hospital measures, evaluation may cover patient education and behavior. Kirkpatrick described a four-level evaluation model for training and education projects (Kirkpatrick and Kirkpatrick, 2005). The effectiveness of an education program might be measured in terms of reaction or satisfaction (level 1), learning or knowledge gain (level 2), behavior change (level 3), and organizational results (level 4). The project question, source of data and level of evaluation is provided in Table 2.14.

COLLECTING AND MANAGING THE DATA

The data needed to answer project questions will come from various sources: hospital quality audits, medical or health records, questionnaires, interviews, and benchmark data. Part of planning a DNP project is also planning how data will be collected and handled. Managing and archiving the data will be critical to assuring its integrity and security. A data codebook is necessary to track the names of variables, sources of data, and abbreviations used. Using password protected documents and files increases the security of the data. For instance, a DNP project required that participants complete an online survey. Two emails were sent to the participants. The first contained the password assigned to the individual participant. In a separate email the DNP student sent the link to the secure online survey. Using such precautions is increasingly important in research or projects using the Internet.

Data must be collected consistently and systematically. If multiple assistants will be collecting data, the DNP student will need to train the team and assure a consistent approach to the process of data collection and recording. Another concern is transferring data from one source to another. Moving data can be wrought with error. There must be a plan for verifying the data and dealing with missing data and outliers (Needham *et al.,* 2009); Osborne, 2013; Polit and Beck, 2012). Guerra-López and Thomas (2011) suggested asking whether the data is relevant, valid, reliable, and complete. For instance, are the data pertinent to the project's goals and questions? Are the data meaningful and accurate?

TABLE 2.15. Tools for Collecting Data.

Content	Source
Data Collection Plan	University of Iowa Hospitals and Clinics https://uihc.org/sites/default/files/documents/asset-3728.doc
Data Collection Check Sheet	American Society for Quality https://asq.org/quality-resources/data-collection-analysis-tools
Collecting Performance Data	National Quality Center http://nationalqualitycenter.org/resources/nqc-quality-academy-collecting-performance-data/
Improvement Tracker	Institute for Healthcare Improvement http://app.ihi.org/Workspace/tracker/

Are the data sources credible? Does the project team have confidence in how the data was collected? Are the data adequate to answer the project questions?

Collecting pertinent, meaningful and credible data requires a clearly articulated data collection plan. Several resources may help the DNP student to create such a plan (Table 2.15).

Managing Timelines and Milestones

Managing a DNP project is all about guiding the people, processes, and time necessary to complete the project and to answer the clinical question. Thus, project management is a merging of skills in communication, time management, and goal-focused support. A sample timeline is offered in Table 2.16.

Tracking milestones and tasks can be as simple as this example or as complex as using a computer spreadsheet, Gantt chart, or other formal project management tracking tool. Additionally, several mobile apps can keep the status of the project at the DNP student's fingertips. These apps include Trello, Casual, OmniPlan, Agantty, Timeweek, and Evernote. Regardless of the tool, a timeline is developed from a careful analysis of the steps and sequences needed to complete a project on time. For a DNP project, these steps make sense: (1) list the major milestones in order of occurring, (2) list the tasks required for each milestone in sequence, (3) assign deadlines working backward from the overall project deadline (end of a quarter, weeks before graduation, etc.), and (4) consider adding a cushion of time at key steps to allow for unexpected delays and snags. In some cases, the student may wish to prepare more than one timeline each reflecting a different scenario. For instance, the time required for acquiring institutional or IRB approval may drive different timelines in the actual project.

As the project progresses and milestones are achieved (or delayed), the DNP student will need to communicate to key stakeholders and constituents. The timing of messages and possible formats are provided in Table 2.17.

The DNP student should consider the frequency of communicating with key project participants. This is often driven by the stakeholder analysis completed early in the project development phase. Some participants will need and want frequent information; others will want less frequent communication. It is wise to anticipate points in the project which might interfere with the intervention, data collection, or analysis.

TABLE 2.16. Project Management Timeline.

Project Milestone	Description	Date
Prepare Complete Proposal	• Seek advice from project mentor and faculty • Complete all required elements of the project proposal • Use project management skills and tools to develop tentative timeline for project	
Build Relationship with Key Stakeholders	• Explore aspects of the project to assess buy-in and support from stakeholders	
Approvals/IRB Submission	• Complete any required human subjects training • Secure necessary approvals from site administrators and from DNP faculty • Secure approval from school IRB and from institution IRB	
Kickoff Meeting	• Introduce project to key participants	
Intervention	• Create implementation checklist • Initiate and monitor activities and processes	
Communication Plan	• Implement communication plan for status and milestone reports	
Collect and Manage Data	• Implement data collection plan • Assure data integrity and security	
Complete Project	• Initiate project completion plan	
Data Analysis/Interpretation	• Implement data analysis plan • Interpret results in terms of project goals	
Close Out Project	• Notify IRB of project completion • Archive all study materials in a secure place	
Disseminate Results	• Implement internal communication plan • Initiate external communication plan • Complete requirements for graduation	
Change Management	• Implement continuity/ sustainability plan	

Such risk analysis includes not only what might happen but who might help. For instance, a DNP student was using data from an outpatient clinic to analyze outcomes after changing the patient appointment reminder system. A change in clinic leadership stalled the project because the necessary forms were not being completed properly under the new management. Fortunately, the student had anticipated such problems in data collection and, after consulting with the project champion, had

TABLE 2.17. *Managing Communications Across the Project.*

Key Message	Timing	Format (example)	Target Audience (example)
Project kickoff	Project introduction	• Announcement by project champion or administrator • Kickoff party • Email blast	• Key stakeholders • Project champion • Project manager • Project team
Planning interventions and evaluation	At start	• Team meeting/webcast	• Project champion • Project manager • Project team
Team support	Throughout and at crisis points	• Email updates • Incentives	• Project manager • Project team • Onsite staff
Project status	Weekly or monthly	• Email updates	• Project champion • Project manager
Milestone achievement	As completed	• Quarterly reports • Stakeholder meeting • Update phone calls or emails	• Key stakeholders
Project completion	End of project	• End of project party • Email update	• Key stakeholders • Project champion • Project manager • Project team • Onsite staff
Summary and lessons learned	End of analysis	• Summation meeting • Reflection survey • Executive summary	• Key stakeholders

implemented an alternative approach to data collection. Because the project timeline was padded with an extra 2 weeks in the data analysis phase, the overall project was completed on time.

Implementing the Data Analysis Plan

DNP projects serve different purposes than PhD research (Melnyk 2013). Yet, each relies on data to describe results. While the research student seeks statistical significance, the DNP student seeks effectiveness and utility of a project. Clinical or practical significance is often the focus of a DNP project. The DNP student should have a working knowledge of descriptive statistics and quality assurance tools. Indeed,

TABLE 2.18. Sample Data Analysis Plan.

Key Success Indicators	Data Source	Handling Missing Data	Data Analysis Strategy	Analytic
Time (days) between refills	Pharmacy records	Report only complete data set	Descriptive; continuous data	Range; Mean number of days
Time (days) between healthcare visit and initial filling of medication	Clinic attendance records Pharmacy records	Report only complete data set	Descriptive; continuous data	Range; Mean number of days
Satisfaction of pharmacy staff	Satisfaction survey	Report available data	Descriptive; ordinal data	Mean score for each question
Number of patients reached with message texting	Phone records	Report all data: Reached, not reached, missing	Descriptive; continuous data	Percentage of patients reached
Number of patients responding to text messaging	Phone records—responses to texts	Report only complete data set	Descriptive; continuous data	Count; Mean number of replies
Nature of patient response to text messaging	Content of text replies	Report available data	Qualitative	Thematic analysis
Patient satisfaction	Satisfaction survey	Report available data	Descriptive; ordinal data	Mean score for each question
Relationship between time to hospital readmission and length of time between refills	Hospital admission data Pharmacy records	TBD	Inferential-measures of association	Compare time to readmission for timely refills versus late refills using t test
Relationship between time to hospital readmission and patient response to text messaging	Hospital admission data Phone records—responses to texts	TBD	Inferential-measures of association	Compare time to readmission for number of replies to texts using t-test

Algase (2010) cautioned that "strong grounding in theoretical, metatheoretical, methodological, and analytic approaches is as essential to both programs [PhD and DNP] as is advanced knowledge and skills in a specialized area of practice." Basic statistics, research, or analytics books such as texts by or Kim and Mallory (2017), Polit and Beck (2017), or Sylvia and Terhaar (2018), will help supplement the DNP student's knowledge and will provide description of the tools needed for analysis and interpretation.

The statistics or analytics used may be as simple as descriptive measures such as mean, percent change, or amount increased or decreased. Charts comparing before and after data can be used effectively to highlight key outcomes. Geary and Clanton (2011) described how run charts might easily demonstrate changes in variables. Run charts visually show trends in variables over time. In the medication adherence project, time between refills and readmission rates could be depicted in a run chart covering the first 6 months of the project.

A data analysis plan helps align the key success indicators and the sources of data to the types and level of measurement and statistical approaches. The CDC (2013) noted that "creating an analysis plan is an important way to ensure that you collect all the data you need and that you use all the data you collect." Further, the data analysis plan articulates strategy for analyzing the results. Should the data be viewed from an exploratory or descriptive stance, or should the data serve to make predictions or inferences? The data analysis plan for the medication adherence project is provided as an example in Table 2.18.

As in other phases of the project development, creating a plan for data analysis will be time well spent. Goals link to interventions which link to type of data collected which ultimately link to an interpretation of the data in terms of the goals. Depending on the nature of the analysis, it may be wise to consult a statistician early in the creation of the data analysis plan.

Creating a Change Management and Sustainability Plan

While it may feel that the project is completed when the last analysis and interpretation are finished, the job of managing change and sustaining the positive outcomes is only beginning. Based on the careful stakeholder analysis and the careful management of stakeholder expectations, the DNP student should have an environment ready for this next phase. Change management strategies include clear communication, dissemination of findings and recommendations, and support of adjustments to processes and roles.

Developing a change management or sustainability plan is much like peering into a crystal ball. The project is completed, there are positive findings, and now the work of applying the change takes over. Several questions may guide the DNP student in this phase of the doctoral project (see Table 2.19). Taking time to develop two or three key messages will help sell the project to others. These key messages should consider the stakeholder's perspective. For example, will this practice change meet resistance from the staff nurses? How might you craft the information about the project to reassures these nurses? How will the project benefit them? What are the easy steps to making this change work? What is the patient-centric message that will resonate for them?

While considering the elements change management/sustainability plan check list, the DNP student should also recognize that the practice environment can play a prominent role in maintaining change. Studer (2014) listed the traits high performing organizations exhibit when ini-

TABLE 2.19. Change Management/Sustainability Plan Check List.

- Key messages
  —Address the stakeholder's perspective (adopters and non-adopters; supporters and non-supporters)
  —Articulate the benefits and challenges of the change
  —Stage the change process by defining the steps toward change
- People
  —Who will be involved in implementing the new state?
  —Who will lead/ supervise/manage the new state?
  —How will impact to workflow and workload be managed/ supported/ sustained?
  —How will changes to jobs and roles be managed/ supported/ sustained?
- Process
  —What processes must continue?
  —Which processes are no longer needed?
  —What policies and procedures are needed to maintain the new state?
- Resources
  —What resources are needed to maintain the new state?
  —What education or training is needed?
- Monitoring
  —How frequently should the program be evaluated?
  —What data will need to be collected (and by whom)?
  —What happens if change processes or practices slip?

tiating change and having that change stick: workers understand the why of change, the organization embraces process improvement, leaders have strong change agent skills, and employees have the knowledge to make change happen. Key to change maintenance is the ongoing communication out to stakeholders and constituents of the project. The Institute for Healthcare Improvement (2004) provides a comprehensive tool, the spread planner, with a series of questions to help the project director plan for informing stakeholders and sustaining the project (see http://www.ihi.org/resources/Pages/Tools/SpreadPlanner.aspx).

SUBMITTING THE DNP PROJECT FOR INSTITUTIONAL REVIEW

While nurses conducting research projects must demonstrate safety to the Institutional Review Boards (IRBs), increasingly, DNP students planning quality improvement projects are also being reviewed by IRBs. As a result, the DNP student must understand the role of the IRB in the student's project planning. IRBs have been established to "assure consistent, safe, ethical behavior of all health professionals and unfailing protection of human subjects" (Terhaar and Taylor, 2018). From 1974 through 1981 several federal rules and guidance documents set the stage for the IRB processes and principles in place today. The Belmont Report (The National Commission for the Protection of Human Subjects of Biomedical and Behavioral Research, 1979), for instance, described ethical principles such as respect, autonomy, beneficence, and justice and provided guidance for the early consent forms and participant selection. By 1981 federal policies protected vulnerable populations and established oversight for the local IRBs (U.S. Department of Health and Human Services, 2018).

To receive approval from the local IRB, the DNP student must do the following: follow all requirements set forth by the IRB and by the student's faculty mentor, complete required training, use only the forms approved by the IRB, complete the forms precisely, and plan sufficient time for the review and possible revisions.

Follow all IRB Requirements

Institutional Review Board have clear expectations and processes in place to assure that reviews are fair and in compliance with federal rules and regulations. For the DNP student this means that application requirements, deadlines, and required communication is non-negotiable. To have a smooth experience with the IRB, thoroughly read the guide or handbook available from the IRB, the nursing program, or the University's research department. Follow all steps in the application process. Consult with your faculty mentor when in doubt.

Complete Required Training

Most IRBs, universities, or project sites require that the DNP student complete an educational program in research ethics and compliance. Courses are produced by the Collaborative Institutional Training Initiative (CITI) and typically available through the student's college or university. Complete the training early in the IRB application process. An IRB will not review the proposal for the DNP project until the training is completed.

Complete Forms Precisely

IRBs must meet federal compliance guidelines. This often means that several documents must be completed by the DNP student. Follow all steps in the application, fully complete each section, and do not exceed the allowed number of words in each section. Often the DNP student completes an IRB application from the more formal proposal presented to a faculty committee. The IRB may want to see this formal proposal as an attachment. However, the IRB will be most interested in the IRB application with the required elements in the required amount of words. An IRB will pay particular attention to how the student plans the following:

- Protecting privacy, autonomy, and dignity of the participants
- Assuring confidentiality of the project data and records
- Describing recruitment and incentive methods
- Assuring that individuals are voluntarily participating
- Providing adequate information which allows participants to make informed decisions
- Identifying and minimizing risks to the participants
- Identifying and protecting vulnerable populations

Supporting materials are typically a required element of the IRB application. The IRB committee will want to see any promotional or advertising materials, the consents or assent forms, data collection tools, and permission to use copyrighted surveys, site approvals, or permission to use existing data.

The types of forms required will depend on the level of review the IRB or university requires. Projects with minimal risk will often require review by a panel of the IRB rather than the full committee. As a project or research study increases in risk, a full review by the entire IRB committee will be required. The IRB staff will determine which level of review will be required by federal law. The required degree of IRB member involvement determines the review timeline.

Pace yourself. Completing an IRB application requires precision and attention detail. Be well rested for each section and complete a few sections at a time.

Plan Sufficient Time

The IRB process is often an iterative one requiring revisions and resubmission. The DNP student should plan for unexpected delays. IRB committee members are volunteers- faculty, community experts, and others. Know the IRB calendar for submissions and reviews. Get to know the administrative colleague who manages the IRB calendar. Know that breaks between academic semesters may also mean breaks for the IRB. IRBs have busy seasons when many doctoral applications are submitted. The IRB administrative colleague can often share this inside information to help the DNP student better plan for a submission timeframe.

Some IRB Tips

Before submitting the application, conduct a checklist. Is the application clear? Would a community member of the IRB understand the project? Could someone else conduct the project simply by reading the application? Are all the documents completed? Are there any pieces missing? Do all the documents tell a consistent story?

Be consistent throughout the application. If you will be recruiting 50 participants, be sure that 50 participants are planned in the data collection and analysis. If participants receive travel expenses, be sure that the budget reflects that. Confirm that numbers are consistent and aligned throughout.

Be ready to safely and confidentially archive all study or project materials (recruitment flyers, consent forms, data files). Depending on the nature of the project and the risk involved, the IRB may require that these materials be retained for seven years beyond the completion of the project.

After approval, any modifications or changes made to the project must be reported to the IRB. Most importantly, the DNP student may NOT conduct any portion of the project without the IRB final approval. That means no recruiting, no consenting, no interventions are allowed until full approval is received.

SUMMARY

Noted visionary, scholar and business guru, W. Edwards Deming (1998) proposed that a System of Profound Knowledge (SoPK) was needed to successfully launch and sustain a change project. He described the interplay among appreciating the interlocking parts of a system, understanding the impact of common and special cause variations, building knowledge from data and repeated cycles of learning and testing, and recognizing the important human element of change. For the DNP student preparing a practice change project, the SoPK serves as a reminder of the components driving change. While Deming provided the theory behind change, this chapter explored the processes to make that change happen through a successful practice change or DNP project.

Practice change projects should afford the DNP student an opportunity to gain expertise in quality improvement (Brown and Crabtree 2013) and should result in knowledge about improving patient care or bettering systems and processes (Waldrop *et al.,* 2014). At the end of a project, the DNP student should have become an expert about a specific problem and its solutions. With these goals in mind, this chapter concludes with several pieces of advice for the DNP student:

- Begin with the problem—not the solution
- Seek strong leadership support and stakeholder involvement
- Communicate throughout the life of the project
- Develop integrals skills in
    - —Quality improvement methods (needs assessment, gap analysis, stakeholder analysis, risk appraisal, evaluation planning)
    - —Project management (milestone and timeline monitoring, communication planning)

—Data management and analysis (data collection and integrity, data analysis and interpretation, use of technology for analysis and presentation)

REFERENCES

Algase, D. L. (2010). Essentials of scholarship for the DNP: Are we clear yet? [editorial]. *Research and Theory for Nursing Practice, 24*(2), 91–93.

Aday, L. A., Begley, C. E., Lairson, D. R., Slater, C. H., Richard, A. J., & Montoya, I. D. (1999). A framework for assessing the effectiveness, efficiency, and equity of behavioral healthcare. *American Journal of Managed Care, 5* (Special issue), S25–S44.

Ahmed, S.W. (Ed.) (2013). *DNP education, practice and policy. Redesigning advanced practice roles for the 21st century*. New York: Springer.

AHRQ. (2002). Systems to rate the strength of scientific evidence. Evidence report/ technology assessment: number 47. AHRQ publication no. 02-E015. Rockville, MD: Agency for Healthcare Research and Quality. Retrieved from http://archive. ahrq.gov/clinic/epcsums/strengthsum.pdf

American Association of Colleges of Nursing (AACN). (2006). *The essentials of doctoral education for advanced nursing practice*. Retrieved from https://www.aacn. nche.edu/publications/position/DNPEssentials.pdf

American Nurses Association. (2009). A message from ANA President Rebecca A. Patton. Retrieved from www.nursingworld.org/FunctionalMenuCategories/MediaResources/PressReleases/2009-PR/President-Patton-Letter.aspx

American Nurses Association. (2010). The nurses's role in ethics and human rights: Protecting and promoting individual worth, dignity, and human rights in the practice setting. Retrieved from http://www.nursingworld.org/MainMenuCategories/EthicsStandards/Ethics-Position-Statements/-Nursess-Role-in-Ethics-and-Human-Rights.pdf

Berry, T. (2014) What is a SWOT analysis? Retrieved from http://articles.bplans.com/ business/how-to-perform-swot-analysis/116

Best, M. and Neuhauser, D. (2006). Walter A. Shewhart, 1924, and the Hawthorne factory. *Quality and Safety in Health Care, 5*(2), 142–143. doi: 10.1136/ qshc.2006.018093. Retrieved from http://www.ncbi.nlm.nih.gov/pmc/articles/ PMC2464836/

Black, K. and Revere, L. (2006). Six Sigma arises from the ashes of TQM with a twist. *International Journal of Health Care Quality Assurance, 19*(3), 259–266. doi:http:// dx.doi.org/10.1108/09526860610661473

Bonnel, W. and Smith, K.V. (2014). *Proposal writing for nursing capstones and clinical projects*. New York, NY: Springer.

Brown, M.A. and Crabtree, K. (2013). The development of practice scholarship in DNP programs: A paradigm shift. *Journal of Professional Nursing, 29*(6), 330-337. doi: 10.1016/j.profnurs.2013.08.003

Bullock, E. (2018). *Blood pressure and heart rate screenings in physical therapy: An interprofessional DNP project* (DNP Scholarly Project, East Carolina University). Retrieved from http://hdl.handle.net/10342/7005

Centers for Disease Control and Prevention (CDC). (2010, April). Individual evaluation plan outline. In CDC, *Learning and growing through evaluation: State asthma program evaluation guide* (pp. E1–E6). Atlanta, GA: Author. Retrieved from http:// www.cdc.gov/asthma/program_eval/guide.htm

Centers for Disease Control and Prevention. (2013). Creating an analysis plan. Atlanta, GA: Centers for Disease Control and Prevention. Retrieved from http://www.cdc.gov/globalhealth/fetp/training_modules/9/creating-analysis-plan_pw_final_09242013.pdf

Centers for Disease Control and Prevention, Division for Heart Disease and Stroke Prevention. (n.d.). *Evaluation guide: Developing and using a logic model.* Retrieved from http://www.cdc.gov/dhdsp/programs/nhdsp_program/evaluation_guides/logic_model.htm

Centers for Medicare and Medicaid (CMS). (2019). Clinical quality measures basics. Retrieved from https://www.cms.gov/regulations-and-guidance/legislation/ehrincentiveprograms/clinicalqualitymeasures.html

Daly, J., Willis, K., Small, R., Green, J., Welch, N., Kealy, M. and Hughes, E. (2007). A hierarchy of evidence for assessing qualitative health research. *Journal of Clinical Epidemiology, 60*(1), 43–49. doi:http://dx.doi.org/10.1016/j.jclinepi.2006.03.014

Deming, W. E. (1998). A system of profound knowledge. In Neef, D., Siesfeld, G. A. and Cefola, J. (Eds.), *Economic Impact of Knowledge* (pp. 161–174). Woburn, MA: Butterworth-Heinemann.

Dissertation. Retrieved from http://www.merriam-webster.com/dictionary/dissertation

Donabedian, A. (1966/2005). Evaluating the quality of medical care. *Milbank Quarterly, 83*(4), 691–729. doi: 10.1111/j.1468-0009.2005.00397.x. Retrieved from http://www.ncbi.nlm.nih.gov/pmc/articles/PMC2690293/pdf/milq0083-0397.pdf (reprinted from "Evaluating the quality of medical care", 1966, *The Milbank Memorial Fund Quarterly, 44*(3, Pt. 2), pp. 166–203.)

Donovan, E. A., Manta, C. J., Goldsack, J. C. and Collins, M. L. (2016). Using a lean Six Sigma approach to yield sustained pressure ulcer prevention for complex critical care patients. *Journal of Nursing Administration, 46*(1), 43–48. doi: 10.1097/NNA.0000000000000291

Duman, B. D., Chyung, S. Y., Villachica, S. W. and Winiecki, D. (2011). Root causes of errant ordered radiology exams: Results of a needs assessment. *Performance Improvement, 50*(1), 17–24. http://dx.doi.org/10.1002/pfi.20192

Duncan, J., Montalvo, I. and Dunton, N. (2011). *NDNQI case studies in nursing quality improvement.* Silver Spring, MD: American Nurses Association.

Dunton, N. and Montalvo, I. (Eds.). (2009). *Sustained improvement in nursing quality: Hospital performance on NDNQI indicators, 2007–2008.* Silver Spring, MD: American Nurses Association.

Evans, D. (2003). Hierarchy of evidence: a framework for ranking evidence evaluating healthcare interventions. *Journal of Clinical Nursing, 12*(1), 77–84. doi:10.1046/j.1365-2702.2003.00662.x

Frye, T.C., Poe, T. L., Wilson, M. L. and Milligan, G. (2018). Evaluation of a postdischarge call system using the Logic Model. *CIN: Computers, Informatics, Nursing. 36*(2), 106–112. doi: 10.1097/CIN.0000000000000397

Geary, M. and Clanton, C. (2011). Developing metrics that support projects and programs. In J.L. Harris, L. Roussel, S. E. Walters and C. Dearman (Eds.), *Project planning and management: A guide for CNLs, DNPs, and nurse executives* (pp. 119–145). Sudbury, MA: Jones and Bartlett.

Godley, M. and Jenkins, J. B. (2019). Decreasing wait times and increasing patient satisfaction: A Lean Six Sigma approach. *Journal of Nursing Care Quality, 34*(1), 61–65. doi: 10.1097/NCQ.0000000000000332

Grundy, S.M., Stone, N.J., Bailey, A.L., Beam, C., Birtcher, K.K., Blumenthal, R.S.,...&

Yeboah, J. (2018). 2018 AHA/ACC/AACVPR/AAPA/ABC/ACPM/ADA/AGS/ APhA/ASPC/NLA/PCNA Guideline on the management of blood cholesterol: A report of the American College of Cardiology/American Heart Association Task Force on Clinical Practice Guidelines. *Journal of the American College of Cardiology.* Advance online publication. https://doi.org/10.1016/j.jacc.2018.11.003.

Guerra-López, I. and Thomas, M. N. (2011). Making sound decisions: A framework for judging the worth of your data. *Performance Improvement, 50*(5), 37–44. http:// dx.doi.org/10.1002/pfi.20219

Guyatt, G.H., Oxman, A.D., Vist, G., Kunz, R., Falck-Ytter, Y., Alonso-Coello, P. and Schünemann, H.J. (for the GRADE Working Group). (2008). Rating quality of evidence and strength of recommendations GRADE: an emerging consensus on rating quality of evidence and strength of recommendations. *BMJ, 336,* 924–926. doi:10.1136/bmj.39489.470347.AD

Hall, M. A., Daly, B. and Madigan, E. A. (2010). Use of anecdotal notes by clinical nursing faculty: A descriptive study. *Journal of Nursing Education, 49*(3), 156–159.

Herold, B., St. Claire, K., Snider, S. and Narayan, A. (2018). Integration of the nurse practitioner into your child abuse team. *Journal of Pediatric Health Care, 32*(3), 313–318. https://doi.org/10.1016/j.pedhc.2018.01.005

Hickey, J.V. and Brosnan, C. A. (2012). *Evaluation of health care quality in advanced practice nursing.* New York, NY: Springer.

Hughes, R.G. (Ed.). (2008, March). *Patient safety and quality: An evidence-based handbook for nurses.* (AHRQ Publication No. 08-0043). Rockville, MD: Agency for Healthcare Research and Quality.

Improvement Science Research Network (ISRN). (2010, July). Research priorities. Retrieved from http://www.isrn.net/sites/improvementscienceresearch.net/files/documents/ISRNSummit_Research_Priorities_508_web_0.pdf

Innovation Network, Inc. (2010). Logic Model workbook. Washington, DC: Author. Retrieved from http://www.slideshare.net/InnoNet_Eval/logic-model-workbook

Institute for Healthcare Improvement. (2004). Spread planner. Retrieved from http:// www.ihi.org/resources/Pages/Tools/SpreadPlanner.aspx

Institute for Healthcare Improvement. (2014). How to improve. Retrieved from http:// www.ihi.org/resources/Pages/HowtoImprove/default.aspx

The Joint Commission. (2014). The Joint Commission's electronic accreditation and certification manuals. Retrieved from http://www.jointcommission.org/standards_ information/edition.aspx

Jung, B.C. (2014a). Evaluation resources on the internet. http://www.bettycjung.net/ Evaluation.htm

Jung, B.C. (2014b). Research resources on the internet. Retrieved from http://www. bettycjung.net/Study.htm

Kim, M., and Mallory, C. (2017). *Statistics for evidence-based practice in nursing* (2nd ed.). Burlington, MA: Jones and Bartlett.

Kirkpatrick, D. and Kirkpatrick, J. (2005). *Transferring learning to behavior: Using the four levels to improve performance.* San Francisco, CA: Berrett-Koehler.

Knowlton, L. W. and Phillips, C. C. (2013). *The logic model guidebook: Better strategies for great results.* Thousand Oaks, CA: Sage.

Lange, P. D. and Coltham, B. (2005). Organizational change management and alignment: A health care case study. *Performance Improvement, 44*(3), 34–45.

Levin, R. F., Keefer, J. M., Marren, J., Vetter, M., Lauder, B. and Sobolewski, S.

(2010). Evidence-based practice improvement: Merging two paradigms. *Journal of Nursing Care Quality, 25*(2), 117–126. doi: 10.1097/NCQ.0b013e3181b5f19f

Liberatore, M. J. (2013). Six sigma in healthcare delivery. *International Journal of Health Care Quality Assurance, 26*(7), 601–626. http://dx.doi.org/10.1108/IJH-CQA-09-2011-0054

Longest, B. B. (2005). Logic models as aids in managing health programs. *Journal of Nursing Administration, 35*(12), 557–562.

Lusardi, P. (2012). So you want to change practice: Recognizing practice issues and channeling those ideas. *Critical Care Nurse, 32*(2), 55–64. doi:10.4037/ccn2012899 20130601061759465080619

Magyary, D., Whitney, J. and Brown, M. (2006). Advancing practice inquiry: Research foundations of the practice doctorate in nursing. *Nursing Outlook, 54*(3), 139–151.

McCoy, T. L. (2018). Implementing high-fidelity simulation to meet undergraduate clinical requirements. *UNLV Theses, Dissertations, Professional Papers, and Capstones*. 3289. Retrieved from https://digitalscholarship.unlv.edu/thesesdissertations/3289

McDonald, K.M., Chang, C. and Schultz, E. (2013, January). Closing the quality gap: Revisiting the state of the science: Summary report. (Prepared by Stanford UCSF Evidence-based Practice Center under Contract No. 290-2007-10062-I.) AHRQ Publication No. 12(13)-E017. Rockville, MD: Agency for Healthcare Research and Quality. Retrieved from http://effectivehealthcare.ahrq.gov/index.cfm/search-for-guides-reviews-and-reports/?productid=1375&pageaction=displayproduct

Melnyk, B. M. (2013). Distinguishing the preparation and roles of doctor of philosophy and doctor of nursing practice graduates: National implications for academic curricula and health care systems. *Journal of Nursing Education, 52*(8), 442–448. doi:http://dx.doi.org/10.3928/01484834-20130719-01

Melnyk, B. M. and Fineout-Overholt, E. (2011). *Evidence-based practice in nursing and healthcare: A guide to best practice* (2nd ed.). Philadelphia, PA: Lippincott Williams and Wilkins.

Mitchell, S.A., Fisher, C.A., Hastings, C.E., Silverman, L.B. and Wallen, G.R. (2010). A thematic analysis of theoretical models for translational science in nursing: Mapping the field. *Nursing Outlook, 58*(6), 287–300.

Montalvo, I. and Dunton, N. (2007). *Transforming nursing data into quality care: Profiles of quality improvement in U.S. healthcare facilities*. Silver Spring, MD: American Nurses Association.

The National Commission for the Protection of Human Subjects of Biomedical and Behavioral Research. (1979, April 18). Ethical principles and guidelines for the protection of human subjects of research (The Belmont Report). Retrieved from https://www.hhs.gov/ohrp/sites/default/files/the-belmont-report-508c_FINAL.pdf

National Organization of Nurse Practitioner Faculties (NONPF). (2007). NONPF recommended criteria for NP scholarly projects in the practice doctorate program. Retrieved from http://c.ymcdn.com/sites/www.nonpf.org/resource/resmgr/imported/scholarlyprojectcriteria.pdf

National Organization of Nurse Practitioner Faculties (NONPF). (2012). Core competencies for nurse practitioners. Retrieved from http://www.nonpf.displacecommon.cfm?an=1&subarticlenbr+14

National Quality Forum. (2004). National voluntary consensus standards for nursing-sensitive care: An initial performance measure set. Washington, DC: Author. Retrieved from http://www.qualityforum.org/Publications/2004/10/National_

Voluntary_Consensus_Standards_for_Nursing-Sensitive_Care__An_Initial_Performance_Measure_Set.aspx

Needham, D. M., Sinopoli, D. J., Dinglas, V. D., Berenholtz, S. M., Korupolu, R., Watson, S. R., Lubomski, L., Goeschel, C. and Pronovost, P. J. (2009). Improving data quality control in quality improvement projects. *International Journal for Quality in Health Care, 21*(2), 145–150. doi:10.1093/intqhc/mzp005

Newhouse, R. P. (2006). Selecting measures for safety and quality improvement initiatives. *The Journal of Nursing Administration, 36*(3), 109–113.

Ogrinc, G. S., Headrick, L. A., Moore, S. M., Barton, A. J., Dolanksy, M. A. and Madigosky, W. S. (2012). *Fundamentals of health care improvement: A guide to improving your patients' care* (2nd ed.). Oakbrook Terrace, IL: The Joint Commission.

Osborne, J. W. (2013). *Best practices in data cleaning: A complete guide to everything you need to do before and after collecting your data.* Thousand Oaks, CA: Sage.

Polit, D. F. and Beck, C. T. (2017). *Nursing research: Generating and assessing evidence for nursing practice* (10th ed.). Philadelphia, PA: Wolters Kluwer.

Reid, A. (2018). Implementing IHI joy in work framework to decrease turnover among unit leaders. *Doctor of Nursing Practice (DNP) Projects.* 143. Retrieved from https://repository.usfca.edu/dnp/143

Richardson, W.S., Wilson, M.C., Nishikawa, J. and Hayward, R. S. (1995). The well-built clinical question: A key to evidence-based decisions [Editorial]. *ACP Journal Club, 123*(3), A12–A3. Retrieved from https://mclibrary.duke.edu/sites/eno.duhs.duke.edu/files/public/guides/richardson.pdf

Roth, E. A. (2018). Improving patients' understanding of their Electronic Medical Record data in order to improve self-management—A quality improvement project. *Doctor of Nursing Practice (DNP) Projects, 174.* Retrieved from https://scholarworks.umass.edu/nursing_dnp_capstone/174

Shearer, G. (2010, October). *Prevention provisions in the Affordable Care Act.* Retrieved from https://www.apha.org/~/media/files/pdf/topics/aca/prevention_aca_final.ashx

Stevens, K. R. and Ovretveit, J. (2013). Improvement research priorities: USA survey and expert consensus. *Nursing Research and Practice, 2013* (Article 695729). http://dx.doi.org/10.1155/2013/695729. Retrieved from http://www.hindawi.com/journals/nrp/2013/695729/

Stillwell, S. B., Fineout-Overholt, E., Melnyk, B. M. and Williamson, K.M. (2010). Evidence-based practice, step by step: Asking the clinical question: A key step in evidence-based practice. *American Journal of Nursing, 110*(3), 58–61. doi: 10.1097/01.NAJ.0000368959.11129.79

Studer, Q. (2014). Making process improvement 'stick'. *Healthcare Financial Management, 68*(6), 90–94, 96.

Stufflebeam, D. L. and Shinkfield, A. J. (2007). *Evaluation theory, models, and applications.* San Francisco, CA: Jossey-Bass.

Sun, G. and Cheery, B. (2018). Using the Logic Model framework to standardize quality and rigor in the DNP project. *Nurse Educator.* Published Ahead of Print. DOI: 10.1097/NNE.0000000000000599

Sylvia, M. L. and Terhaar, M. F. (2018). *Clinical analytics and data management for the DNP* (2nd ed.). New York, NY: Springer.

Talsma, A., McLaughlin, M., Bathish, M., Sirihorachai, R. and Kuttner, R. (2014). The quality, implementation, and evaluation model: A clinical practice model for sustainable interventions. *Western Journal of Nursing Research, 36*(7), 929–946. doi:10.1177/0193945914537121

Terhaar, M. F. and Taylor, L. A. (2018). Best practices for submission to the Institutional Review Board. In M.L. Sylvia and M. F. Terhaar (eds.). Clinical analytics and data management for the DNP (2nd ed.). New York: Saunders.

Titler, M.G., Kleiber, C., Steelman, V., Goode, C., Rankel, B., Barry-Walker, J., Small, S. and Buckwalter, K. (1994). Infusing research into practice to promote quality care. *Nursing Research, 43*(5), 307–313.

Titler, M.G., Kleiber, C., Stee lman, V.J., Rakel, B. A., Budreau, G., Everett, ... Goode, C. J. (2001). The Iowa model of evide nce-based practice to promote quality care. *Critical Care Nursing Clinics of North America, 13*(4), 497–509.

United Nations. (2013). Millennium development goals and beyond 2015. Retrieved from: http://www.un.org/millenniumgoals/pdf/MDG_FS_4_EN.pdf

U.S. Department of Health and Human Services. (2010, November). *Healthy People 2020* [ODPHP Publication No. B0132]. Retrieved from http://www.healthypeople. gov/sites/default/files/HP2020_brochure_with_LHI_508_FNL.pdf

U.S. Department of Health and Human Services. (2018, July 19). Electronic Code of Federal Regulations, Part 46: Protection of human subjects. Retrieved from https:// www.ecfr.gov/cgi-bin/retrieveECFR?gp=&SID=83cd09e1c0f5c6937cd9d7513160 fc3f&pitd=20180719&n=pt45.1.46&r=PART&ty=HTML

U.S. Department of Health and Human Services, Centers for Disease Control and Prevention (CDC). Office of the Director, Office of Strategy and Innovation. (2011, October). *Introduction to program evaluation for public health programs: A self-study guide*. Atlanta, GA: Centers for Disease Control and Prevention, Retrieved from http://www.cdc.gov/eval/guide/CDCEvalManual.pdf

U.S. Preventive Services Task Force (USPSTF). (2012, July). Grade definitions. Retrieved from http://www.uspreventiveservicestaskforce.org/uspstf/grades.htm

University of Wisconsin-Extension, Program development and evaluation. (2014). Evaluation logic model templates. Retrieved from http://www.uwex.edu/ces/ pdande/evaluation/evallogicmodelworksheets.html

Van Tiem, D. M. (2004). Interventions (solutions) usage and expertise in performance technology practice: An empirical investigation. *Performance Improvement Quarterly, 17*(3), 23–44.

Waldrop, J., Caruso, D., Fuchs, M.A. and Hypes, K. (2014). EC as PIE: Five criteria for executing a successful DNP final project. *Journal of Professional Nursing, 30*(4), 300–306. http://dx.doi.org/10.1016/j.profnurs.2014.01.003.

Whelton, P.K., Carey, R.M., Aronow, W.S., Casey, D.E. Jr, Collins. K.J., Dennison Himmelfarb, C.,Wright, J.T. Jr. (2018). 2017 ACC/AHA/AAPA/ABC/ACPM/ AGS/APhA/ASH/ASPC/NMA/PCNA guideline for the prevention, detection, evaluation, and management of high blood pressure in adults: A report of the American College of Cardiology/American Heart Association Task Force on Clinical Practice Guidelines. Hypertension, 7(6), e13–e115. DOI: 10.1161/HYP.0000000000000065.

Whittington, J. W., Nolan, K., Lewis, N. and Torres, T. (2015). Pursuing the Triple Aim: The first 7 years. *The Milbank quarterly, 93*(2), 263–300. doi:10.1111/1468-0009.12122

W.K. Kellogg Foundation. (1998/2004a). *Logic model development guide*. Battle Creek, MI: Author. Retrieved from http://www.wkkf.org

W. K. Kellogg Foundation. (1998/2004b). *Evaluation handbook*. Battle Creek, MI: Author. Retrieved from www.wkkf.org

Preparing to Write Your DNP Project Example-Faculty Incivility: Implementation of Civility Policy and Procedures

JENNIE PATTISON, DNP, RN

Although the beginning stages of developing an evidenced-based project proposal for the DNP program can seem daunting at first, it will end up being one of the most rewarding educational experiences. The ability to follow a passionate subject from the discovery of a gap between research and practice to planning and implementation of the project is an extraordinary experience. It is important for DNP students to find a topic that they deeply care about because an enormous amount of time will be spent turning this topic into a quality evidence-based practice project.

When exploring topics for the DNP project, do not hesitate to contact specific stakeholders, colleagues, peers, and scholars to discuss the potential topic or concern. LaRose (2016) emphasizes the need for collaboration with significant stakeholders when researching an evidence-based practice change. The collaboration process helps to validate the gaps in practice and the need for the evidence-based practice change. The information received throughout this collaboration process will add to the success of your project.

PROBLEM IDENTIFICATION

The first step in developing the DNP proposal is identifying an issue or concern in nursing that ignites passion. I recommend identifying more than one topic/concern that sparks interest and passion. Explore each of the concerns further through an extensive literature review. This is an excellent way to discover the current research on the topic, what intervention works, and what intervention does not work. Remember that the librarian is a great resource within the university. Please do not hesitate to ask the librarian for help if there is difficulty finding the necessary literature. In addition, continue to collaborate with stakeholders, colleagues, peers, and scholars.

When exploring the topics that generate passion, stay within the setting in which you are most familiar and comfortable. For example, if the work experience of the DNP student concentrated in a traditional ground campus, choosing an online setting would most likely be unfamiliar and uncomfortable. I stayed within the post-licensure online environment since I was most familiar with this setting.

Initially, the three nursing education issues I identified were faculty/student incivility, poor rubrics, and communication issues within the online environment. I recommend staying organized with this process and report the articles and findings on a spreadsheet or table. I had several research articles on each topic but decided to settle on an area that exuded the most excitement and passion—faculty incivility.

When I was in nursing school, incivility was rampant. The common metaphor phrase, "nurses eat their young," resonated throughout nursing school. I could not help but wonder how this was possible. Nursing was supposed to be a caring profession; yet, incivility prevailed. I felt that I was one of the most kind and considerate nursing students. However, my kind nature turned into fear of nurses and doctors alike. My passion developed over the years to discover a way to eradicate incivility in nursing. I felt nursing faculty were role models to future nurses. If nursing instructors were uncivil, student nurses may follow with the same behavior; students may think it was acceptable behavior since their nursing instructor conveyed incivility. According to Del Prato (2013), faculty incivility creates a negative image of nursing, which should be a caring environment, which will lead to disillusionment of student nurses. I realized that I have a passion to fix the problem of faculty incivility, so students have civil, caring faculty role models. Consequently, faculty incivility in nursing school was a great place to focus my DNP project.

As a nursing instructor, I witnessed both student and faculty incivility in traditional and online environments. It is imperative that nurses develop solutions based on evidence to prevent incidences of incivility. Incivility in the academic environment can significantly increase the stress load on the student and decrease learning (Clark, Nguyen and Barbosa-Leiker, 2014). My personal experience, the existing research on the topic of incivility, and my passion to eliminate incidences of incivility helped to establish my DNP project.

It is essential to explore the most current research on the topic. Questions to ask oneself include: (a) which type of setting is affected by the nursing concern?; (b) which population group is affected the most by the nursing concern?; and (c) what interventions based on evidence helps improve outcomes? The setting that came up repetitively during the literature was nursing schools, both the traditional classroom and distance learning. I decided to apply my DNP project to the post-licensure online environment. I was currently working in this area, so it felt most comfortable. According to Atmiller (2012), faculty behavior can stimulate uncivil behavior in students. This helped to spark my interest in faculty incivility. Students' uncivil responses can be a reaction to an uncivil remark or behavior from the faculty.

Students perceived faculty incivility in such behaviors as not posting a syllabus, untimely grades, and unavailability of the instructor (Clark, Ahten, and Werth, 2012). Faculty may not realize some of the behaviors that students perceive as uncivil. For example, faculty may be late in posting a syllabus, but would never think to consider the behavior as uncivil. Atmiller (2012) stressed the need for policy and procedures regarding the prevention of incivility in faculty. Since the literature showed decreased incidences of faculty incivility when education of faculty and policy and procedures were instituted, my DNP project intervention involved developing civility policy and procedures for online faculty and measuring their effectiveness through case studies. Anthony and Yastik (2011) and Mott (2014) stressed the need for a zero-tolerance policy for bullying behaviors in nursing schools. Consequently, the purpose of my DNP project was to improve online faculty (a) knowledge, (b) skills, and (c) attitude to maintain civility and avert faculty uncivil behaviors.

PROJECT FOCUS AND OBJECTIVES

The identification of the problem and purpose statement for the DNP project helps with formulating the DNP project objectives. The project focus is to develop a civility policy and outline the procedure all new faculty will follow. Once the project focus is determined, the objectives are easier to develop. The main project focus was to operationalize faculty and university standards regarding civility between faculty and students. This became the first objective. Knowing that I wanted to create civility policy and procedures for faculty in the online environment helped to establish my second objective. To develop the next objective, I concentrated on my ultimate goal, which was to improve faculty's knowledge, skills and attitudes concerning the recognition of uncivil behaviors. I had to ask myself—how will I know faculty improved? This helped to establish the evaluation process and include with the third objective—completion of case studies before and after the intervention, which includes signed documentation of faculty reading the three assigned peer-reviewed research articles and agreeing to the civility policy and procedures. The fourth and final objective to the DNP project was examining the difference in knowledge acquisition, skills, and attitude based on the pre- and post-reading case studies. The objectives supported the ultimate goal of my DNP project, which is the development of Civility policy and procedures that support a kind, safe, and caring environment.

The determination of the project approach and design is the next step. The case studies involved both multiple choice and open-ended questions. Since I planned to obtain both quantitative and qualitative data, I planned my DNP project around a mixed method research design. Hall and Roussell (2014) discuss qualitative data as helpful in gaining the feedback necessary in a case study approach. When a DNP project includes a pre- and post-intervention case study, a paired samples t-test is the appropriate data analysis method (Pallant, 2013). The comparison of the mean value of the paired sample t-test helps to determine if there was improved knowledge acquisition, skills, and attitude regarding the recognition of uncivil behavior. The chosen DNP project approach and design helps align the data collection and analysis with the project objectives.

DESCRIPTION OF PROBLEM/TARGET POPULATION

It is important to provide a clear description of the identified problem. Providing examples from the literature will help to validate the problem. Faculty incivility is the problem identified for my DNP project. The target population is faculty in a post-licensure online environment. The online environment was chosen as the target population because this environment is very popular and, in many cases, lacks face-to-face interaction. This lack of face-to-face interaction can breed miscommunications when the main source of communication is in the written form. For example, students may perceive a faculty member as being uncivil due to misinterpretation of the written communication; however, faculty had no uncivil intention. Once the target population and problem are identified, an intervention is formulated to resolve the problem.

INTERVENTION

Establishing the evidence-based intervention for the DNP project is a critical element to the proposal. The first step is the literature review. The literature review validates the need for the intervention and positive outcomes. Delving into the literature requires the use of several databases. Identifying the key search words and phrases to successfully gather appropriate literature can be somewhat challenging. I began with incivility. I then found that I needed to narrow the search to faculty incivility. Adding the online classroom to the search helped to narrow the search further. I also used the word caring since this identified research on caring behaviors. Always remember that the librarian at the university where the DNP student is enrolled can assist with the literature search process. Do not hesitate to use resources provided by the university where the DNP student is enrolled as needed.

Be sure to allow plenty of time for the literature review as these findings are critical to the DNP project. I recommend using an excel spreadsheet to identify the pertinent literature and separate the literature into specific themes. The columns designated in the literature review spreadsheet include a breakdown of each article—purpose, design, data collection, analysis, and findings. This kept the literature organized and easy to find the appropriate article when writing the DNP proposal. I discovered three themes during my review of literature—faculty incivility, faculty/student interactions, and caring. Synthesizing the information helps to build the evidence needed for the DNP project. Organization is key to a successful review of literature. It is important to find the best strategy to stay organized. This leads to organized thoughts and an increased ability to analyze and synthesize the information from the nursing research articles.

The evidence-based practice intervention for my project involved the development of civility policies and procedures. All newly hired faculty within the online post-licensure nursing courses read and agreed to abide by the civility policies and procedures. The civility policy and procedures consist of completing pre-reading case studies. Then the faculty are required to read the following three peer-reviewed journal articles pertaining to faculty incivility:

- Clark, C. M., Werth, L. and Ahten, S. (2012). Cyber-bullying and incivility in the online learning environment part I: Addressing faculty and student perceptions. *Nurse Educator*, 37(4), 150–156. doi: 10.1097/NNE.0b013e31825a87e5
- Clark, C. M., Ahten, S. & Werth, L. (2012). Cyber-bullying and incivility in the online learning environment part 2: Promoting student success in the virtual classroom. *Nurse Educator*, 37(5), 192–197. doi: 10.1097/NNE.0b013e318262eb2b
- Sitzman, K. L. (2016). What student cues prompt online instructors to offer caring interventions? *Nursing Education Perspectives*, 37(2), 61–71. doi: 10.5480/14-1542

After the faculty read the three required articles, they took the post-reading case study. Lastly, the faculty signed a document agreeing to the established Civility Policy and Procedures.

Another critical element in establishing the intervention is identifying an appropriate theoretical framework. The theoretical framework helps to guide the DNP project. I felt that prevention of faculty incivility required an element of caring. I knew that I wanted to use a caring theory. I looked at Jean Watson's theory of human caring and Kristen Swanson's theory of caring.

It is important to consider the type of nursing theory. I decided to go with Swanson's theory of caring due to the ease of applying the middle range theory as compared to a grand theory such as Watson's theory of human caring. The tenants of Swanson's (1991) theory of caring (knowing, being with, doing for, enabling, and maintaining belief) incorporate the central themes of my DNP project, which include faculty incivility, faculty/student relationships, and caring. The project is now well underway in the planning phase. The problem has been identified, objectives formulated, and interventions based on best evidence have been explored and narrowed.

DATA COLLECTION

The next step is deciding the best way to collect the data. Keep in mind that confidentiality and anonymity of participants is essential throughout the project. It is also important to identify a valid and reliable tool that can ensure the quality of data. For my DNP project, I used Qualtrics®, an online survey, to house the answers to the pre- and post-reading case studies. This outside online survey guarantees anonymity and confidentiality. The case studies are a mixture of multiple choice and short answers to various incivility scenarios. The Kirkpatrick and Kirkpatrick (2006) model also guided the collection of data. Utilizing the four levels of evaluation (reaction, learning, behavior, and results) helped to guide the development of the pre and post-reading case studies.

Be sure to state the data collection method clearly and succinctly within the DNP project proposal. The participants need clear communication regarding each step of the project. This helps to decrease miscommunications. I recommend numbering or sequencing the steps within the data collection procedures to help increase clarity for participants. For example, I stated the expectations for the participants in short, easy-to-read phrases such as: (a) read the policy, (b) complete the pre-reading case studies, (c) read the assigned peer reviewed journal articles, (d) complete the post-reading case studies, and (e) sign and return the required document.

To protect the rights and privacy of the participants, the DNP project proposal needs to go to the Institutional Review Board (IRB) at both the university and the implementation site. In this case, the project was a quality improvement project and determined to be IRB exempt. The IRB process can take time. It is important to prepare the IRB documents early in the project timeline and submit through the appropriate process. Once the IRB exemption or approval is granted, the DNP project can be implemented.

Another important consideration is the development of a timeline. This is crucial to the success of the DNP project. A good location for the timeline in the proposal is as an appendix. A simple table adding each row as week 1, 2, etc. works well. Add tasks to each week in a labeled column as this helps keep the project on task and prevents missed items.

ANALYSIS OF THE DATA

Whichever way is chosen to collect the data, be sure to store the data in a safe, confidential location. It is important to identify exactly who has access to the data. For example, I collected data through a secure, reliable online survey tool—Qualtrics®. I was the creator of the account and held sole ownership of the data.

Using a statistical software can help to accurately analyze data. The Statistical Package for the Social Sciences (SPSS) served as a tool for the descriptive statistics and paired sample t-tests on the data gathered from the case studies. The goal was to show improvement from the pre-reading case studies to the post-reading case studies in knowledge acquisition, potential to develop skills, and attitudes to maintain civility and avert faculty uncivil behaviors. After compilation and analysis of the data retrieved from the pre- and post-reading case studies, it was determined that civility policy and procedures improved faculty's ability to identify uncivil behaviors and provide civil behaviors in the online environment.

CONCLUSION

Overall, the DNP project is an incredible experience. The ability to develop an intervention based on the best evidence provided in literature and implementing the intervention at the practice setting is the epitome of scholarliness. Determining a nursing concern, developing an intervention based on best evidence, planning, implementing and analyzing the data benefits the nursing profession extensively. Remember to disseminate your DNP project findings. I was able to present a poster at an education summit in my home state. I also hope to publish the project in a nursing education journal. As you embark on this incredible journey, please do not be afraid to ask the professor questions. As you write your DNP project proposal, keep your information clear and succinct. Pick a topic that you are passionate about, ask questions, keep it simple and enjoy the experience.

REFERENCES

Anthony, M. & Yastik, J. (2011). Nursing students' experiences with incivility in clinical education. *The Journal of Nursing Education, 50*(3), 140–144. doi:10.3928/01484834-20110131-04

Atmiller, G. (2012). Student perceptions of incivility in nursing education: Implications for educators. *Nursing Education Perspectives, 33*(1), 15–20. Retrieved from http://search.proquest.com/docview/923246002?accountid=14375

Clark, C. M., Ahten, S. and Werth, L. (2012). Cyber-bullying and incivility in an online learning environment, part 2: Promoting student success in the virtual classroom. *Nurse Educator, 37*(5), 192–197. doi: 10.1097/NNE.0b013e318262eb2b

Clark, Nguyen, Barbosa-Leiker (2014). Student perceptions of stress, coping, relationships, and academic civility: A longitudinal study. *Nurse Educator, 39*(4), 170–174. DOI: 10.1097/NNE.0000000000000049

Clark, C. M., Werth, L. and Ahten, S. (2012). Cyber-bullying and incivility in the online learning environment, part 1: Addressing faculty and student perceptions. *Nurse Educator, 37*(4), 150–156. doi: 10.1097/NNE.0b013e31825a87e5

Del Prato, D. (2013). Students' voices: The lived experience of faculty incivility as a barrier to professional formation in associate degree nursing education. *Nurse Education Today, 33*(3), 286–290. doi:10.1016/j.nedt.2012.05.030

Hall, H. R. & Roussel, L. A. (2014). *Evidence-based practice: An integrative approach to research, administration, and practice.* Burlington, MA: Jones & Bartlett Learning

Kirkpatrick, D. L. and Kirkpatrick, J. D. (2006). Evaluating training programs: *The four levels* (3rd ed.). San Francisco, CA: Berrett-Koehler Publishers, Inc.

LaRose, P. (2016). An education exemplar: E-mentoring: Confidence intervention for senior nursing students preparing for readiness to practice. In M. Bemker & B. Schreiner (Eds), *The DNP degree & capstone project: A practical guide* (pp. 135–155). Lancaster, PA: DEStech Publications, Inc.

Mott, J. (2014). Undergraduate nursing student experiences with faculty bullies. *Nurse Educator, 39*(3), 143–148. doi: 10.1097/NNE.0000000000000038

Pallant, J. (2013). *SPSS survival manual: A step by step guide to data analysis using IBM SPSS.* (5th ed.). New York: McGraw Hill.

Sitzman, K. L. (2016). What student cues prompt online instructors to offer caring interventions? *Nursing Education Perspectives, 37*(2), 61–71. doi:10.5480/14-1542

Swanson, K. M. (1991). Empirical development of a middle-range theory of caring. *Nursing Research, 40,* 161–166. Retrieved from http://nursing.unc.edu/files/2012/11/ccm3_032548.pdf

CHAPTER 4

Dissemination and Sharing of the DNP Project

CHRISTINE M. RALYEA, DNP, MBA, MS-NP, NE-BC, CNL, OCN, CCRN
BARB SCHREINER, PhD, APRN, CDE, BC-ADM
MARY BEMKER, PhD., Psy.S. MSN, RN, LPCC, CADC, CNE

You have worked hard completing your DNP project. The American Association of Colleges of Nursing (AACN) identified in 2006, *The Essentials of Doctoral Education for Advanced Nursing Practice* including:

I. Scientific Underpinnings for Practice

II. Organizational and Systems Leadership for Quality Improvement and Systems Thinking

III. Clinical Scholarship and Analytical Methods for Evidence-Based Practice

IV. Information Systems/Technology and Patient Care Technology for the Improvement and Transformation of Health Care

V. Health Care Policy for Advocacy in Health Care

VI. Interprofessional Collaboration for Improving Patient and Population Health Outcomes

VII. Clinical Prevention and Population Health for Improving the Nation's Health

VIII. Advanced Nursing Practice (AACN, 2006).

Reading the 8 essentials, one is inclined to say dissemination of your project is in alignment with these essentials and a professional priority to showcase your work. Telling your story about your evidence-based project is essential. In this chapter, we will look at dissemination and how to get started.

WHY IS DISSEMINATION ESSENTIAL AS A DNP?

Dissemination according to the Webster dictionary is the process of

97

sharing and spreading information widespread (Webster, 2019). You selected an evidence-based practice project for your DNP project, and it is important to spread your findings and outcomes. Others will be able to learn from and spread your work. This can be possibly replicating the project or revising it to better fit the interested party's practice environment and situations. Dissemination starts the domino effect of evidence-based, and in direct alignment with the essentials II, III, IV, V, VII above, and soft alignment with essentials I, VI, and VII. Completing evidence-based projects and retaining the information does not support the spread and improvements necessary in healthcare today. As we deliver our story of our DNP project, the key messages should be: "What should I care about? How will I apply these findings to my practice or job?" (Bemker and Schreiner, 2016, 86). See Chapter 7 in this book (p. 149), which shows how Dr. Kotaya Griffith proudly sought dissemination opportunities.

NECESSARY SKILLS FOR DISSEMINATION

As a doctorate level student, you have also been developing strong communication skills. These skills include scholarly writing, visual presentations, and oral presentation skills. Looking back through your DNP journey, you have developed professionally in each of these communication areas.

Writing

As DNP prepared nurses, it is essential that strong communication skills are part of the overall professional repertoire. This communication dynamic supports professional credibility and supports scholarly work. Writing can be challenging but organizing your thoughts and developing an outline can help build the structure for a clear and concise article for publication, developing a poster presentation, or even starting the preparation for a podium presentation. Shirey (2013) wrote "scholarly writing is no longer a skill set that should exist exclusively within the professoriate; it is a competency required of all nurses and is needed to elevate nurse's voice within broader health policy arenas" (139).

Quality writing does not mean use of sophisticated language and lengthy sentences (Bemker and Schreiner, 2016, 77). Scholarly writing includes accurate use of American Psychology Association (APA) or whichever reference citation is required for the publication source you select. It is always important to use the latest reference source, so you are following the most current guidelines. For example: The 7th edition for APA was published in 2020. APA style includes more than proper citations and referencing. Additionally, it supports proper use of headers, presentation of tables and labels, writing of numbers, punctuation, abbreviations and more. Times have changed since the first version of APA in 1929 when it was a 7-page guideline. If you do not have access to the current APA manual, a great reference is Purdue OWL for checking the formatting and reference style. You can verify APA and Modern Language Association (MLA) using Purdue Online Writing Lab (Purdue OWL).

Coffin (2001) shared "professional success and image are also in part determined by writing ability" and writing "may determine whether you are invited to be a conference speaker or you are interviewed for a new

TABLE 4.1. Writing Resources.

Source	Content
Purdue Online Writing Lab http://owl.english.purdue.edu/owl/	Writing tips, citation help, style, formatting guides (APA, MLA)
U.S. Copyright Office http://www.copyright.gov/	U.S. copyright laws and resources
American Psychological Association, APA Style http://apastyle.org/	Formatting style, APA blog
Strunk and White's The element of style http://www.bartleby.com/141/index.html	Free access to a classic book on rules of composition and writing style
Grammar Girl http://www.quickanddirtytips com/grammer-girl	Useful site for questions about grammar, punctuation, and usage.
Wordcounter http://www.wordcounter.com/	Free program that counts words and frequency of their use in your document
Writing Coach http://www.academiccoachingandwriting.org/	Tips, tools, and resources for academic writing
Improve your writing http://www.grammarly.com	Tips and tools for improving your writing

(Bemker and Schreiner 2016, 78)

TABLE 4.2. Slide Presentation Resources.

Resources for Designing	Presenting Slides
Clip art, photographs, images (some free, others fee-based)	www.istockphoto.com www.fotolia.com www.everystockphoto.com www.shutterstock.com www.images.com www.presentermedia.com
Presentation advice and tips	www.indezine.com www.betterppt.com
Design tips	www.thinkoutsidetheslide.com/colorcontrast.htmcolor www.billiondollargraphics.com www.thinkoutsidetheslide.com

(Bemker and Schreiner 2016, 79)

position" (81). Your scholarly writing needs to be clear and concise. Grammar is critical. Even understanding the use of the comma is an important skill. For example, these are two very different sentences: Let's eat, Jamie or Let's eat Jamie. The use of a comma adds very different meaning and understanding to each sentence. The suggestion is to have someone else read your work and afterwards, ask them to explain their understanding of the content and material. They can correct the grammar but also assure your message was delivered. Ask them, what else do you need to explain further?

TABLE 4.3. Resources and Tools for Creating Infographics.

Resources for Developing Infographics	Presenting slides
Infographic Creation Tool	http://visual.ly/ http://piktochart.com http://infogram/ http://www.easel.ly/
Instruction Guide for Making Infographics	http://www.marketingtechblog.com/infographic-do-it-yourself-guide-toinfographics/ http://www.thewire.com/technology/2011/07/few-rules-making-homemade-infographics/39918/ http://www.visioncritical.com/blog/pretty-and-useful-how-create-awesome-inographics

(Bemker and Schreiner 2016, 79)

Visual Presentations: Slides

You will often plan for dissemination of your DNP project by providing an oral presentation or poster. This sharing can be at a conference at your facility, local, state, regional, national, and international levels. Your presentation must be concise, sharing the critical elements of the project, telling your story. "The slides must be clear, easy to read, and visually appealing . . . three to four points is about hat the viewer can grasp without the information starting to get muddled" (Bemker and Schreiner, 2016, 79). Be sure your select an appropriate background, all fonts and information on the slide is readable to the audience with consideration of the size of the room. There is nothing worse than a room of 150 participants and only the first 6 rows can clearly view the slides. Each of these concepts add or subtract from your credibility as a DNP.

Your message delivery in the slides should also reflect the audience to whom you are speaking. How can you grab the attention of the audience? The use of cartoons must be carefully selected. You can add clip art or pictures to provide visual appeal and aligns with the message you are delivering on a slide, but be sure it is not a distraction. Be sure the use of pictures, clip art, and graphics are following copyright laws. The copyright laws can be viewed at U.S. Copyright Office (http://www.copyright.gov/). Considerations for colors on the slides are also important for the viewers to read the slides and not lose the message delivery.

Your slides are a linear representation of your DNP project's story. They will include the purpose, interventions, and the outcomes. Remember to include your references and supporting documents to add credibility to your presentation. There are other presentation formats, such as Prezi (http://prezi.com) that supports a creative flow of information being shared with your audience. Other novel styles of presentation, such as Pecha Kuchamay, may be most attractive for younger, digital savvy audiences (Breyer, 2011; Masters and Holland, 2012). "Pecha Kucha relies on simple slide design and concise delivery of information using 20 slides, each displayed for 20 seconds" (Bemker and Schreiner, 2016, 80). Infographics support a visual storytelling for the dissemination of your DNP project. Infographics will capture the viewer's attention and is appealing (Arcia *et al.,* 2013; Bemker and Schreiner, 2016). See Chapter 13 in this book (p. 247), where Dr. Veronica Rankin highlights her presentations and dissemination of the scholarly work of her DNP project.

Visual Presentations: Posters

Often a poster presentation may be your first steps in the dissemination of your DNP project. Submitting an abstract for an appropriate upcoming conference is the first step in the process for dissemination plans. Once you are accepted, pay attention to deadlines for acceptance, registering for the conference, and more. Read the notification details and do not miss any steps. The excitement of acceptance can send you down a wrong path missing essential deadlines. Poster presentations create a "relaxed, informal, interactive and social context" (Ranse and Aitken, 2008, 3) for dissemination of information. During poster sessions, the opportunity for networking is strong and a positive experience for the DNP.

Creating a visual abstract that captures the essence of your DNP project in an appealing form with critical elements to inform and explain (Desilets, 2010). The top banner for the poster will include the title, author, and your affiliation. The title will be read first and catch the poster session attendee's attention, making the decision whether they stop to hear your story. The next sections include introduction,

TABLE 4.4. Resources for Production of Academic Posters.

Resources for Selecting Appropriate Effective Color Palettes	Content
Scientific poster design http://www.cns.cornell..edu/documents/ScientificPosters.pdf	Attractive tutorial on creating the effective scientific poster
Poster Perfect http://www.the-scientist.com/?article.view/articleNo/3107/title/Poster-Perfect/	Tips for designing and printing a poster
Designing Conference Posters http://colinpurrington.com/tips/academic/posterdesign	Dos and Don'ts, templates and tips
Poster Presentation http://libweb.lib.buffalo.edu/guide/guide.asp?ID=155	Extensive list of resources and links for creating academic posters
Faculty of 1,000 posters http://f1000.com/posters/browse?docTypeSearch=Poster	

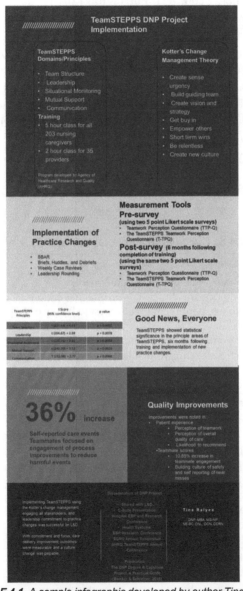

FIGURE 4.1. A sample infographic developed by author Tina Ralyea related to her DNP Project: *For Labor and Delivery Staff: How does the implementation of TeamSTEPPS compare to current practice impact quality indicators over a 6-month period? (Ralyea 2013).*

background, objectives of the project, methodology/interventions, discussion, recommendations, and references. "Like links in a chain, each of these sections should be cohesive and consistent, yet concise" (Bemker and Schreiner, 2106, 82). Purrington (2014) suggests limiting the poster to 800 words maximum. This will limit your review of literature in the introduction and background sections. Limiting your content to three pages single-spaced, 12-point font as you prepare content for the enlarged poster printing is a guideline for success (Writing Center at CSU, 2012). A successful poster should be read in less than 10 minutes (Pontin and Albarran, 2008). Hedges (2010) suggests views should be able to read all font at a five-foot distance. Remember to maintain some white space on the poster.

Do not delay preparing your poster in an organized fashion, as often printing of the poster can take several weeks. Most poster sizes will be printed 4 × 6 feet or 4 × 8 feet, so be sure to validate the correct size

TABLE 4.5. Checklist for Scholarly Poster Presentation.

Appearance of Poster
• Size and format meet conference requirements
• Images and graphics are attractive and attract attention
• Color, white space, harmony of sections, and balance are pleasing and attract attention
• Title is visible from 10 feet and more
• Content in sections visible from at least 3–5 feet
• Font style and size are consistently and appropriately used
• Content is well organized and flows easily (vertical columns)
Content of Poster
• Title is consistent with project
• Purpose and objectives of project are clearly stated
• Methods and interventions are consistent with stated objectives
• Outcomes are clearly presented and consistent with methods
• Conclusions and recommendations are consistent with outcomes
• Images and graphs are clear and easy to read and interpret
• Content of sections is concise, cohesive, and clear
• Content is free from errors in grammar and spelling
• Project's relevance or implications is clearly articulated
Presence of Author
• Demonstrates professional appearance
• Demonstrates knowledge of project and subject matter
• Interacts with conference attendees in a professional and attentive manner
• Provides contact information, supplemental information, or handouts

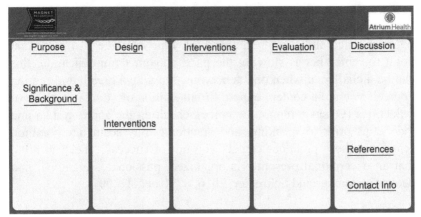

FIGURE 4.2. *Sample of a Poster Template.*

based on the conference guidelines. Make a timeline to assure you do not have unanticipated delays leading to no final poster to take to the conference. When you attend the conference, Hedges (2010) strongly recommends taking a handout with references to share with the audience.

Sample of a Poster Template

The template in Figure 4.2 is an example of the Atrium Health Poster template. Check with your organization or school, as they may have a standard template to be used for dissemination of a poster. This helps organizations assure professional presentation and lay out of content that reflects their institution.

Oral Presentations Skills

Public speaking can be stressful, yet this is an essential skill for DNPs and in disseminating your project. You are the content expert and practicing help to assure the delivery of your content is clear for the audience. Use an outline for content you want to cover based on the allotted time you have to speak. Be aware of your audience, paying attention to cultural, gender, professional make up, and other variables. Speaking to administrators from the C-suite will be very different than speaking to bedside clinical nurses. Whenever possible, engage the audience with questions and save time for questions and answers at the end of your presentation.

According to Starver and Shellenbarger (2004), maintaining eye contact with the audience and your positive body language will engage your audience and support delivery of your message. An important point to remember is slowing the pace of your communication, this can be a challenge when one is nervous, but take a breath and remind yourself you are a content expert. Pronunciation of your words, use of inflections (versus a monotone voice), checking the audio system and videoclips prior to speaking, and practicing may seem like common sense, but these practices can set you up for success. "Keep in mind that an exceptional presenter is organized, passionate, engaging, and neutral" (Bemker and Schreiner, 2016, 87; Koegel, 2007).

INTERNAL DISSEMINATION

Your organization when you implemented your DNP project will expect you share the results, outcomes and next steps. This can be an executive summary to the leadership team, sharing with clinical nurses at staff meetings or committee meetings, a poster at your organization's professional nursing days or poster sessions, or organizational wide quality sharing events. You should explore what opportunities can be available to showcase your DNP project within your school, your organization, or healthcare system.

EXTERNAL DISSEMINATION

Often your school and/or organization will suggest you seek ways to disseminate your DNP project beyond the school setting and your place of employment. Going beyond the walls to external broader venues can produce a wider spread of your work. If you share your information at a conference, it will reach the number of attendees. Seeking successful publication can reach a broader audience and opens your DNP project to access via search engines.

WRITING FOR PUBLICATION

Oermann, Turner, and Carman (2014) suggests that writers of practice-based initiatives use the guidelines from the Standards for Quality Improvement Reported Excellence (SQUIRE). SQUIRE is aligned with the DNP evidence-based practice projects and process improvement interventions. "SQUIRE forces you to clarify your thinking, verify your observations, and justify your inferences. Hastens the spread of important and useful innovations. Reduces the waste scarce of resources in confirming findings that are already firmly established" (http://squire-statement.org, 2019). Additional writing tips and resources can be found at https://library.frontier.edu/writingresources/style.

Finding the correct journal and audience is essential. One can seek out a peer reviewed journal for publishing in or read several volumes of the journal that you are thinking about publishing in. Is the journal publishing evidence-based practice and DNP projects? If they are research focused, the suggestion will be to find a more appropriate journal. An effective early step is to send a letter of interest to the editor, asking about the need for your topic for future publications. If you receive a not interested in topic from the editor, that does not mean give up. Seek a new journal and there will be someone out there interested in your project topic. If you receive a yes, stay focused and pull the journal writing guidelines. Even the number of words for the abstract will vary for each journal. Follow the guidelines closely. Your writing must be clear and concise, tables must follow the guidelines and use the journals' citation referencing (APA vs. AMA as examples).

Having a message from the editor of interest in your topic does not assure 100% that your article will be published. You may submit your article, and you may have multiple responses as the article get reviewed. Accepted after major revisions, accepted with revisions, accepted without revisions, and declined (with reasons) are several of the messages you may receive from the journal. Know that most authors are not accepted for publication with the first submission. Often there are rewrites and point of clarity needed prior to publication. First time authors often give up at this time. Find support to reread and help you with the revisions. You can and will be successful if you take the peer review feedback and align with the publishing guideline to set yourself up for success. There is such a proud and humbling moment when you know the article is finally accepted and will be published, so stay focused on the goal for publication and external dissemination. Due to copyright laws and conflicts of interest, once you receive an acceptance of your publication topic for one journal, you will not be able to submit to other journals. You now have a commitment to follow through for publication with your accepted journal.

Already shared is the posters and presentation that can be external dissemination. If your project supports a new nursing practice and policy, you can also participate in legislative events (Day on Capitol Hill as an example) to articulate and share your story promoting a health policy change. Often external dissemination can be a domino effect. For example, you published your article and another reader contacts you and asks you to speak at their organization or health system to spread your work. I have seen DNPs speak at various conferences and then asked to present at other conferences and/or at other healthcare systems across the nation. Sharing my personal DNP project related to TeamSTEPPS implementation in Labor and Delivery, I first had a poster presentation at the hospitals poster day during nurse's week, then accepted for the poster presentation at the TeamSTEPPS conference, hosted by Agency for Healthcare Research and Quality (AHRQ), and a presentation at Society of Gynecological Nurse Oncologist (SGNO). From the contacts made during the AHRQ conference, I then had a podium presentation at the Clinical Nurse Leader Conference. The poster was the same, but by the time I gave the podium presentation to a different audience, the message and story told was different. So, the best advice is to start your journey and stay focused to share your hard work and DNP project.

REFERENCES

American Association of College of Nurses (AACN). (2006). The essentials of doctoral education for advanced nursing practice. Retrieved from http://www.aacn.nche.edu/publications/position/dnpessentials.pdf

American Psychological Association (APA). (2020). Publication manual of the American Psychological Association (7th edition). Washington, DC: Author.

Arcia, A, Bales, M.E., Brown, W. Co., Gilmore, M., Lee, Y. J., et al, (2013). Method for the development of data visualizations for community members with varying levels of health literacy. *AMIA Annual Symposium Proceedings*, 2013, 51–60. Retrieved from http://www.ncbi.nlm.nih.gov/pmc/articles/PMC3900122/pdf/amia_2013_symptoms-051.pdf

Bemker, M. and Schreiner, B. (2016). *The DNP Degree & Capstone Project: A Practical Guide*. Lancaster, PA: DEStech.

Breyer, A. M. (2011). Improving student presentations: Pecha Kucha and just plain PowerPoint. *Teaching of Psychology*, 38(2), 122–126. Doi:10.1177/0098628311401588

Coffin, C. (2001). The scientific journal article: Approaching the first draft. In S. Barnard, P.J. Casella, C. Coffin, K.T. Hughes, J.W. Hurst, J.S. Rasey, D. Redding, R. J. Robillard, D. St. James, and S.C. Ullery, *Writing, speaking, and communication skills for health professionals* (p. 70–90). New Haven, CT: Yale University Press.

Desilets, L.D. (2010). Poster presentations. *Journal of Continuing Education in Nursing, 41*(10), 437–438. Doi: 10.3928/00220124-201009244-02

Hedges, C. (2010). Poster presentations: A primer for critical care nurses. *AACN Advance Critical Care*, 21(3), 318–321. Doi: 10.1097/NCI.0b013e3181e138da

Koegel, T.J. (2007), The exceptional presenter. Austin, TX: Greenleaf Book Group Press.

Masters, J. C. and Holland, B. E. (2012). Rescuing the student presentation with Pecha Kucha. *The Journal of Nursing Education*, 51(9), 536. Doi: 10.3928/01484834-20120822-02

Oermann, M.H., Turner, K. and Carman, M. (2014). Preparing quality improvement, research, and evidence-based practice manuscripts. *Nursing Economic$, 32*(2), 57–69.

Purdue Online Writing Lab (OWL). (2019). Retrieved from https://owl.purdue.edu/owl/purdue_owl.html

Purrington, C, (2014). Designing conference posters [Web log]. Retrieved from http://colinpurrington.com/tips/academic/posterdesign

Ralyea, C. M. (2013). *For Labor and Delivery staff, how does the implementation of TeamSTEPPS compare to current practice impact quality indicators over a 6-month period?* (Doctorate dissertation). Retrieved from ProQuest Dissertations and Theses. (Order No. 3587159).

Ranse, J. and Aitken, C. (2008). Preparing and presenting a poster at a scientific conference. *Journal of Emergency Primary Health Care 6*(1) 1-9. Retrieved from http://ro.ecu.edu.au/cgi/viewcontent.cgi?article=1277&context=jephc

Shirey, M.R. (2013). Building scholarly writing capacity in the Doctor of Nursing Practice program. *Journal of Professional Nursing, 29*(3), 137–147. Doi: 10.1016/j.profnurs.2012.04.2019

Starver, K. D. and Shellenbarger, T. (2004). Professional presentations made simple. *Clinical Nurse Specialist, 18*(1), 16–20.

Webster (2019). Dissemination Definition. Retrieved from https://www.merriam-webster.com/dictionary/dissemination

Writing Center at Colorado State University (CSU). (2012). *Writing guide: Poster sessions*. Retrieved from http://writing.colostate.edu/guides/pdfs/guide78.pdf

Part 2: Education Exemplars

The Application of a Simulation Model in an Ambulatory Surgery Center: Developing from Novice to Expert Practitioner

NICHOLAS GREEN, DNP, RN, ALUMNUS CCRN

PROBLEM IDENTIFICATION/STATEMENT

Deterioration of clinical exposure has steadily increased over the years. While many variables contribute to the lack of clinical experience a student nurse to which may be exposed, one recurrent theme emerges. Surrounding the phenomenon of clinical scarcity, students often find themselves competing for clinical placement with graduate nurses within a unit to allow for orientation of newly hired nurses to occur. Understandably, hospital education has always and will continue to demonstrate preference towards the hospital's direct investment of training the registered nurse (RN). Spector and Odom (2012) note "major changes in the U.S. healthcare system and practice environments will require equally profound changes in their education of nurses both before and after they receive their licenses" (40).

Due to increased demands of mentorship being placed onto staff nurses, many facilities not associated with a healthcare organization are embracing the opportunity to acquire a newly graduated registered nurse (RN). The hiring organization's other alternative is to employ an individual who possesses experience in healthcare but not in the area of specialty in which they have been offered a position of employment. The uneducated versus inexperienced nurse poses numerous concerns with regards to the knowledge and skill set of the RN who may be prematurely placed at the bedside. One area of concern is the freestanding ambulatory surgery center (ASC), which frequently lacks an association with a larger healthcare system.

With the stable pool of experienced nurses declining, the ability to assess an individual's knowledge base concerning the population of interest has witnessed an increase in the popularity of commencing the utilization of simulation, providing for an appraisal of nursing staff knowledge of item-specific processes. The following Doctor of Nursing Practice (DNP) project appraised current evidence-based literature and implemented the development of an organizational policy while evaluating the feasibility and functionality by utilizing a simulation-based method of delivery to enforce knowledge obtained from the new policy. Enhancing the development of an organizational policy through simulation allowed information to be reinforced at the selected project site. Through the development and implementation phase of the project, identification of knowledge gap deficits was identified to aid the organization in evaluating the need for remediation, further reinforcing the new policy.

DEVELOPING PROJECT FOCUS AND OBJECTIVES

The absence of experience stems from many sources, i.e., newly graduated nurse, mean length of experience of nurses found working on desired unit or institution, and decreased time spent during orientation, lends itself to an identified need. Schools of nursing are being pressured to produce a graduate nurse who can implement the fundamental skills of nursing care through the adversity of decreased clinical exposure.

The ability to perform a knowledge-based assessment of either the graduate or experienced nurse needs to be addressed. Capacity to do so exists through conducting a simulated experience. The identified practicum site, which is recognized as a free-standing ASC specializing in vein and vascular care, currently has five locations throughout the Phoenix area with nursing staff, both experienced and novice who rotate through each location. After meeting with the practicum site's Assistant Director, the needs of the ASC were discussed exposing the necessity to develop an organizational policy to advance staff's knowledge base. The following DNP project was discussed with a key stakeholder of the practicum site who granted permission for utilization and implementation of the proposed project. The following project was implemented through the development of an organizational policy used to enhance staff's foundational knowledge of at-risk conditions within the ASC setting.

Through collaboration with a small university and simulation center, Bednarek *et al.* (2014) determined "simulation does facilitate learning in medical education under certain conditions" (27). When conducted, the simulated experience will focus its foundational program on four key components of professional growth. Bednarek *et al.* (2014) describes the elements as being, "(1) Recognizing a change in condition; (2) Performing an assessment of that situation; (3) Identification of interventions for that status; (4) Evaluating the effectiveness of said intervention" (27). The chosen simulated experience to assist in the facilitation of the new policy will incorporate the emergent condition of malignant hyperthermia crisis (MHC).

Hospitals are seeing an increase in the number of rapid responses being utilized while freestanding centers are witnessing increased transfers to higher levels of care based on lack of critical assessments of the patient due to being discovered in an appropriate length of time. With the acuity of patients increasing, the amount of knowledge an RN is expected to know exponentially grows regardless if they received specific training or not. To foster a healthy learning environment and not one of fear and intimidation, the utilization of simulated experiences has proven beneficial in establishing quality care while providing knowledge gap assessment.

The DNP project sought to see if evidence exists to suggest the implementation of an organizational policy founded upon the application of a simulation model will improve nursing knowledge and comfort levels among ambulatory surgery center staff.

The implemented project established an organizational policy utilizing the simulation methodology to conduct a knowledge and skills assessment among ambulatory surgery center (ASC) staff. A simulated experience involving low-volume, high-risk scenarios such as malignant hyperthermia crisis (MHC) was utilized as an exemplar for evaluative purposes to address the proposed project question. With implementing the policy which centered on the simulated experience, the leadership of the ASC was able to utilize an evaluative tool allowing outcomes to be measured based on individual performance.

After conducting a need-based approach, the design of the policy established the ability to evaluate and enhance the ASC staff member's knowledge towards patient care which was carried out to indicate achieved objectives at the conclusion of the DNP project (Table 1).

An example in which the provided tool would be used to educate nurses incorporates the implementation of ASC's malignant hyperthermia protocol before the patient's condition deteriorates. According to Sheldon (2014), "the evaluation of policy implementation, the development of systems models to explain the multiple factors that influence policymaking, and the advancement of knowledge within specific policy areas, are redefining the field of policy analysis" (102). During the implementation of the DNP project, the leadership of the ASC had the opportunity to view a simulated scenario to reinforce the implementation of the proposed policy. Application of such a policy allows for increased retention of staff should leadership look towards the policy as a means of a staff nurse's return-on-investment. Lapkin and Levett-Jones (2011) state, "it is important that decision-makers have an economic analysis that considers both the costs and outcomes of simulation to identify the approach that has the lowest cost for any outcome measure or best outcomes for a particular cost" (3543).

The capability to conduct simulated scenarios lies in the capacity to emulate as closely as possible to an identified situation in which an area of healthcare is underdeveloped. As an example—ensuring patient safety is of the utmost concern—a patient who undergoes treatment which is seen to be labeled as low-frequency, high-risk can now be examined by a nurse who has been taught utilizing the simulated experience. According to Frick *et al.* (2014), "simulation use has escalated in nursing education programs as well as clinical practice institutions, which use it for the interview process, orientation, and annual competency review" (9).

Equal to the circumstance in which the ASC finds itself, many hospitals are finding themselves stretched thin due to budgetary restraints, resulting in an inability to orientate new staff correctly. Specialty areas such as the intensive care unit, cardiovascular critical care unit, and emergency departments are finding themselves with employees who are providing care to patients with minimal knowledge of how to care for the critically ill patient. Hospitals have found a lack of an established knowledge base through new graduate orientation programs or how experienced nurses perform during competency reviews. The potential legal implications of an individual possessing a knowledge deficit regarding patient safety can be detrimental to the organization.

It is in this respect that the need for development and implementation of a policy addressing the needs of staff to promote patient safety through knowledge gap analysis was established to enhance an individual's baseline knowledge. The application of simulation allows staff members of the ASC to be placed in a simulated scenario in which staff performance can be evaluated and critiqued. The importance of this lies in the fact that staff is being hired with little to no experience within the acute surgical/post-anesthesia setting, necessitating the need for performance evaluation.

Organizational policy formation within the ASC was developed to establish standards which lie in congruence with those found within the hospital setting and are in line with the Arizona State Board of Nursing standards. The predominant goal of the project addressed patient safety while increasing the prospect of staff retention due to the visible support of the leadership team. Each participant who volunteered to be part of the project acquired the ability to increase patient safety when positive feedback was utilized. As the ASC leadership evaluated staff based on ability to perform within the clinical area, the focus was not based on previous skill levels or level of degree obtained (i.e., Associated Degree, Bachelor of Science in Nursing) but rather on the employee's ability to think critically. McGaghie *et al.* (2014) state, "measured outcomes [through simulation] have been achieved in [various] educational laboratories, and has improved patient care practices, patient outcomes, and collateral effects" (375). Prior to implementation, measurable goals included the voluntary participation of 100% of staff members working in the identified project site.

DESCRIPTION OF PROBLEM/TARGET POPULATION

The progression of utilizing simulation to assess for clinical knowledge competency has increased based on various needs of nursing staff. To further give authority to this developmental tool, what was initiated as an advisory opinion from the State Board of Nursing will be integrated as part of the Nurse Practice Act with more stringent protocols. Inconsistencies among the utilization of simulation currently exist as hospital systems seek to integrate more simulated (low, mid, and high-fidelity) experiences within the healthcare arena. Exemplars range from conducting mock code blues to maintaining staff's proficiency during an emergent situation inclusive of scenarios which deal with how to call the physician to obtain orders based on a need's assessment.

Other uses of simulation have included how to administer and provide care during the acute phase of the patient who receives thrombolytic therapy such as tissue-plasminogen activator (tPA). Patients who receive tPA are considered low-frequency, high-risk causality due to reperfusion injury increasing an individual's risk of developing a hemorrhage causing the implementation of stringent administration guidelines. The prevalence of community-wide education towards stroke prevention along with national patient safety goals such as door-to-needle time practiced through simulation has significantly impacted the care of the acute stroke patient. Exemplars such as the one provided have allowed continued growth in the American Heart Association's use of the evidence-based practice of recommending the treatment time frame from three (3) to four and a half (4.5) hours regarding receipt of thrombolytic therapy.

As positive exposure continues, nurse leaders within hospital systems are enthusiastic about the opportunity to utilize simulation as it allows for real-time feedback based on learner responses. To assist in advancing the technology which has impacted patient care through the development and implementation of simulated scenarios, the International Nursing Association for Clinical Simulation and Learning (INACSL) was established in 2011.

The standards set forth by INACSL for best practice regarding simulation saw "the original seven standards published in 2011 revised in 2013 [to] include two new standards" (Sittner *et al.,* 2015, 294). With the revision of standards, numerous opportunities for the implementation of the simulated experience have allowed leadership to evaluate a nurse or nurse's strengths and weaknesses through content analysis in conjunction with evaluating debriefing sessions of the simulated experience with the nursing staff.

A comprehensive literature review has shown increased utilziation of simulated practices among hospital leadership as its use increases among schools of nursing. One downfall to the integration of simulation among a hospital system incorporates the financial construct of the need to develop a dedicated simulation center. Schools of nursing and other teaching facilities often possess the funds to implement the technology. In an ironic twist, those who stand to benefit most from the utilization of simulation lack the capacity to afford such equipment. Numerous hospital organizations, including freestanding clinics and ASCs, are unable to afford the cost, maintenance, and training of staff or a particular member of the team to maintain the upkeep of the simulation equipment.

Should a healthcare system wish to obtain a high-fidelity simulator along with supportive material, inclusion into the unit's or hospital system's capital budget must be calculated for each fiscal year. A quote for start-up costs for a high-fidelity mannequin averaged more than $85,000, less the cost of yearly maintenance and staff (A. Sinyay, personal communication, September 9, 2016). As a result of constraints within the healthcare system, hospitals are often unable to validate the purchase of simulation equipment based on current healthcare costs and reimbursement rates.

Due to the limitations mentioned above, it may prove to be beneficial for a healthcare system, especially freestanding centers, to establish a partnership with a school of nursing or other approved simulation center that has established equipment. Based on wants versus needs assessment of hospital leadership, forming an affiliation could work in both interests of the hospital and nursing school/simulation center.

The importance of feedback demonstrated through a review of the literature, staff discussion, and administration, lends itself to the importance of establishing a project such as the one implemented. Through establishing an organizational policy by incorporating the utilization of simulation within an ASC, the care of the patient can be drastically increased. Due to the nature of the proposed system change, collaboration among nursing staff will be paramount in providing productive nursing results, positively affecting patient outcomes.

The population of interest studied was comprised of volunteers who were RNs currently working at the identified project site within the peri-operative and post-anesthesia care unit areas of the practicum site. Individuals who hold an associate, bachelor's, or master's degree in nursing, aged 18 to 75 years, and either male or female were asked to participate in the project voluntarily. Inclusion criteria for participants also included individuals who hold a current unencumbered Arizona nursing license issued by the Arizona State Board of Nursing and possess a current advanced cardiac life support (ACLS) certificate.

Volunteers must also not have had limitations placed on their ability to work; have worked within an ASC peri-operative and PACU area for at least six months, and have not been recently trained in MHC within the past three months. All participants must be able to read, write, and speak English. Volunteers provided consent to participate and understood they could stop participating at any time without penalty.

Therefore, exclusionary criteria of the targeted population consisted of individuals who did not hold a current ACLS card or were in the process of obtaining a current ACLS card due to a lapse between renewal. Registered nurses holding an unencumbered license who work within the ASC were not included in the project proposal due to inconsistent time spent at the practicum site. Limitations of the project were restricted to RNs and excluded other healthcare providers, i.e., physicians, surgical technicians. Individuals who do not have a current basic life support card, are unable to perform cardiopulmonary resuscitation, or have physical limitations due to being placed on active light duty by a healthcare provider were also excluded from the project.

Due to the small size of the ASC, an estimated four to seven staff members will be informed of the organizational policy along with criteria to participate in the MHC simulation project. The setting of the simulated experience occurred in one of the identified ASC's five post-anesthesia care unit (PACU) recovery stations to mirror the environment in which the staff could encounter a patient undergoing MHC.

Through dialogue with the stakeholders (staff and administration), the utilization of the simulated experience was discussed in how it could be applied as both a learning and evaluative tool. Apprehensive feelings towards involvement in clinical trials and project development characteristically exist through a lack of knowledge of what it means to participate in a clinical trial or project implementation (Chu *et al.,* 2015). Feelings of anxiety, fearfulness, etc. allowed for assessment of therapeutic communication, which provided supportive evidence to the nursing process with regards to critical thinking while encouraging open communication.

DNP PROJECT INTERVENTIONS

One of the significant components an individual must assess when steering change among clinical practice is to consider the dissemination of the project to determine if results yielded an outcome favoring the intended intervention. Through continued literature review, the role of the DNP has an impact on healthcare by utilizing existing literature while translating it into a clinical platform which is patient-centric. According to Ingham-Broomfield (2016), "nurses need to be competent in evaluating the strengths and weaknesses of . . . studies and the applicability of them about their working environment" (41). As the DNP prepared nurse begins to formulate change; the individual must continually evaluate the intervention for efficacy and its effects on different areas of the healthcare system including knowledge acquisition and patient care. If evaluative efforts find the intervention not to be well received or needing adjustment, it becomes the obligation of the DNP prepared nurse to notify key stakeholders (i.e., leadership) while reexamining which phase of the intervention may need to occur.

Permission from the site administrator to perform the implementation project was granted after discussing the benefits of how a simulated experience allows for enhanced learning opportunities. Also discussed were evaluative measures of the staff who participate in the simulated experience, as well as return-of-investment opportunities, including increased retention of staff while maintaining evaluation of annual competencies based on low-volume, high-risk scenarios.

After permission was granted and prior to implementation, the proposed DNP Project was submitted to the Institutional Review Board (IRB) at Touro University Nevada located in Henderson, Nevada, which determined the proposed DNP Project to be exempt from full IRB review. The project involved little to no risk of the participant in accordance with statute §46.101(b) of 45 CFR 46; activities which involve human subjects will be deemed as exempt status if the project involves minimal to no risk. Further examples of exempting a study/project from IRB review include "research involving the use of… survey procedures" (Health and Human Services 2009, para. 4).

The project involved the application of an organizational policy change which utilized simulation to implement and enforce the new policy which encompassed MHC protocols developed by the ASC. Voluntary participation in the project included distribution of a multiple-choice pretest to establish participants baseline knowledge of MHC. At the conclusion of the simulation, an identical multiple-choice posttest questionnaire with the inclusion of open-ended questions was provided to allow participants to offer feedback on the execution of the project. Both pretest and posttests were administered online via a survey tool which did not ask for or contain any personal, identifiable information.

At the conclusion of the simulation and debriefing session, an end-of-course evaluation (reflective of the subject's feelings regarding the implemented organizational change through simulation to reinforce the organizational policy) was provided. Due to the project being voluntary, compensation for participating in the project did not result in monetary payment to the DNP student or affiliated school. Since the project did encompass an organizational policy change, compensation was determined at the discretion of the leadership of the ASC as the date for project implementation occurred during ASC staff members scheduled work time, in which surgical cases were not conducted on a weekly basis.

DATA COLLECTION, MEASUREMENT TOOLS, ANALYSIS

Utilizing standards set forth by the Arizona State Board of Nursing Advisory Opinion, it is recommended, but not mandatory, for each simulated experience to be video recorded to allow for review during the debriefing session (AZBN, 2015). Due to the introduction of the new organizational policy, utilization of a new methodology to reinforce said policy (simulation) in conjunction with utilizing debriefing techniques, this author chose to omit video recording of the simulated experience to decrease potential anxiety among ASC staff members. If utilized in the future, language incorporated in the policy does reflect the option to use video recording during a simulation should the project site wish to use the option in agreement with the standards set forth by the Arizona State Board of Nursing.

On the day of the scheduled simulation, a "Confidentiality Agreement for Simulation" was presented to members of the ASC staff who, a week prior, met the inclusion criteria and signed voluntary consent forms to participate in the project. The agreement allows for accountability on the learner's part to act as if the simulation scenario focused on a real patient. The agreement also discusses the Health Insurance Portability and Accountability Act to maintain 'patient' confidentiality, along with consent to be video-recorded. The latter section was discussed with each individual as not being utilized during the implementation of the project.

EVALUATION

Individuals who voluntary participated were provided a copy of the newly developed policy while the concept behind clinical simulation was explained. Although the simulation took place in the staff member's place of work, time was permitted for each individual to inspect and familiarize themselves with the location of equipment before beginning the simulation. Each was also reminded of the voluntary consents they signed and were each reminded that they reserved the right to choose to stop participation at any time during implementation of the project.

Formative and summative evaluation of the individual's knowledge and retention of a new policy regarding MHC was to be conducted online through the utilization of SurveyMonkey. Done one week prior and two weeks after project implementation, a questionnaire consisting of 10 multiple-choice questions was given to staff members who met inclusionary criteria in the ASC and provided consent to participate in the project. The 10 multiple-choice questions provided after the implementation phase of the project included open-ended questions to allow individuals to provide thoughts and opinions regarding the reasoning in choosing a specific answer. Fit-for-purpose competency tools are typically utilized during the application of simulation to evaluate staff learning needs about improved recognition of the deteriorating patient, which need continual development (Waldie, Tee, and Day, 2016).

After the first questionnaire has been conducted, answer choices will be discussed with staff during the discussion of the new organizational policy. Utilization of the Plus Delta Debriefing Tool as well as the Promoting Excellence & Reflective Learning in Simulation tool will be applied to allow all participants to contribute feelings while providing feedback during debriefing. Both tools allow for individuals to reflect on how they felt they performed during the simulated experience. Questions include areas the participants felt they needed to improve on based on their experience throughout the simulation.

DATA COLLECTION PROCEDURES

During the consent process, it was emphasized to the participants that no personal identifiers would be collected during the pre- and post-test analysis, nor from post-implementation surveys. A 10-question, multiple-choice, pre-simulation questionnaire was provided via SurveyMonkey to participants the week prior to the scheduled simulation scenario, testing the individual's baseline knowledge of MHC. A post-simulation questionnaire consisting of 10 multiple-choice questions based on the same pre-test questions along with the ability to offer a narrative for each question was provided to participants while remaining open for two weeks. Immediately after the debriefing session, utilizing a Likert scale, surveys were provided to each individual, which elicited participant opinions regarding if they felt objectives were met, improvements needed, etc.

The pre- and post-test questionnaire tool consisted of 10 multiple-choice questions inclusive of four select all that apply questions and one rank order question to evaluate the participant's knowledge of dantrolene, a first-line medication used in MHC, as well as other components of the patient experiencing MHC. Throughout the simulation phase of the project, correct answers were incorporated to assess retention of material learned and assessed through the post-test questionnaire to evaluate if cognitive growth occurred.

Upon completion of the simulated experience and in a combination of the pre- and post-test questionnaire, all participants were requested to complete a "Participant Evaluation of the Simulation Experience" survey. Results provided feedback allowing for determination of areas for improvement, development, and proposed methodology in the implementation of the new organizational policy to the key stakeholder(s).

A Likert scale was utilized, where scoring of the tool implemented a system of allocating a score of 1, equating to not at all, through 5, equating to extremely. During the consent process, each participant was informed they would be asked to complete essentials of the project which consisted of pre-test, post-test, and post-implementation surveys. Provider knowledge before and after the simulation was evaluated to assess for areas of improvement based on the proposed organizational policy. The goal was to have all ASC staff members participate in the project. If voluntary consent was not obtained, the individual was still allowed to take part in the simulated experience and debriefing session but was not provided access to the questionnaire delivered via SurveyMonkey for pre- and post-test feedback analysis of informational knowledge obtained.

Six (n=6) individuals currently working in the ASC PACU who met inclusionary criteria provided voluntary consent to participate in the project to further develop organizational change through the implementation of simulation. Of the six individuals, four participants were female (66.7%). Utilizing SurveyMonkey, the pre-test was opened for a period of one week (March 22, 2017–March 29, 2017) prior to the implementation of the simulated activity (March 30, 2017), allowing individuals who chose to participate in the project time to answer the pretest, which consisted of 10 questions about MHC. Before the implementation of the project, a 100% pre-test response rate was obtained.

At the conclusion of the scenario, participants were asked to anonymously complete two survey tools consisting of a Likert scale scoring system utilizing a value structure of 1–5 (1 equating to strongly disagree/not at all to 5 equating to strongly agree/extremely), which focused on how the participant felt the simulated scenario was perceived. The "Simulated Scenario Observer," "Participant Evaluation," and "Evaluation of Organizational Objectives" questionnaires were collected by having participants place the documents into a manila envelope, anonymously and unwitnessed. Upon review of the collected documents, 100% of participants (n=6) completed all three forms.

Utilizing descriptive statistics, analysis of the three forms was conducted. Organizational objectives yielded a mean score of 4.91 out of a 5-point Likert Scale with participant evaluation of the simulated experience yielding a mean score of 4.90 out of a 5-point Likert Scale. Upon closing of the post-test questionnaire, five of the six individuals had completed the post-test resulting in an 83.3% response rate. Upon review of the ten questions asked, five questions saw an increase in the percentage of change to the correct answer choices from the pre-test.

The ability of the participant to take the same pre-test and post-test allowed this student to evaluate if cognitive development encompassing MHC had changed through the implementation of an organizational transformation with specified goals and objectives through simulation. In doing so, the primary goal of the analysis conducted was to evaluate whether the implementation of simulation answered the clinical question, "Is there evidence to suggest the implementation of an organizational policy founded upon the application of a simulation model will improve nursing knowledge and comfort levels among ambulatory surgery center staff?"

CONCLUSIONS

The ability to implement a project such as the one proposed possesses the capacity to influence change not only at the organizational level but acts as a catalyst in which policy formation is utilized as an exemplar in how staff will be evaluated based on clinical proficiency within other outpatient centers. At the conclusion of the project, sustainability must be maintained to allow AAAASF to witness how continuing education is occurring. Similar to any organizational restructuring of policy and procedure, the possibility may arise for the project to experience pitfalls. Learning from these mistakes and continually improving the process will allow the identified ASC to act as a model for freestanding surgical centers.

With simulated clinical experience increasing to 50% among nursing schools or greater, it could be argued the Arizona State Board of Nursing, in combination with its mission statement, witnessed a deficiency in the ability to provide care at the fundamental level. Should this be the case, does one cast blame onto the school, the organization (hospital, clinic, etc.), or the healthcare system as a whole? This author feels all of the above play an integral part in not providing a quality orientation process for the new graduate or experienced nurse transferring to a new department.

Due to the increasing acuity of patients being cared for, many nurses are often left to utilize little knowledge of how to care for critically ill individuals. Through the establishment of a partnership which positively affects both stakeholder(s) and DNP students, the proposed intervention will serve as a model allowing for continued growth to occur in the practicum site as well as in other ASCs.

REFERENCES

Arizona State Board of Nursing. (2015). Advisory opinion: Education use of simulation in approved RN/LPN programs. Retrieved from https://www.azbn.gov/media/2053/ao-use-of-simulation-in-pre-licensure-programs.pdf. *Note*: The second line - and all remaining- are indented per APA format.

Bednarek, M., Downey, P., Williamson, A., & Ennulat, C. (2014). The use of human simulation to teach acute care skills in cardiopulmonary course: A case report. *Journal of Physical Therapy Education*, (28)3, 27–34.

Chu, S., Kim, E., Jeong, S. and Park, G. (2015). Factors associated with willingness to participate in clinical trials: A nationwide survey study. *BMC Public Health*, 10(10), 1.

Frick, K., Swoboda, S., Mansukhani, K. and Jeffries, P. (2014). An economic model for clinical simulation in prelicensure nursing programs. *Journal of Nursing Regulation, (5)*3, 9–13.

Health and Human Services. (2009). Public welfare and protection of human subjects. (HHS publication of 45 CFR 46 Code of federal regulations Title 45). Washington, DC: U.S. Government Printing Office.

Ingham-Broomfield, R. (2016). A nurse's guide to the hierarchy of research designs and evidence. *Australian Journal of Advanced Nursing, 33*(3), 38–43.

Lapkin, S. and Levett-Jones, T. (2011). A cost-utility analysis of medium vs. high-fidelity human patient simulation manikins in nursing education. *Journal of Clinical Nursing, 20*, 3543–3552. doi: 10.1111/j.1365-2702.2011.03843.x

McGaghie, W., Issenberg, S., Barsuk, J. and Wayne, D. (2014). A critical review of simulation-based mastery learning with translational outcomes. *Medical Education, 48*, 375–385. doi:10.111/medu.12391

Sheldon, M. (2016). Policy-making theory as an analytical framework in policy analysis: Implications for research design and professional advocacy. *Physical Therapy, (96)*,1, 101–110.

Sittner, B., Aebersold, M., Paige, J., Graham, L., Schram, A., Decker, S. and Lioce, L. (2015).

INACSL standards of best practice for simulation: Past, present, and future. *Nursing Education Perspectives, 36*(5), 294–298 doi: 10.5480/15-1670

Waldie, J., Tee, S. and Day, T. (2016). Reducing avoidable deaths from failure to rescue: A discussion paper. *British Journal of Nursing, 25*(16), 895–900.

CHAPTER 6

Exemplar for Educational Practice: A Collegial Mentoring Program

LAURA M. SCHWARZ, DNP, RN, CNE

IDENTIFYING THE AREA OF NEED

The first step to creating a DNP project is determining an area in need of a practice change or clinical problem. Often this is not difficult to ascertain as all one generally needs do is monitor trends or for nuances in their given practice area to determine any number of needs. Choosing an area of greatest need for practice change is a good place to start. Do not worry if you have more than one need area because you can probably use other topics for other papers or projects in your DNP program. I myself had a second idea for the DNP project (comparing associate degree with baccalaureate degree education), but this was not a practice project topic, and so I could not use it. While I did not use this idea for my DNP project, I did use it for other projects including a concept analysis.

My practice area is nursing education and the area of need at my place of work, an Associate Degree Nursing Program, was obvious. In the fall I began my DNP program, eight of twenty-four (1/3) of our faculty members in the AD program in which I taught were new hires. The new faculty members had very little to no teaching experience. To compound the lack of experience, we had no formal mentoring program in place which caused new faculty to struggle. Some new faculty members did seek help from current faculty members, and some current faculty members did reach out to new hires. Reaching out was often dependent upon new faculty teaching the same courses as more seasoned faculty, as well as willingness to mentor or be mentored. Mentoring was largely happenstance with no formal structure. Some new faculty members bonded together to be each other's

127

informal mentors. As it went, a rift formed between the new faculty members and the more seasoned faculty causing job dissatisfaction. Job satisfaction and intent to stay are highly correlated, and the converse is true (Derby-Davis, 2014; Jeffers and Mariani, 2017; Lee *et al.,* 2017). The shortage of nursing faculty is a practice problem and compounds the overall nursing shortage (AACN, 2017; NLN, 2014). My practice change, therefore, was to develop an evidenced based mentoring program for new faculty members to help retain them, particularly in light of the faculty shortage.

FORMULATING THE PRACTICE QUESTION

I first needed to obtain approval for my mentoring program idea from my two DNP project professors to begin my project. This was done at the first meeting of spring semester of my first year of a two-year, five-semester program. Spring of year one was the semester the planning part of the project was commenced. My professors were enthusiastic about my project idea and helped my peers and I to each develop a practice question for our project. My DNP program utilized the PICOT Model: Problem/Patient/Population, Intervention or Issue of interest, Comparison and Timeline. My PICOT question was formulated as: What is the difference in new faculty job satisfaction and intent to stay employed with the school of nursing in those participating in a formal mentoring program versus those who did not experience the formal mentoring program? To answer the question of interest, I proposed to develop a formal evidence-based mentoring program.

P	Population	New faculty members in the school of nursing who experienced the mentoring program
I	Intervention	Formal mentoring program
C		New faculty members who did not experience the mentoring program
O	Outcome	Job satisfaction and intent to stay
T	Timeline	Semester (not written into the question but under stood as the length of the project implementation).

Significance

I reasoned that if job satisfaction and intent to stay are greater in new nursing faculty who take part in a formal mentoring program than those who do not, that formal faculty mentoring programs should be standard in schools of nursing. Furthermore, I reasoned that if there was no difference in job satisfaction and intent to stay between those faculty who took part in a formal mentoring program and those who did not, that efforts should be concentrated in determining what else may contribute to job satisfaction and intent to stay in nursing faculty. This ascertainment is of significance to nursing because if job satisfaction and intent to stay are increased, then the nurse faculty shortage may be attenuated, thus helping to decrease the nursing shortage.

LITERATURE REVIEW

I began with the literature review rather than project design for the mentoring program because the literature review would inform the project design. It is important to search a variety of data bases because while they overlap, one will find that some data bases have publications the others do not. I used CINAHL, Medline, ERIC, Google Scholar, and others. The literature review had many facets. First, it consisted of documenting the problem which encompassed the nursing faculty shortage including antecedents and consequences. The literature review informed the theoretical definitions of the variables: mentoring, job satisfaction and intent to stay. Likewise, I procured literature on the relationships between mentoring and intent to stay, mentoring and job satisfaction, and job satisfaction and intent to stay, as well as other potential outcomes of mentoring, both positive and negative. I used the *Canadian Task Force on Preventive Health Care Levels of Evidence and Grades of Recommendations* to rate the evidence from the literature for support of the implementation of the mentoring program. I also searched for the best tools, that is, those with the best fit, reliability, and validity, to measure the outcomes of job satisfaction and intent to stay. To measure perceived job satisfaction, I chose the Index of Job Satisfaction (Brayfield and Rothe, 1951), a very tried and true tool. This tool is an 18-item questionnaire using a five-point Likert Scale. The authors reported a reliability of 0.87 and concurrent validity of 0.92 through correlation with the Hoppock Job Satisfaction tool (Brayfield and Rothe). I chose a six-question survey developed by Garbee and Killacky (2008), specifically for use with nursing faculty to measure intent to stay. The six questions were tested by the authors for internal reliability. The correlation was: $r(313) = -0.467, p < 0.001$ between intent to stay and intent to leave. Lastly, I identified gaps in clinical knowledge that might be addressed, at least in part, through the project.

APPROVALS

There were three major areas of approval that I needed for the project. The first was to gain permission from the authors of the job satisfaction and intent to stay tools. I contacted the authors of the *Intent to Stay* tool via e-mail and they agreed that I could use their tool. The *Hoppock Job Satisfaction* tool was a little more interesting in that both authors were deceased, therefore, I could not ask them for permission. The fortunate aspect was that the tool was developed in 1951, and copyright laws only apply to documents created on or after January 1, 1978. Secondly, because I would be conducting a research study, I needed IRB permission. In my case, I would be using two sites and hence needed to create and submit two different proposals because each IRB had slightly different guidelines. Lastly, My DNP program required both a DNP project proposal paper and oral defense with my two professors and my project advisor. The paper included an abstract, introduction, the background of the problem, literature review, project implementation plan that included the theoretical model and application of stages, significance, methodology including subjects and setting, data collection instruments, data analysis plan, human subjects' considerations, references and appendices for the actual instruments to be used, budget, and timeline. For the defense, I gave a presentation with an accompanying PowerPoint and handout. I included the background and significance of the problem, purpose of the project, PICOT question, very brief review of the literature, theoretical framework, participants (mentors and mentees as well as control group), how participants would be invited, overview of the mentoring program and design, risks of participation, how outcomes would be evaluated, risks of the survey, how I would perform data analysis, and time for questions and suggestions. My DNP project professors and project advisor asked several questions about the project and DNP essentials. I was then sent out in the hall for a few minutes while they discussed whatever it is that is discussed behind closed doors. Then I was invited back in, congratulated and notified that I had passed the exam and could proceed with my project.

Tips for Oral Defense

I received these in an e-mail prior to my oral defense from one of my very seasoned professors (Dr. K. Willette-Murphy, personal communication, July 14, 2008).

- Prepare PowerPoint.
- Very briefly touch on the lit review—include only salient points because the committee members will have read your paper.
- Very briefly discuss reasons the study is important—one or two sentences.
- Very briefly the theoretical framework for the study—a few sentences.
- Describe in depth and detail the design of the study subjects/ participants, measures, interventions, analysis, etc. Focus on what you will do and why and how you will analyze it.
- Focus on what is your planned outcome. Spending most of the time on this will allow time for questions, answers and suggestions.
- Bring a copy of your IRB proposal and an electronic copy of your proposal in case you need to change something before it is signed.
- A handout may facilitate this process.

TIMELINE

The timeline for the project included three semesters: summer semester of year one, fall semester of year two, and spring semester of year two. The summer outcomes were to develop the project to address the practice problem and consider a clinical context. Fall semester outcomes focused in implementing clinical project. I planned to evaluate and disseminate the clinical scholarship knowledge Spring semester. This very ambitious timeframe was written into the DNP curricula. See Table 6.1 for a more detailed timeline that I developed for my project.

TABLE 6.1. Timeline.

Course/Semester	Product/Product Contents	Timeline
Clinical Scholarship II	Contact school(s) of nursing and discuss the project, get buy-in for the project and approval to work with them.	By June 10
Summer Year 1	Interview leaders and faculty regarding mentoring needs	By June 30
	Develop mentoring project including mentoring packet and guidelines and gain buy-in and approval from school leaders/faculty.	By June 30
	Gain permission from authors to use their well-developed tools for measurement of the outcomes (intent to stay & job satisfaction).	By June 13
	IRB Proposal	Submit by July 25, gain approval by July 18
	Qualifying exam	By June 18
	Written Paper	Submit by July 25
Clinical Scholarship III	Present the project to any new faculty who were not present to hear about it previously, gain their buy-in	By August 29
Fall Year 2	Host a seminar on mentoring to be held with mentors, mentees, and anyone else who may be interested. Distribute mentoring handbook.	By September 5
	Survey newer faculty who did not have the benefit of mentoring using the intent to stay & job satisfaction and tools.	By September 19
	Touch base with the mentors and mentees and keep a log of the feedback, make and take weeks from suggestions as needed	Every 2–3 weeks from Septembe 5–November 21
	Send intent to stay & job-satisfaction surveys to the new faculty who were mentored.	By November 1
	Send "reminder" to any new faculty members who did not return the survey.	By November 7
	Begin to analyze survey data	By November 14
	Data analysis write-up complete	By November 21
	Submit DNP Project Manuscript paper	By November 25
Clinical Scholarship III	Choose journal and write final manuscript in publishable format Submit Manuscript to Research Journal	By February 28
Spring Year 2	Defense of DNP Project	By May 1

PROJECT IMPLEMENTATION PLAN

The Theoretical Base

The collegial mentoring program required careful design and that began with my consideration in choosing a theoretical base. I had studied many middle range theories the first semester in the program. Middle range theories are more practical for a practice project than grand theories. I chose a change theory as the most fitting, specifically *Diffusions of Innovations Theory* (Rogers, 1995). The sequential stages of this theory informed the project and include:

(1) Knowledge; person becomes aware of an innovation and has some idea of how it functions, (2) Persuasion; person forms a favorable or unfavorable attitude toward the innovation, (3) Decision; person engages in activities that lead to a choice to adopt or reject the innovation, (4) Implementation; person puts an innovation into use, (5) Confirmation; person evaluates the results of an innovation-decision already made (Rogers, 1995).

Further informing the project implementation were what Rogers (1995) describes as categories of behavior frequently seen as individuals respond to change. They are innovators, early adopters, early majority, late majority, laggards, and rejecters. Early adopters are useful in rallying for and speeding the diffusion process and will be helpful in assisting with buy in on the change. The leader should be cautious of the late majority, who are skeptical of change, of laggards who slow the change process and often do not adopt it until it is replaced by something else, and of rejecters who will likely never adopt the change. Peer pressure is often helpful in persuading late adopters to accept the change. Laggards and rejecters may not be appeased, so it may be best to steer clear of them and respectfully disagree with their traditional views of the way things should be done.

Knowledge and Persuasion-Stakeholders

Background information should be provided to stakeholders as a way to gain buy-in through persuasion. The mentoring project could not be implemented without proper support. During the persuasion stage, I shared background knowledge from the literature review on both the nurse faculty shortage and on mentoring as a way to attenuate this shortage through increasing intent to stay, job satisfaction, job confidence in the knowledge. Further, I disseminated information regarding the other benefits for mentors, mentees, the program, and profession. Getting support of leadership and faculty, who are the key stakeholders, was fundamental for success in implementation of my project. I needed to include these persons upfront in the persuasion because they are the people who could support or reject the project. The settings for the mentoring project included one private and one public baccalaureate school of nursing. The reason for my choosing two schools was to increase the sample size, to diversify the sample, and to increase anonymity. The reasons for choosing these schools of nursing were both accessibility and representativeness of schools of nursing in Minnesota. I gained permission from the school of nursing leadership of the two different baccalaureate nursing programs. I then submitted proposals to the two different universities' IRBs.

After leadership and IRB approval, I recruited a convenience sample of voluntary participants from lists provided by nursing departmental leaders. Eligible participants who were recruited to be mentees and who served as the experimental group for this study were newly hired nursing faculty teaching in the schools of nursing. The experimental group included five nursing faculty hires new to the schools of nursing. The participants of the control group were four relatively new nursing faculty members in the same schools of nursing and who had been hired within the past two years. Experimental group and control group participants included both permanent and adjunct nursing faculty who had previously taught in a different setting, but were new to these settings, and those who had never taught anywhere else.

Mentors were recruited on a voluntary basis by me with help from departmental leaders in each school of nursing. Leaders' judgment of inclusion criteria was used to select mentors. These criteria included: generosity, competence, self-confidence, commitment to the mentor relationship, camaraderie, approachability, and good interpersonal skills (Smith and Zsoshar, 2005) understanding of tenure and promotion, and skill at teaching and research. The mentors must have also been at the proficient or expert level described by Benner (1982). I provided all participants with human subjects' protection information and completed informed consent procedures prior to participation and data collection.

TABLE 6.2. Mentoring Seminar Agenda in Consecutive Order.

1. Self-introductions of researcher/program leader, mentors, and mentees including experience, background, and teaching assignment for the semester.
2. Explanation of why a researcher became interested in mentoring and development of a mentoring program.
3. Participants were given a handbook which explained the collegial mentoring program and guidelines.
4. Researcher reviewed the handbook page-by-page with participants.
5. Time for participants to ask questions about the program.
6. Informed consent forms distributed, signed, and returned to researcher
7. E-mail and phone number contacts of participants as well as best days and times for researcher to contact them taken by researcher.
8. Mentors and mentees paired.
9. Mentor and mentee pairs discussed goals for the program and set up meeting time.
10. Researcher informed participants she would contact them in two-three weeks, took any last questions from participants, and closed the seminar meeting.
11. Departure.

Decision Stage

Preparing the potential mentors and mentees for their roles was part of the decision stage. I sent an e-mail with an informational letter to potential mentors and mentees inviting them to participate in the mentoring program and study. In the email, I explained the project as well as the potential benefits and associated risks. Mentors and mentees were invited to participate in a mentoring seminar whereby the collegial mentoring program and guidelines would be explained. Five mentors and five mentees agreed to participate, as well as 4 control-group (non-mentored) faculty members. See Table 6.2 and *Implementation Stage* below for further explanation of the mentoring seminar agenda.

Implementation Stage

The implementation stage planning began with careful matching of the 5 mentors and 5 mentees who had agreed to participate in the mentoring program. Proper matching of the pairs based on personality, goals, and expectations is suggested by the literature (Nick *et al.*, 2012; Potter and Tholen, 2014). The leaders, mentor, and mentees all worked together to match pairs based on geographic location, courses taught (mentors and mentees taught the same course[s]), and desire to work with one-another. The program I developed was based on a collegial mentoring model (Thorpe and Kalischuk, 2003) as opposed to a more authoritarian-based mentor-protégé model. The literature suggested orienting mentors on how to mentor and offering a workshop or seminar to do so (Nowell *et al.*, 2017). The seminar with a mentoring handbook containing guidelines for the mentorship process is the method I chose to prepare the faculty for this project. I surmised that a seminar would encourage faculty interaction, dialog, and networking. Each participant received a mentoring handbook which I developed and included descriptions of the formal collegial mentoring intervention and evidence-based guidelines for the program. The handbook was used during the seminar to help guide explanation of the mentoring program. The mentoring handbook was a valuable accompanying tool to which faculty could refer. The seminar and handbook contained the best evidence-based recommendations from the literature and became part of the implementation stage. I incorporated the implementation elements into the mentoring handbook. These included meeting early, generational differences, culture and policies, mentor assets, characteristics and responsibilities, NLN core competencies, and strategies to promote change as well as a reference list. See Table 6.3 for a complete description of handbook contents which explain the intervention and program guidelines.

Confirmation

The specific recommendations for evaluation of mentoring during this project would consider both the mentors-mentee pairs' accomplishments and the overall project success. Specifically, the pairs should meet weekly for the first month and then at least every two weeks following. They should evaluate whether the goals are being met and how the relationship is functioning. The mentors shall provide verbal feedback to the mentees regarding performance. The pairs should revise goals and roles as deemed necessary by themselves and or the project leader who will touch-base every two to three weeks with each of the program participants to evaluate the performance, goals and roles.

I would evaluate the outcomes of intent to stay and job satisfaction for the new faculty mentees at the end of the semester as measured by survey. These outcomes were to be compared to the same outcomes of a comparison group of newer faculty members who did not have the benefit of the mentoring program. The comparison group was surveyed at the beginning of the implementation semester.

TABLE 6.3. *Contents of Collegial Mentoring Project Program Guidelines Handbook in Chronologic Order. (Note that the table indicates current updated references which differ from the original publication).*

- Abstract
- The nurse faculty shortage: background of the problem (AACN, 2017; NLN, 2014)
- Causes of the nurse faculty shortage (AACN, 2017; NLN, 2014)
- The purpose of the mentoring program (Hadidi, Lindquist, and Buckwalter, 2013; Jacobson and Sherrod, 2012; Jeffers and Mariani, 2017).
- The possible benefits of the mentoring program (Eller, Lev, and Feurer, 2014; Hadidi, Lindquist, and Buckwalter, 2013; Jeffers and Mariani, 2017; Nick *et al.,* 2012).
- Possible negative outcomes of mentoring (Hadidi, Lindquist, and Buckwalter, 2013; Jacobson and Sherrod, 2012)
- Participants and setting: review IRB proposal
- The design of the program: formal collegial mentoring with a carefully chosen, assigned mentor (Jacobson and Sherrod, 2012; Nick *et al.,* 2012; Thorpe and Kalischuk, 2003)
- Meeting (Eller, Lev, and Feurer, 2014; Hadidi, Lindquist and Buckwalter, 2013; Nick *et al.,* 2012; Potter and Tolson, 2014):
  —Can take place in many formats: on or off campus, in person, over the phone and/or through e-mail
  —The first meeting should include discussion of: roles, goals for the relationship (such as learning how to grade clinical paperwork and performance, learning how to lecture and or formulating a professional/faculty development plan); responsibilities and ground rules: history, culture, political environment, and decision-making of the school; policies and procedures of the program
  —Pairs should weekly the first month and then at least every two weeks to discuss whether goals are being met and how the relationship is functioning, and revise goals and roles as necessary
- Mentor and mentee responsibilities (Eller, Lev, and Feurer, 2014; Jacobson and Sherrod, 2012)
- Communication with the researcher/program leader
- Project time involvement of participants: total time 12–14 hours total, lasting one semester
- Using generational differences in mentoring to facilitate understanding of mentors/ mentees (Gibson, 2009; Nick, 2015, Popkess and Frey, 2016)
- The NLN Core Competencies of Nurse Educators© as a guide for mentoring and formulating mentoring goals (NLN, 2012; NLN, 2018).
- *From Novice to Expert* (Benner, 1982) as a guide for defining current and outcome teaching proficiencies of mentees and used as criterion in selecting mentors
- Helpful references (Billings and Halstead, 2019; Caputi, 2015; NLN, 2018)
- Potential risks of participation in the mentoring program-review IRB proposal
- Evaluation of the mentoring program-review IRB proposal
- Limitations: review IRB proposal
- Protection and confidentiality: review IRB proposal
- Researcher and IRB contact information: review IRB proposal
- References

MEASURES

I combined the 18-item job satisfaction and 6-item intent to stay quantitative survey research instruments and a demographics survey into one instrument. I administered the survey online via SurveyMonkeytm to both control group and experimental group participants. I collected Quantitative online survey data from the mentees three separate times and from the experimental participants once (see Table 6.3 for timeline). Both mentors and mentees were asked to complete verbal surveys which included ten open-ended questions asked by the researcher. I conducted these interviews every two-three weeks throughout the mentoring program and at the conclusion of the program via phone calls and e-mail. I asked participants how well the mentoring relationship functioned, about goals and roles, and also asked them to identify the positives and negatives of the program. I kept field notes regarding the program throughout the duration of the program.

Four out of the five of the mentees completed the online surveys. Four control group participants completed the online surveys which were used as a comparison to data reported in the surveys completed by the mentees.

Job Satisfaction and Intent to Stay Surveys

Independent t-test results from the study did not show a statistical difference in either job satisfaction or intent to stay between the mentored and non-mentored group. I believe this may have been due to the small sample size and also to the fact that two of four control group participants reported having a nursing faculty mentor previous to the study. The mentored group's mean scores did, however, indicate a greater mean intent to stay employed with the school of nursing and less intent to leave by at least one-point difference on five of six questions measuring intent to stay/leave. Additionally, mentees scored high on the intent to stay, low on the intent to leave, and positively on job satisfaction. Repeated measures of job satisfaction and intent to stay over time for experimental group do not show statistical significance. This may have been due to both the small sample size and the short length of program and measurement time period.

All five mentors and mentees actively participated in the program and provided verbal participant feedback periodically when contacted by the researcher. Three out of five mentoring pairs were actively engaged in the mentoring relationship and met in person on a weekly or near weekly basis. Two pairs met only two to three times in person during the semester but used phone calls and e-mails to communicate on mentoring topics in between face-to-face meetings. In these cases, it seemed that the mentor served as more of a resource or safety net on an as-needed basis. Some participants experienced no obstacles to meeting while others experienced few to several obstacles. Obstacles described included illness, busy, and/or mismatched schedules, lack of time, second jobs, expanded faculty responsibilities, living or having clinical a distance from campus, and mentees' lack of time spent on campus due to adjunct status. Participants reported that planning the next future meeting at the end of the current meeting, making a date ahead of time around mutual schedules, and e-mail all helped to facilitate future meetings.

Examples of participants' goals included learning about how to organize; departmental culture; grading assignments/performance; giving students feedback; dealing with student performance issues; building self-confidence; and creating a faculty/career development plan. Mentors often gave mentees examples to follow which they found beneficial. The majority of the participants reported that they were actively engaged in working on and had good accomplishment of the goals, though some participants felt they could have accomplished more.

Participants reported being pleased with the mentoring program and relationship, and that it was a positive, worthwhile experience. Overall, participants reported feeling connected with good rapport and that the relationship was open, honest, and beneficial. All mentees stated that they benefitted from having an experienced faculty member assigned directly to them. Mentors served as a safety net and were there for advice and affirmation. The experience was confidence-building for mentees who felt comforted by having an assigned mentor. Mentors expressed that they felt valued in their role and enjoyed sharing their expertise. Two of the mentees said they would not have continued in their role as nursing faculty if it had not been for their mentor. One mentee stated that she would enjoy serving as a mentor in the future and that serving as a mentor appeared to be an effective method for advancing mentors' expertise in the faculty role. Participants acknowledged that they felt that having one person set up and coordinate the program and touch base regularly was a benefit and that the program was well organized.

Few negatives regarding the mentoring program were reported but some included frustration that the program did not last longer, difficulty in scheduling meeting times, constraints due to lack of time, and about the difficulty of not meeting before the start of the semester. Not being given a release time was negatively reported by one mentor and one mentee. Lack of recognition for serving as a mentor and a limited number of mentors compared to the mentoring need were also stated as drawbacks.

There were a few barriers to project implementation encountered. First and foremost, I found that it was difficult to recruit participants and response rate was relatively low. Potential participants who declined to partake in the study cited lack of time as the reason. Interestingly, I had the most difficulty recruiting control group participants, and needed to expand the pool of potential recruits including sending four separate sets of invitations. Tight schedules made it difficult to find a time when all participants were available at the same time for the mentoring seminar. My intent was to host the seminar at the start of the school year, but the seminar was delayed until the second and third weeks of the semester. I held three separate seminars to accommodate participant schedules. Finally, contacting participants reliably via phone, as suggested by my lead professor, was a challenge for me and I found e-mail to be more effective.

Facilitators of the mentoring program were threefold. My hosting the mentoring seminar at the kickoff of the program helped to clarify the goals and expectations and was an opportunity for a question and answer session. The seminar provided a useful forum for the mentors and mentees to become acquainted with one another as well as with me as the researcher/program host. The mentoring handbook was beneficial as a guide for participants to follow along as I explained the program in the seminar, and as a reference throughout the program.

DISCUSSION

Three out of the five mentoring pairs met on a weekly basis as recommended by me, the researcher. These pairs reported the most accomplishment of goals and benefits from the program. Two of the mentoring pairs met in person only two to three times during the program, and though they did report benefit from the program, the relationship may not have fully operationalized. The collegial mentoring program as an intervention was found to increase faculty retention since two participants stated that they would not have continued on to pursue teaching in nursing if it were not for their mentors. These findings are consistent with those of the literature

Based on project findings, use of a mandatory formal collegial mentoring program for all new nursing faculty members, regardless of previous experience seems prudent. Recommendations for mentoring programs included: having one person in charge of the program; use of a mentoring handbook to guide the program; hosting of a mentoring seminar to introduce the program and scheduling it at the start of the semester with the assistance of the departmental leader to enhance participation; formulation of goals during the mentoring seminar; having mentoring pairs set up a standing meeting time at the beginning of the semester and/or plan the next meeting at the end of the current meeting; mentors and mentees should both share responsibilities and accountability in the mentoring relationship; and having mentors share school culture, policies and procedures early in the program. Finally, offering honoraria or recognition for mentors and release times for mentors and mentees may help with increase program participation.

This project has several implications for nursing faculty as well as the profession of nursing. If mentoring programs are effective in retaining nurse faculty, the nurse faculty shortage and hence the nursing shortage may be reduced. Additionally, faculty retention may perhaps decrease frequency of new faculty hiring and subsequent orientation. This could in turn result in decreased burden on seasoned faculty who serve to orient them and often pick-up additional duties to lessen the workload of novice faculty. Retaining faculty increases overall faculty experience, which in turn may increase the quality of nursing education and enhance student learning creating benefits for both patient care and the profession. Collegial mentoring programs may serve as a safety net for novice nurses. Mentoring may also serve as a catalyst to developing comfort through caring for novice faculty. Caring, a central value of nursing may deserve more attention as applied to nursing faculty. Finally, mentoring may possibly increase faculty job satisfaction and be a positive and friendly method of socializing new faculty.

Limitations of the project include the small sample size and short time of the formal mentoring program. The sample size decreases the reliability and validity of the results as well as statistical power. The short time frame may have decreased the amplitude of impact of the program. Because the mentoring program was conducted during one semester of a school year only, it did not allow for examination of changes over time. A possible confounding factor was that two of four control group participants had the benefit of being mentored in nurse faculty positions prior to the study.

RECOMMENDATIONS

The sample size of this study was small with two schools of nursing participating. Though useful, the study has limited statistical power and more work is needed to confirm the extent to which these results could be extrapolated to other programs. A similar study of collegial mentoring programs using a larger sample size, a variety of schools of nursing in different locations, and investigation of outcomes over an extended period of time should be conducted with careful use of both qualitative and quantitative measures of outcomes.

PROJECT CONCLUSIONS

In light of the dire and worsening nurse faculty shortage and its impacts on the nursing shortage and the profession as a whole, the field of nursing needs interventions now more than ever, to attenuate this crisis. This project demonstrates the benefits of a formal collegial mentoring program on new nursing faculty retention. Mentors are a safety net, resource, and guide for new faculty. It is recommended that all schools of nursing consider budgeting for and implementing similar programs as a potential method to enhance nurse faculty retention.

DISSEMINATION

Dissemination took the form of three arenas. The first was a DNP project manuscript to be submitted to my professor and project advisor, written according to the specifications of my program. The paper was similar to how I have outlined the project above. The next was creation of a poster and accompanying handout presented at a DNP symposium with all DNP students and faculty as well as invited guests with over 100 attendees. The poster was a challenge for me because (1) I had never created a poster before; (2) I had no poster examples to model as I was part of the first cohort in my DNP program; and (3) too many things were asked to be placed for on the poster and it was difficult to fit without scrunching the words or making font too small. The poster content included title, authors, clinical problem PICOT question, review of literature, key literature, review of literature table, synthesis statement, theoretical base, purpose, methodological basis, review of findings, practice implications, and references. We were also asked to choose a professional journal and revise our manuscripts to fit with the journal criteria. Choosing a journal was not an easy task as I needed to find the right fit and to keep with APA formatting (some journals had other types of formatting such as AMA). I submitted my revised journal manuscript to my professors and also to the journal for possible publication. My manuscript was not chosen for publication. I was disappointed, but looking back, the sample size was very small with low generalizability. I also was a little lofty in choosing a very top-notch education journal. Lastly, I defended my project at my DNP defense. I prepared by reviewing my project and reviewing the Essentials of DNP Nursing Education. The defense went well, due mostly to all I had learned while in my program, as well as preparing myself. Again, I was asked to step out, and this time I waited in another room. After what seemed like forever (in reality probably no more than five or ten minutes), my lead DNP project professor invited me to come back to the room with a "Congratulations Doctor!" What an exhilarating feeling!

PERSONAL TAKEAWAYS AND CONCLUSIONS

My DNP program and DNP project encompassed some of my greatest learning experiences in my personal and professional life. Firstly, and maybe my most precious takeaway, were the life-long friends I made with my four cohort peers. I keep in touch with all of them through social media and we plan to have a reunion soon. One of my DNP program friends is now an adjunct professor in the RN-Baccalaureate Completion Program in which I teach and of which I am the coordinator. I learned to not give up. There were times I really wanted to quit, especially the first semester in the program when I was spending 40+ hours a week on the statistics course alone (not to mention the other 4-credit course, plus teaching full time, being a mom, and becoming a new grandmother that semester). It was undenounced to me that my peers were also spending 40 hours a week on statistics homework (I thought I was just slow or dense). I learned to both provide and ask my peers for emotional support and advice during the tough times as we were all in the same boat after all and no one understood the struggles better. I learned that I could endure just about anything for two years; lack of sleep, mountains of reading, a multitude of data base searches, writing, and re-writing. I am a lot stronger than I thought. I learned to expect the unexpected; changes of plan, subjects not following through, being asked to do something different than what was asked originally, added assignments, and meeting in person even though it was an all online program (because faculty and students wanted to do so). To save time, I learned to give up some things, as least temporarily (regular hair appointments, coupon-cutting, having a perfectly clean house, doing laundry on a regular basis, updating my students' assignments every single semester, lunches, or happy hour with my friends, and even time with my family). It had to learn to say no and to explain the best I could to friends and family that I was too busy to spend much time with them. Keeping a calendar and checklist of things to do every day was very important to staying on track and not falling behind, but I also found I could not check off every single thing on the list each day. Some things (maybe a reading here or there) simply did not get done, and some tasks were prioritized and shifted to another day because there was simply not enough time or energy in a day to do it all. I learned that I had outgrown my (14-year) career as a nursing instructor at a community college where I thought I would stay forever and found myself ready for and actualizing teaching at the University level. I found that I enjoy research, writing, and presenting at conferences much more than I had anticipated and now do so as part of my career. Most importantly, I found that I am a changed person, in a good way. It's hard to explain, but I look at the world quite a bit differently now, through a new set of Doctor glasses if you will.

REFERENCES

American Association of Colleges of Nursing. (2017). Nursing faculty shortage fact sheet. Available from https://www.aacnnursing.org/News-Information/Fact-Sheets/Nursing-Faculty-Shortage.

Benner, P. (1982). From novice to expert. *American Journal of Nursing*, 402–407.

Billings, D. M. and Halstead, J. A. (2019). Teaching in Nursing: A guide for faculty (3rd ed). St. Louis: Saunders Elsevier.

Brayfield, A. H. and Rothe, H. F. (1951). An index of job satisfaction. *Journal of Applied Psychology, 35*(2), 307–311.

Caputi, L. (2015). *Certified Nurse Educator review book: The official NLN guide to the CNE Exam.* Philadelphia: Wolters Kluwer.

Derby-Davis, M. J. (2014). Predictors of Nursing Faculty's Job Satisfaction and Intent to Stay in Academe. *Journal of Professional Nursing, 30*(1), 19–25. doi: 10.1016/j.profnurs.2013.04.001

Eller, L. S., Lev, E. L. and Feurer, A. (2014). Key components of an effective mentoring relationship: A qualitative study. *Nurse Education Today, 34*(5), 815–820. doi: 10.1016/j.nedt.2013.07.020

Garbee, D. D. & Killacky, J. (2008). Factors influencing intent to stay in academia for nursing faculty in the Southern United States of America. *International Journal of Nursing Education Scholarship, 5*(1), 1–15.

Gibson, S. E. (2009). Enhancing intergenerational communication in the classroom: Recommendations for successful Teacher-Student Relationships. *Nursing Education Perspectives, 30*(1), 37–39.

Hadidi, N. N., Lindquist, R. and Buckwalter, K. (2013). Lighting the fire with mentoring relationships. *Nurse Educator, 38*(4), 157–163. doi:10.1097/NNE.0b013e318296dccc

Jacobson, S. L. and Sherrod, D. R. (2012). Transformational mentorship models for nurse educators. *Nursing Science Quarterly, 25*(3), 279–284. doi:10.1177/0894318412447565

Jeffers, S. and Mariani, B. (2017). The effect of a formal mentoring program on career satisfaction and intent to stay in the faculty role for novice nurse faculty. *Nursing Education Perspectives, 38*(1), 18–22. doi:10.1097/01.NEP.0000000000000104

Lee, P., Miller, M. T., Kippenbrock, T. A., Rosen, C. and Emory, J. (2017). College nursing faculty job satisfaction and retention: A national perspective. *Journal of Professional Nursing, 33*(4), 261–266. doi:10.1016/j.profnurs.2017.01.001

National League for Nursing. (2012). *The scope of practice for academic nurse educators 2012 revision.* Philadelphia: Wolters Kluwer.

National League for Nursing. (2014). *Nurse educator shortage fact sheet.* Available from http://www.nln.org/docs/default-source/advocacy-public-policy/nurse-faculty-shortage-fact-sheet-pdf.pdf?sfvrsn=0.

National League for Nursing. (2018). *Certified Nurse Educator (CNE®) 2018 candidate handbook.* Available from http://www.nln.org/docs/default-source/default-document-library/cne-handbookb203c85c78366c709642ff00005f0421.pdf?sfvrsn=0

Nick, J. M. (2015). Chapter 1 Facilitate learning. In L. Caputi (Ed). *Certified Nurse Educator review book: The official NLN guide to the CNE Exam* (1-31). Philadelphia: Wolters Kluwer.

Nick, J. M., Delahoyde, T. M., Prato, D. D., Mitchell, C., Ortiz, J., Ottley, C., . . . Siktberg, L. (2012). Best practices in academic mentoring: A model for excellence. *Nursing Research & Practice,* 1–9. Doi:10.1155/2012/937906.

Nowell, L., Norris, J. M., Mrklas, K. and White, D. E. (2017). A literature review of mentorship programs in academic nursing. *Journal of Professional Nursing, 33*(5), 334–344. https://doi-org.ezproxy.mnsu.edu/10.1016/j.profnurs.2017.02.007

Popkess, A. M. & Frey, J. L. (2016). Chapter 2 strategies to support diverse learning needs of students. In D. M. Billings & J. A. Halstead (Eds.) *Teaching in nursing,* 5th ed. (15-34). St. Louis, MO: Elsevier.

Potter, D. R. and Tolson, D. (2014). A Mentoring Guide for Nursing Faculty in Higher Education. *International Journal of Caring Sciences, 7*(3), 727–732. Retrieved from

https://search-ebscohost-com.ezproxy.mnsu.edu/login.aspx?direct=true&db=rzh&
AN=103900081&site=ehost-live

Rogers, E. M. (1995). *Diffusion of Innovations* (4th ed.). New York: The Free Press.

Smith, J. A. & Zsoher, H. (2005). Essentials of neophyte mentorship in relation to the
faculty shortage. *Journal of Nursing Education, 46*(4), 184–186.

Thorpe K and Kalischuk RG. (2003). A collegial mentoring model for nurse educators.
Nursing Forum, 38(1), 5–15. doi:10.1111/j.1744-6198.2003.tb01198.x

Part 3: Clinical Exemplars

Increase Advance Directives Knowledge Among African Americans in the Faith-Based Organization

KOTAYA GRIFFITH, DNP, MSN, APRN, AGPCNP-C, CNL

PROBLEM IDENTIFICATION/STATEMENT

Upon entry into the Doctor of Nursing Practice (DNP) program, you must identify a clinical problem for your quality improvement (QI) project. As a nurse practitioner working in the long-term care setting, I examined some of the problems that occurred in my practice environment. One problem that I encountered was the lack of completed advance directives (AD) found among the African American (AA) residents. Many of the residents and their family members were also not knowledgeable about AD. Advance directives are legal paperwork, which allows an individual to select a healthcare agent to communicate decisions about end-of-life (EOL) care in the event that a person is unable to communicate his or her own wishes (National Library of Medicine, 2016). Advance directives are important tools for communicating patients' EOL wishes and are associated with many benefits, such as reducing the burden for both the surrogate decision-makers and families, reducing EOL costs, stress and depression reduction, increasing quality of care, and higher patient satisfaction scores (Brinkman-Stoppelenburg, Rietjens, and Van, 2014; Detering *et al.* 2016; Wholihan and Pace, 2012). Therefore, in the absence of an AD it poses many challenges for the patient, family, and healthcare team.

For my QI project, I was interested in increasing AD completion rates among AAs but had limited insight about the evidence regarding AD completion rates or any interventions. My primary assumption was that AAs were not knowledgeable about AD. The main reason was thought to be due to a lack of AD education. Therefore, it was assumed that a community education intervention regarding AD would increase awareness and ultimately lead to completed AD. So, my initial clinical question was what the effect would community AD educational intervention among AAs participants upon AD completion rates? After constructing the clinical question my next step was to perform a literature search. For my literature review I used multiple electronic databases; CINAHL, PUBMED, PsycINFO and a hand search of Journals. The key terms used were advance directives, advanced care-planning, living wills, healthcare power of attorney, healthcare proxy, Ulyssess contracts, AAs, blacks, faith-based programs, church, end-of-life care, education, community, and do not resuscitate orders. In an effort to narrow my search, I used inclusion criteria which was in the English language, online journals, and a date range from 2006 to 2018 with a focus on the last five years. The search yielded 83 articles of which 21 were found to be specific, useful, and relevant to my selected topic.

LITERATURE SYNTHESIS

Barriers to AD Completion

African Americans (AAs) were found to have lower AD completion rates compared to whites (Ko and Lee, 2014; Koss and Baker, 2017; Portanova et al., 2017; Rao et al., 2014). The literature suggests several reasons for decreased use of AD among AAs (Huang et al., 2016; Rhodes et al., 2015). Rhodes et al. (2015) examined provider experiences working with AA patients and families at the EOL. Barriers identified were conflict with spiritual belief, family difficulties, desire for aggressive care, medical mistrust, illness hastens death, and lack of knowledge (Rhodes et al. 2015). Huang et al. (2016) reported similar barriers, including mistrust of doctors and avoidance of death discussions. Sanders, Robinson, and Block (2016) found similar barriers in their systematic review, which added life sustaining treatment preferences and poor health literacy. However, Sanders et al. (2016) highlighted that these barriers were connected to the historical context of AAs in America. Belisomo (2017) wrote that racial barriers to advance care planning (ACP) existed among AAs. Such barriers were acknowledged among some physicians as challenges when discussing EOL concerns. Additionally, Ramsey (2013) examined the attitudes of young AA adults toward AD. The researcher found that a lack of knowledge contributed to low AD.

Ladd (2014) found several explanations for AAs' EOL preferences. Mistrust of healthcare providers, social structure and dynamics, religion, education and health literacy impacted AAs' EOL preferences (Ladd, 2014). Ladd (2014) highlighted that education level had the strongest association with life-sustaining measures and use of hospice care. Koss (2017) examined religion as it influenced AD completion rates. The findings indicated no significant difference in religious practice between blacks and whites.

Even though the literature identified many compounding barriers, the lack of knowledge was the chief barriers in most studies (Ladd 2014; Huang *et al.*, 2016; Ramsey, 2013; Rao *et al.*, 2014; Rhodes *et al.*, 2016). Due to the knowledge deficit about AD, individuals are unaware of its benefits. Therefore, community-based ACP education programs are a strategy used to potentially increase AD awareness and to inform patients of their rights to make EOL decisions to guide their care.

AD Benefits

Several benefits are associated with completion of an AD. Main intentions are to (1) communicate patients' EOL preferences and (2) ensure their wishes are met (Brinkman-Stoppelenburg *et al.*, 2014; Detering *et al.*, 2016; Wholihan and Pace, 2012). According to Detering *et al.* (2016), benefits for completing ACP and AD include: (1) ensuring that care aligns with patient wishes, (2) improving communication among families and the healthcare team, (3) reducing hospital costs, and (4) achieving "a higher satisfaction with the quality of care" (para. 10). Brinkman-Stoppelenburg, Rietjens and Van (2014) conducted a systematic review on ACP's impact on EOL care. Advanced care-planning was associated with an increased compliance with patients' wishes and an increased satisfaction with quality of patient care (Brinkman-Stoppelenburg *et al.*, 2014). Several studies showed hospitalization reduction rates associated with having Do Not Hospitalize (DNH) orders (Brinkman-Stoppelenburg *et al.*, 2014). Advanced care-planning discussions were found to reduce stress, depression, and anxiety (Brinkman-Stoppelenburg *et al.*, 2014). Rocque *et al.* (2017) found that patients who had started or completed an ACP conversation had a significantly lower hospitalization rates than patients who had not (46% vs. 56%, $p = 0.02$).

Multiple components associated with EOL care are expensive for patients and their family from direct and indirect costs. Rao *et al.* (2014), stated that "healthcare costs are greatest during the final years of life" (66). Evidence suggests that ACP and AD have significant impacts on reducing patient health care spending during EOL (Wholihan and Pace, 2012; Rao *et al.*, 2014). Rao *et al.* (2014) stated evidence have shown "advance directives were associated with significantly lower levels of Medicare spending and lower in-hospital deaths" (66). Klinger, In der Schmitten, and Marckmann (2016) conducted a systematic review on care costs with ACP compared to standard without ACP costs. Six studies demonstrated a "cost saving ranging from $1,041 to $64,830 per patient" (Klinger, In der Schmitten, and Marckmann, 2016, 429). Wholihan and Pace (2012) highlighted an ACP program Respecting Choices®, which showed costs reduction during the final two years of life with "13.6% of deaths associated with a stay in intensive care" (174).

Education Intervention Effects on AD Completion Rates

Advanced care planning is a complex topic that warrants public education. Lack of education is one of the main barriers to ACP (Ladd, 2014; Huang *et al.*, 2016; Ramsey, 2013; Rao *et al.*, 2014; Rhodes *et al.*, 2015). Rao *et al.* (2014) identified racial and education disparities about AD completion. The researcher noted the need for ACP education. Findings indicated that education interventions increased AAs participants' knowledge and completion of AD (Huang *et al.*, 2016; Pecanac *et al.*, 2014).

Hinderer and Lee (2014) assessed a nurse-led AD and ACP community seminar using Fives Wishes. There were 82.6% of participants ($n = 71$) found the seminar practical and 97.7% ($n = 84$) reported an increased likelihood to complete an AD and ACP participation (Hinderer and Lee 2014). Although this study did not measure AD completion rates, it found that participants were willing to engage in the ACP process. The evidence suggests that education interventions may facilitate ACP conversations in the community. In a similar study, a nurse practitioner led a community-based Five Wishes workshop that resulted in ACP discussions with 15 of 22 participants completing AD one-month post workshop (Splendore and Grant, 2017). Bonner *et al.* (2014) created an education intervention, ACT-Plan (Advance Care Treatment Plan) using group sessions to improve self-efficacy of ACP among AA caregivers. The intervention group showed a significant improvement in self-efficacy to make EOL decisions when compared to control group ($p = 0.02$) (Bonner *et al.*, 2014).

Bullock (2006) used a faith-based model to promote AD among AA participants in North Carolina. The intervention was an AD education module based upon Emmanuel's medical directive for focus groups (Bullock, 2006). Emmanuel's medical directive is a comprehensive advance care document that outlines four paradigmatic scenarios, proxy of designation, organ donation, and a personal statement to communicate EOL care decisions (Emanuel and Emanuel, 1989). Bullock (2006) reported that only 25% of participants were willing to complete AD following the intervention. She concluded that the education intervention had minimal impact. Although this study found only a small percentage of participants completed AD, dissemination of ACP education increased AD awareness among the AA populations.

Litzelman *et al.* (2017) conducted a study using lay community health workers care coordinators to initiate ACP discussions with patients and to document the discussion in the electronic medical record. The care coordinators received ACP training workshops, simulation sessions, and clinical decision support tools. ACP documentations were measured pre-and post-intervention. The results showed that 392/818 patients had an ACP discussion, in which 64% participants signed the health care designee form, 22.7% recorded their goals of living, and 18.4% completed a Living Will (Litzelman *et al.*, 2017). The study findings indicated ACP discussions could lead to AD completion.

Hamayoshi (2014) developed an education program using the situation of EOL care to facilitate AD completion among persons with dementia. A quasi-experimental design was used with 81 participants in the intervention group and 60 participants in the control group. The education intervention consisted of lectures on EOL combined with an AD booklet explaining how to complete an AD (Hamayoshi, 2014). Fourteen participants completed AD in the intervention group and two participants in the control group post-intervention.

Markham *et al.* (2015) conducted a study of AA participant's usage of a computer program on ACP. The education intervention was a computer-based decision aid of complex problems about EOL medical decisions (Markham *et al.*, 2015). Eighteen participants completed the program. The findings revealed significantly increased knowledge with ACP scores increasing from 44.9% to 61.3% ($p = 0.0004$). Follow-up interviews found that 88% of participants had shared the AD with their family (Markham *et al.*, 2015). The findings in this study suggested an interactive computer program may increase knowledge of AD and its completion rates.

An ACP evidence-based program, Respecting Choices®, received national recognition for ACP initiatives increasing community awareness of AD and a reducing hospital costs (Wholihan and Pace, 2012). The Respecting Choices® program was used among racial and ethnic populations showing "increased prevalence of AD for racial and ethnic minorities from 25.8% to 38.45%" (Pecanac *et al.*, 2014, 285). Pecanac *et al.* (2014) stated that the Respecting Choices® program "provided the means to alleviate barriers for racial and ethnic minorities to complete advance directives" (285). Huang *et al.* (2016) included the Respecting Choices® in a multi-component ACP intervention among 30 AAs participants. Findings showed a significant increase in knowledge about AD among the participants in the intervention group ($p = 0.01$) (Huang *et al.*, 2016). An increase in participants completing an AD post- intervention was also reported (Huang *et al.*, 2016). Additionally, Mackenzie *et al.* (2017) conducted a systematic review on Respecting Choices® and related models. The researchers reported a high level of evidence of AD completion among the Caucasians with a lower level of evidence among AAs.

The studies included in this literature review used qualitative or quantitative methods and represent a range of levels of evidence. A commonality found in multiple studies was education interventions used in community settings. The evidence suggests education intervention increases knowledge about AD.

Faith-based Setting Utilization for ACP Discussions

Churches have always served as one of the primary places for education among AAs, dating back to Dr. Martin Luther King's work during the Civil Rights Movement. During King's era, churches were the primary platforms for dissemination of information. Rowland and Isaac-Savage (2014) discussed the role of the black church in promoting health and fighting disparities, stating that the "black church has been the epicenter and have served as the education institution and a vehicle for healthcare and health promotion" (19). Rowland and Isaac-Savage (2014) advocated for adult educators to create healthcare programs with the black churches to reduce the impact of disparities. Due to the social, racial, and historical context of AAs in America, there remains a level of distrust of healthcare systems and healthcare providers. Therefore, ACP is a sensitive topic of discussion for this population and as a result, conversation must start in a familiar environment that is non-threatening.

The IOM report *Dying in America* (2015) strongly recommended ACP in community settings among minority populations. Literature suggests that community settings, such as a churches or clinics, are less threatening environments than acute settings for AAs and are suitable places for ACP discussions (Belisomo, 2017; Bonner *et al.*, 2014; Bullock, 2006; Hendricks Sloan *et al.*, 2016; Ramsey, 2013). Hinderer and Lee (2014) stated that community settings were ideal for addressing AD because individuals had more time to discuss EOL wishes. Splendore and Grant (2017) found community-based workshops prompted participants to be proactive in ACP discussions and completion. Rhodes *et al.* (2016) emphasized collaborating with faith-based organizations to provide ACP education to equip AAs with making EOL decisions.

Hendricks Sloan *et al.* (2016) surveyed blacks' parishioners about ACP and received 930 responses of 2500 attendees with a 30% response rate. Hendricks Sloan *et al.* (2016) reported 93% ($n = 865$) of the respondents welcomed "church-based information on ACP and believes that good EOL care is important" (192). There were 40% ($n = 372$) of parishioners that had never completed an ACP. Therefore, Hendricks Sloan *et al.* (2016) pointed out the need for a church-based program providing education on ACP and suggested involving clergy in the implementation of ACP programs.

Bullock (2006) reported 74% of participants in the study "believed that a faith-based promotion of ACP was an effective method of mobilizing community members to come together to learn about ACP" (191). Bullock (2006) wrote that participants were unwilling to receive EOL information if the church didn't support the program. Johnson *et al.* (2016) partnered with AA churches to conducted seven focus groups on EOL care and decision-making from spiritual perspectives. Faith beliefs were found to influence AAs decision-making about EOL, palliative and hospice care (Johnson *et al.*, 2016). However, Johnson *et al.* (2016) urged health providers to welcome faith beliefs of AA patients and view it as an asset, not a barrier. In these studies, the church was identified as a venue for increasing awareness and knowledge among AAs and called for new models to prepare church members and clergy in overcoming communication challenges about EOL care (Bullock, 2006; Johnson *et al.*, 2016).

Developing Project Focus and Objectives

Once my literature synthesis was completed, I was able to narrow down my project focus and reformulated my clinical question based upon the evidence. The 21 articles were separated into four themes: barriers to AD completion, AD benefits, educational intervention effect on AD completion rates, and faith-based setting utilization for ACP discussions. The use of the themes was a great strategy to categorized articles and was instrumental in redefining the project.

My project focus remains on AD rates among AAs, however, I shifted my focus to assessing the readiness level to completing AD through use of a Readiness Ruler (RR). The RR was developed by Stephen Rollnick based on the Transtheoretical Model (TTM) stages of change. The RR assesses an individual's readiness or willingness to change a specific behavior (Rollnick, Heather, and Bell, 1992). The educational intervention selected was from Respecting Choices®, an ACP evidence-based program that had received national recognition for increasing community awareness of AD and was used among racial groups. Additionally, a post-survey evaluating the effectiveness of the education session, required as part of Respecting Choices®, was used. The project site was changed from the long-term care facility to three faith-based organizations due to the evidence showing churches were viewed as a non-threatening environment. My clinical question was changed to what is the impact of an AD education intervention within faith-based organizations among AA participants? I was also interested in the readiness level to completing AD per- and post-educational sessions.

The main objectives of the project were to provide an education intervention to AAs participants in the faith-based community, to assess participants' readiness level to enact an AD by increasing their knowledge of EOL care and offering support for completion of the proper documentation, administered a post evaluation survey to assess the effectiveness of the education sessions, and lastly, to see the impact of an AD education intervention within faith-based organizations among AA participants.

Description of Problem/Target Population

Advance directive utilization was found to be low nationally (Koss and Baker, 2017; IOM, 2015). However, when examining the various factors, race was noted to impact AD completion rates. Particularly, AAs' completion rates were found lower compared to whites (Ko and Lee, 2014; Koss and Baker, 2017; Portanova, *et al.,* 2017; Rao *et al.,* 2014). One of the top reasons for AAs decreased utilization of AD is the lack of awareness (Rao *et al.,* 2014). Consequently, this project provided an education session aimed at increasing AAs knowledge and awareness of AD an ultimately increase completion rates. The target population were AAs participants aged 21 or older within three faith-based organizations.

Project Interventions

The Transtheoretical Model (TTM) of behavior change was used to guide this project (Prochaska, 2008). The TTM uses five stages to assess individual's readiness and willingness to make behavior changes (Prochaska, 2008). The five stages of change are precontemplation, contemplation, preparation, action, and maintenance (Prochaska, 2008). Applying the TTM to the phenomenon of deciding to complete an AD provided a better understanding of an individual's decision-making process regarding AD and helps to identify a reference point for their readiness for change. This model provides a framework to help assess individual's readiness for AD completion. A customized RR based upon TTM was used to assess participant's self-reported readiness levels about completing an AD before and after attending an education session.

This project included an education intervention by the project leader during which AD were discussed using handouts written and provided by Respecting Choices® and a PowerPoint presentation. In preparation, the project leader received a coaching session regarding the PowerPoint presentation by the Respecting Choices® educator. A readiness ruler (RR) was prepared to assess the participants' self-perceived readiness to complete AD pre-and post-education, as well as to document participants self-reported readiness level to complete AD. An anonymous post-evaluation survey, required by Respecting Choices®, was administered after the education session. The post-survey asked participants to provide feedback about the education session. Handouts were provided to participants, including an AD information sheet, AD forms, and a listing of the various workshops in Charlotte, NC about AD education or assistance with completing the formal paperwork. The total time for the education intervention, RR administration pre-and post-education, and an anonymous post-evaluation survey took approximately 90 minutes to complete at each of the three venues. The project was implemented in three faith-based organizations in Charlotte, NC. The duration of the project spanned over a four-month period with potential make-up dates pre-selected in the event of bad weather. The recruitment

process consisted of announcements, via a flyer, along with an information sheet. Participants' attendance implied consent. The project leader
collaborated with other certified ACP facilitators who assisted to provide one-on-one discussions with participants interested in completing
AD. Notaries were available for those interested in completing AD on
site. To facilitate ongoing conversations within the community, leaders
within the faith-based organizations were provided information to attend a future AD workshop to help guide individuals in completing AD.

Data Collection, Measurement Tools, Analysis

The three educational sessions were conducted over a timespan of
four months. Data was collected from participants by the project leader.
A data collection tool was created in Microsoft Excel© which was used
to document participants' responses to the RR and post-evaluation survey. A sealed box was used by participants to return the completed RR
and post-surveys. Data analysis included the tabulation of each response
from the RR and post-survey completed by the participants. Descriptive statistics, frequencies, percentages, means, and standard deviations
were calculated using the data. Calculations of the data were recorded
as site-specific, allowing comparisons of data, as well as aggregates of
all responses, using SPSS version 25 software.

The project had a total of 74 participants ($n = 74$) with 58 participants ($n = 58$) completing the post-evaluation survey and the pre-and
post-RR. Aggregate data indicated a change in participants readiness
to complete AD. The post-evaluation survey indicated that the use of
Respecting Choices®, an evidence-based education program to raise
participants' awareness of AD, was beneficial in communicating with
persons voluntarily attending one of three education sessions at the
faith-based organizations.

Overall, the goal of increasing participants' knowledge related to
AD was met, with 91.4% ($n = 53$) indicating that they strongly agreed
that the ACP education sessions were useful and would help them to
plan for their future healthcare choices. Thirty-four participants (68%)
self-selected, "I will write down my medical choices using an advance
directive" after completing the education session. However, the AD
completion rates were found to be low with only four of the 50 participants (8%) completing an AD onsite. After the education session,
many of the participants shared their desire to complete an AD. But as
highlighted during the presentation, their prioritized need to identify a

health care agent stymied their ability to complete the AD at that time. This was an important point provided during the session. Therefore, although 68% of the participants self-reported their readiness to complete an AD, they were not prepared to do without more preparation of sharing their wishes with their loved ones or and established health agent.

CONCLUSIONS

Advance directive (AD) remains a national topic of discussion due to poor utilization since the passing of PSDA in 1990. African Americans (AAs) were found to have lower AD completion rates compared to whites. The absence of AD utilization is associated with prolonged hospitalization and increased economic burden for both the patient and the healthcare system at the EOL. After completing a thorough literature review on AD barriers, benefits, and educational intervention effects on completion rates, it was determined to use Respecting Choices® to increase AD awareness and completion rates among the AA population.

This evidence-based project provided AD education sessions to participants in three faith-based organizations in Charlotte, North Carolina. Participants completed RR to self-assess readiness to complete an AD pre-and post-education session and a post-survey. Aggregate data indicated a change in participants readiness to complete AD. Post-evaluation survey results showed the use of the Respecting Choices® evidence-based program was successful in increasing participants awareness of AD. This project has the potential to increase AD awareness and improve completion rates.

SCHOLARLY DISSEMINATION

Dissemination of project findings is a way to diffuse information to other professionals to help improve outcomes and the discovery of new ideas. It is important that these findings are shared for multiple reasons such as to provide baseline data, to highlight potentials gaps in care or to improve outcomes. For this project, the dissemination plans included presenting to the supporting organization, "Your Care, Your Choice" to share findings for future advance directives community project. I also presented findings through a poster and podium presentation at the College of Nursing at East Carolina University. I submitted an abstract and was selected as a podium speaker at the Doctor of Nursing Practice Education Symposium by North Carolina Nurses Association. Additionally, the findings from this project were used as data to apply for a grant to provide AD education in an underserved community to engage in ACP discussion. The grant was awarded, to offer AD education sessions within the AA community in Charlotte, North Carolina. The education intervention consisted of a game called "Hello" that was developed by the Philadelphia-based company Common Practice and has been found to promote meaningful EOL discussions among participants. The goal of this initiative was to increase AD conversations among AA participants. I was asked to assist the project leader, which provided another opportunity to disseminate project findings. Dissemination of findings can be beneficial for future project development and to improve health outcomes for the vulnerable population.

REFERENCES

Belisomo, R. (2017). Reversing racial inequities at the end of life: A call for health systems to create culturally competent advance care planning programs within African American communities. *Journal of Racial and Ethnic Health Disparities*, 1–8. http://dx.doi.org/10.1007/s40615-017-0360-2

Bonner, G. J., Wang, E., Wilkie, D. J., Ferrans, C. E., Dancy, B., & Watkins, W. (2014). Advance care treatment plan (ACT-plan) for African American family caregivers: A pilot study. *Dementia, 13*(1), 79–95. http://dx.doi.org/doi:10.1177/1471301212449408

Brinkman-Stoppelenburg, A., Rietjens, J. A. and Van, D. H. (2014). The effects of advance care planning on the end of life care: A systematic review. *Palliative Medicine, 28*(8), 1000–1025. http://dx.doi.org/10.1177/0269216314526272

Bullock, K. (2006). Promoting advance directives among African Americans: A faith-based model. *Journal of Palliative Medicine, 9*(1), 183–195. http://dx.doi.org/doi:10.1089/jpm.2006.9.183

Detering, K., Silveira, M., Arnold, R. and Savarese, D. (2016). Advance care planning and advance directives. *UpToDate*. Retrieved from http://www.uptodate.com/contents/advance-care-planning-and-advance-directives

Emanuel, L. L. and Emanuel, E. J. (1989). The medical directive: A new comprehensive advance care document. *Jama, 261*(22), 3288–3293. http://dx.doi.org/10.1001/jama.1989.03420220102036

Hamayoshi, M. (2014). Effects of an education program to promote advance directive completion in local residents. *General Medicine, 15*(2), 91–99. http://dx.doi.org/10.14442/general.15.91

Hendricks Sloan, D., Peters, T., Johnson, K. S., Bowie, J. V., Ting, Y. and Aslakson, R. (2016). Church-based health promotion focused on advance care planning and end-of-life care at black Baptist churches: A cross-sectional survey. *Journal of Palliative Medicine, 19*(2), 190-194. http://dx.doi.org/doi:10.1089/jpm.2015.0319

Hinderer, K. and Lee, L. C. (2014). Assessing a nurse-led advance directive and advance care planning seminar. *Applied Nursing Research, 27*(1), 84-86. http://dx.doi. org/doi:10.1016/j.apnr.2013.10.004

Huang, C. S., Crowther, M., Allen, R. S., DeCoster, J., Kim, G., Azuero, C., Kvale, E. (2016). A pilot feasibility intervention to increase advance care planning among African Americans in the deep south. *Journal of Palliative Medicine, 19*(2), 164–173. http://dx.doi.org/10.1089/jpm.2015.0334

Institute of Medicine [IOM] (2015). *Dying in America: Improving quality and honoring individual preferences near the end of life.* Washington, DC: The National Academics Press.

Johnson, J., Hayden, T., True, J., Simkin, D., Colbert, L., Thompson, B., Martin, L. (2016). The impact of faith beliefs on perceptions of end-of-life care and decision-making among African American church members. *Journal of Palliative Medicine, 19*(2), 143–148. http://dx.doi.org/doi:10.1089/jpm.2015.0238

Klingler, C., In der Schmitten, J. and Marckman, G. (2016). Does facilitated advance care planning reduce the costs of care near the end of life? Systematic review and ethical considerations. *Palliative Medicine, 30*(5), 423–433. http://dx.doi.org/ doi:10.1177/0269216315601346

Ko, E. and Lee, J. (2014). Completion of advance directives among low-income older adults does race/ethnicity matter? *American Journal of Hospice & Palliative Medicine, 31*(3), 247–253. http://dx.doi.org/10.1177/1049909113486170

Koss, C. S. (2017). Does religiosity account for lower rates of advance care planning by older African Americans? *The Journals of Gerontology: Series B*, 1–9. http://dx.doi. org/doi:10.1093/geronb/gbw155

Koss, C. S. and Baker, T. A. (2017). Race differences in advance directive completion: The narrowing gap between white and African American older adults. *Journal of Aging and Health, 29*(2), 324–342. http://dx.doi.org/10.1177/0898264316635568

Ladd, S. C. (2014). Systematic review of research literature on African Americans' end-of-life healthcare preferences. *Journal of African American Studies, 18*(4), 373–397. http://dx.doi.org/doi:10.1007/s12111-013-9276-z

Litzelman, D. K., Inui, T. S., Griffin, W. J., Perkins, A., Cottingham, A. H., Schmitt-Wendholt, K. M. and Ivy, S. S. (2017). Impact of community health workers on elderly patients' advance care planning and health care utilization: Moving the dial. Medical Care, 55(4), 319–326. http://dx.doi.org/10.1097/MLR.0000000000000675

MacKenzie, M. A., Smith-Howell, E., Bomba, P. A. and Meghani, S. H. (2017). Respecting choices and related models of advance care planning: A systematic review of published evidence. *American Journal of Hospice & Palliative Medicine*, 1–11. https://doi.org/10.1177/1049909117745789

Markham, S. A., Levi, B. H., Green, M. J. and Schubart, J. R. (2015). Use of a computer program for advance care planning with Africans American participants. *Journal of the National Medical Association, 107*(1), 26-32. http://dx.doi.org/doi:10.1016/ S0027-9684(15)30006-7

National Library of Medicine (2016). Advanced directives. Retrieved January 21, 2017, from https://medlineplus.gov/advancedirectives.html

Pecanac, K. E., Repenshek, M. F., Tennenbaum, D. and Hammes, B. (2014). Respecting choices® and advance directives in a diverse community. *Journal of Palliative Medicine, 17*(), 282–287. http://dx.doi.org/10.1089/jpm.2013.0047

Portanova, J., Ailshire, J., Perez, C., Rahman, A. and Enguidanos, S. (2017). Ethnic differences in advance directive completion and care preferences: What has changed in a decade? *Journal of the American Geriatrics Society, 65*(6), 1352–1357. http://dx.doi.org/doi:10.1111/jgs.14800

Prochaska, J. (2008). Decision-making in the transtheoretical model of behavior change. *Medical Decision-making, 28*(), 845–849. http://dx.doi.org/10

Ramsey, C. (2013). Young adult African Americans family matters' perceptions, knowledge, attitudes, and utilization toward advance directives. The ABNF Journal: Official Journal of the Association of Black Nursing Faculty in Higher Education, Inc, 24(2), 51–59.

Rao, J. K., Anderson, L. A., Lin, F. C. and Laux, J. (2014). Completion of advance directives among U.S. consumers. American Journal of Preventive Medicine, 46(1), 65–70. http://dx.doi.org/doi: 10.1016/j.amepre.2013.09.008.

Rhodes, R. L., Batchelor, K., Lee, S. C. and Halm, E. A. (2015). Barriers to end-of-life care for African Americans from the providers' perspective: Opportunity for intervention development. *American Journal of Hospice and Palliative Medicine, 32*(2), 137–143. http://dx.doi.org/doi:10.1177/1049909113507127

Rocque, G. B., Dionne-Odom, J. N., Sylvia Huang, C., Niranjan, S. J., Williams, C. P., Jackson, B. and Kvale, E. A. (2017). Implementation and impact of patient lay navigator-led advance care planning conversations. *Journal of Pain and Symptom Management, 53*(4), 682–692. http://dx.doi.org/10.1016/j.jpainsymman.2016.11.012

Rollnick, S., Heather, N. and Bell, A. (1992). Negotiating behaviour change in medical settings: The development of brief motivational interviewing. *Journal of Mental Health, 1*(1), 25–37. Retrieved from https://phe512.files.wordpress.com/2011/03/04-rollnick.pdf

Rowland, M. L. and Isaac-Savage, E. P. (2014). The black church: Promoting health, fighting disparities. *New Directions for Adult and Continuing Education, 142*, 15–24. http://dx.doi.org/doi:10.1002/ace.20091

Sanders, J. J., Robinson, M. T. and Block, S. D. (2016). Factors impacting advance care planning among African Americans: Results of a systematic integrated review. *Journal of Palliative Medicine, 19*, 202–227. http://dx.doi.org/doi:10.1089/jpm.2015.0325

Splendore, E. and Grant, C. (2017). A nurse practitioner-led community workshop: Increasing adult participation in advance care planning. *Journal of the American Association of Nurse Practitioners*, 1–8. http://dx.doi.org/doi:10.1002/2327-6924.12467

Wholihan, D. J. and Pace, J. C. (2012). Community discussions: A vision for cutting the costs of end-of-life care. *Nursing Economics, 30*(3), 170–176. Retrieved from http://go.galegroup.com.jproxy.lib.ecu.edu/ps/i.do?p=HRCA&u=gree96177&id=GALE|A291496702&v=2.1&it=r&sid=summon

Exploring the Effectiveness of Sepsis Protocol in the Emergency Department: A Quality Improvement Project

JAYANTHI HENRY, DNP, MSNCH, MSNIPC, GNED, RN-BC, CIC

INTRODUCTION

Sepsis is a worldwide problem. According to Dellinger *et al.* (2013), as per Surviving Sepsis Campaign, a critical component of reducing the death rate and preventing multiple organ failures is through routine screening, which enables early identification, diagnosis, and protocol implementation. According to Schetter in 2013, empowering nurses with decision-making capacity by providing nurse-driven protocols, in guiding nurses to take decisions on their own, recognize the situations in which the protocols are used for certain conditions. Scatter, the senior consultant at Joint Commission Resources, further stated in 2013 that nurse-driven protocols must be developed and implemented as recommended by the national evidence-based guidelines. The protocol needs to be formulated and reviewed by the medical board, nursing leadership and is by any state of federal laws or regulations such as state boards of nursing, pharmacy, and medicine.

PROBLEM STATEMENT

As a Doctor of Nursing Practice (DNP) student, I identified the goal of exploring the sepsis protocol in one of the acute care hospital emergency department (ED) and to recommend measures to improve future outcomes. This posed many challenges such as identifying the key issues, opportunities for improvement, and concerns of the registered nurses in the ED and the ED physicians.

Patients with sepsis develop multiple complications, thereby requir-

163

ing a longer stay at the hospital. According to the Center for Disease Control, the patients hospitalized due to sepsis-related problems were 727,000 in 2010, and this figure was twice the number reported ten years earlier (Michael *et al.,* 2013). Referable to the disabling nature of sepsis, prompt identification followed by rapid response is important in preventing further effects of the shape. To better the outcomes of hospitalization while reducing the incidence of deaths associated with sepsis, it is important that nurses follow the sepsis protocol. The recommended sepsis protocol is 4-hour and 6-hour Bundles. Health care facilities that have gone through these elements of care have seen significant improvement in the sepsis outcome (Tromp *et al.,* 2011). A nurse-driven sepsis protocol is dependent on the power of nurses to spot early signs of sepsis in a patient so that they can initiate life-saving interventions.

According to the Joint Commission Center for Transforming Healthcare (2016), sepsis is the primary cause of death in patients admitted to the hospital and, sepsis has a mortality rate of 30 to 50 percent. Every year, 740,000 Americans are diagnosed with sepsis and of those, 210,000 die. Also, sepsis is the costliest disease to treat in the hospital; the approximate monetary value is $17 billion dollars per year. Early recognition and effective treatment of sepsis can decrease the death rate, improve patient outcomes, and reduce the length of stay in hospitals.

PURPOSE STATEMENT

According to Moser (2014), there are total failures at the starting time of recognition and implementing timely interventions in emergency departments. It was identified that patients with SIRS/sepsis were not handled according to the guidelines for one to six-hour time frames. Prompt recognition and treatment are essential in reducing the death rate related to sepsis. Moser (2014) implemented the educational program for nurses in emergency triage, and the findings revealed a change in retention of the educational program information. Still, sepsis is a direct cause of mortality worldwide, and continued education for nurses is critical. According to Chism (2013), the Doctor of Nursing Practice (DNP) graduates practicing in the clinical area set an environment to develop and utilize skills in evaluating, integrating, and establishing the evidence-based practice. According to Conner (2014), the purpose of quality improvement is to use systematic, data-guided approach to improving processes or outcomes.

As per the American Association of Colleges of Nursing (AACN) in 2016, it is critical to expanding collaborative opportunities with healthcare, higher education, and other stakeholders to improve health and enhance quality outcomes. This DNP student as a leader wanted to collaborate with the sepsis committee in the hospital in facilitating the sepsis protocol in the emergency department and orient the nurses to the sepsis protocol. Also, the DNP student wanted to guide the nursing practice in the emergency department to promote positive outcomes. This DNP student tried to identify the barriers in using sepsis protocol and recommend measures to improve the sepsis outcomes.

TOPIC AND PROJECT QUESTION

The topic is "Exploring the Effectiveness of Sepsis Protocol in the Emergency Department: A Quality Improvement Project."

In this project, the PICOT question is: Does the exploration of the sepsis protocol in the emergency department identify the barriers in six to eight weeks to recommend measures to improve the future outcomes?

The population (P) of interest is adult patients treated for sepsis in an acute care hospital emergency department. The adult is defined as 18 years of age or older. The intervention (I) is the administration of the survey questionnaire to the health care workers in the ED. The outcome (O) is to identify the barriers in using sepsis protocol in the emergency department (ED) and recommend measures to improve sepsis outcomes. The time (T) is from six to eight weeks. The comparison (C) is the present situation.

PROJECT OBJECTIVES

- To identify the sepsis protocol used in the ED
- To explore the outcomes of the sepsis protocol utilized in the ED
- To identify the barriers in using the sepsis protocol in the ED
- To recommend measures to improve sepsis bundle outcomes in the ED

AACN ESSENTIALS IN NURSING PRACTICE

According to American Association of Colleges of Nursing (2006), doctoral education in nursing is designed to prepare nurses for the highest level of leadership in practice and scientific inquiry. The DNP is a degree designed specifically to prepare individuals for specialized nursing practice, and *The Essentials of Doctoral Education for Advanced Nursing* (AACN) *Practice* articulates the competencies for all nurses practicing at this level. This quality improvement project is based on the following AACN essentials. This DNP student focus is utilizing the ANCC essentials in the project.

Essential I: Scientific Underpinnings for Practice

The scientific foundations of this education reflect the complexity of practice at the doctoral level and the rich heritage that is the conceptual foundation of nursing. The need for positive outcomes related to sepsis protocol is identified in the facility, the nursing action and processes will be developed to bring out positive changes in the health condition of the patients. The DNP student developed the new practice approaches based on nursing theories and from other disciplines.

Essentials II: Organizational and Systems Leadership for Quality Improvement and Systems Thinking

Organizational and systems leadership are critical for DNP graduates to improve patient and healthcare outcomes. Through this quality improvement practice, the DNP student assessed the practice, ongoing improvement of health outcomes, and ensuring patient safety by reducing the sepsis mortality in the practice area. The DNP student used the advanced communication skills with the sepsis committee, course instructor, academic mentor, project mentor, content expert, and stakeholders lead quality improvement, and patient safety initiatives related to sepsis outcomes in the practice area.

Essential IV: Information Systems/Technology and Patient Care Technology for the Improvement and Transformation of Health Care

DNP graduates are distinguished by their abilities to use information systems/technology for supporting and improving patient care and healthcare or academic settings. This DNP student coordinated with the facility informatics, and analyst using the information system to collect data from the hospital data analyst the pre and post protocol findings and recommended appropriate measures to improve sepsis bundle outcomes.

Essential VIII: Advanced Nursing Practice

The DNP graduate is prepared to practice in an area of specialization within the larger domain of nursing. This DNP student conduct a comprehensive and systematic assessment of health and illness related to sepsis and design, implement, and evaluated the outcome measures based on nursing science. This DNP student identified the importance of guidance, mentoring, and supporting the other nurses to achieve excellence in nursing practice and use conceptual and analytical skills in evaluating the links among practice, organizational, population, fiscal, and policy issues related to sepsis.

APPLICATION OF SIX SIGMA MODEL TO DNP PROJECT

Application of the Six Sigma model in this quality improvement project will have a positive impact on outcomes. According to Conner (2014), the goal of quality improvement (QI) is to use a systematic, data-driven guidance to make positive changes in better outcomes. Principles and methods in QI have risen from organizational philosophies of total quality management and continuous quality improvement. While the idea of quality can be subjective, QI in healthcare mainly focuses on positive patient outcomes. So, the key is to define clearly the issues that need to be improved, identify how the outcome is measured and develop a plan for implementing an intervention and collecting data before and after the intervention. Quality improvement projects are site specific. This DNP student practice site is the acute care hospital ED.

In this DNP project defines refer to identifying the goals and stakeholders. The goal is to improve the sepsis outcome regarding the short length of stay, reducing the sepsis mortality and reducing the cost associated with sepsis complications. Also, to identify and improve the effectiveness of sepsis bundle elements and decrease septic shock and the severe sepsis mortality rate in an acute care facility ED. The stakeholders in this project are the quality management director, market director of clinical compliance, nurse educators, content expert, project mentor, physicians, nurses, laboratory, and pharmacy staff. In this project, measure refers to collecting the data on sepsis outcomes in the past and identifies the process in recognition and treatment of sepsis patients in the ED and identifies the change needed in practice.

In this DNP project, analyzes refer to the data analyzed from the sepsis outcome data collection and based on the deficiencies, plan for appropriate measures with the leadership and the interdisciplinary team to improve the practice. In this DNP project, improve refers to using the results to inform improvement, make changes, and put into practice the chosen measures of sepsis code algorithm, early recognition, and sepsis bundle alert in Cerner. In this DNP project, control refers to the on-going monitoring and improvement. Also, to measure the outcome by the physician notified within the given time of positive sepsis screen, the percentage of sepsis screens completed correct, and sepsis bundle elements completed within three hours. Based on the outcome, reevaluate the practice, and give recommendations to sustain the gains and improvements, and further plans to correct deficiencies in the future.

POPULATION OF INTEREST, SETTING, AND STAKEHOLDERS

In this project, the population of interest is adult patients 18 years and older who are identified in the ED with severe sepsis or septic shock. The setting is the ED at one of the Acute Care Hospitals in NV. The facility is the Joint Commission on Accreditation of Healthcare Organizations (JCAHO) accredited, 50 bedded emergency department. Staff within the ED includes full and part-time employees: 10 physicians, 4 nurse practitioners, 90 registered nurses, and 7 monitor technicians/ unit coordinators. According to Grove, Burn, and Gray (2013), the student should develop a plan for research participants, which involves identifying, assessing, and communicating with potential study participants who are a representative of the target population. Exclusion criteria include those who are identified as non-septic patients in the ED triage and children below 18 years. In this project, immediate stakeholders include ED physicians and ED registered nurses. Other stakeholders include the quality assurance director, Nevada clinical compliance officer, data analyst, project mentor, and the content expert. The DNP student established rapport with the stakeholders during sepsis committee meetings and communicated with the stakeholders every week through personal meetings and email. The hospital administration had given permission to this DNP student to utilize ED as a practice area to explore the effectiveness of the sepsis protocol.

RECRUITMENT METHODS

According to Grove, Burns, and Gray (2013), students should develop a plan for research participants, which involves identifying, assessing, and communicating with potential study participants who are a representative of the target population. Recruitment strategies differ, depending on the type of study, population, and setting. The Electronic Medical Record (EHR) was used by the data analyst to abstract sepsis protocol outcome data for all patients who visited the ED identified as having severe sepsis with septic shock from January 2016 to April 2016, and they are considered as "before—protocol group." During the month of May 2016, sepsis protocol was modified and implemented by the hospital sepsis team. The after-protocol group included patients who visited the ED with severe sepsis and septic shock from June 2016 to September 2016. For the survey portion of the project, the ED physicians and the ED nurses were approached to complete the survey and the convenient sampling method was used.

TOOLS/INSTRUMENTATION

According to Goldstein (2011), the Greater New York Hospital Association (GNYHA) and the United Health Fund (UHF) provided support for participants through monthly conference calls, data collection, and assistance with data-reporting. Also, they provide assistance through site visits with the other clinical experts. The focus of the sepsis collaborative is to foster a protocol-based approach to identifying and treating patients with sepsis. The survey instrument was used for the ED Physicians and the ED nurses, published originally by New York-Presbyterian Hospital, and adapted for the STOP Sepsis Collaborative by the Greater New York Hospital Association (GNYHA)/United Hospital Fund Quality Initiatives (GNYHA, 2015). The GNYHA and the United Hospital Fund (UHF) launched the STOP Sepsis Collaborative in 2015 to support hospitals' efforts to improve care and reduce mortality. It also was to implement standardized processes for the recognition and treatment of sepsis, and to enhance communication and patient flow between the emergency department and other areas of the hospital. Both the RN and MD versions of this instrument were utilized in the present project in the ED. The ED health care providers, such as ED physicians and the ED nurses, were requested to answer the short questionnaire and demographic data. The DNP student got permission to use the GYNHA tool from the vice president the regulatory and professional affairs, GYNHA.

DATA COLLECTION PROCEDURES

According to Grove, Burns, and Gray (2013), data collection is the precise, systematic gathering of information relevant to the research purpose or the specific objectives, questions, or hypotheses of a study. The data collected in quantitative studies are usually numerical. Patient data abstracted from medical records were de-identified (i.e., have all 18 protected health information identifiers removed) to protect the privacy and confidentiality of the patients involved in this study. The patient data included the sepsis bundle management outcomes from January 2016 to April 2016 related to severe sepsis with initial lactate management, broad spectrum antibiotic and blood cultures in three hours, and repeat lactate level measurement in six hours. Also, the septic shock data the sepsis resuscitation with colloid fluids, vital signs, bedside cardiovascular ultrasound, and leg raise and fluid challenge in six hours was compared after protocol implementation in May 2016 from June 2016 to September 2016. The data were entered in a password-protected spreadsheet (excel sheet) for eventual analysis. Survey data was transferred from the survey forms to a separate password-protected spreadsheet (excel sheet) for eventual analysis. The names of the participating practitioners were not recorded anywhere in the survey, although their discipline was noted.

According to Moran, Burson, and Conrad (2014), DNP projects can involve the collection of new data via surveys and interviews or evaluation of stored data from repositories such as electronic health records and national registries. The primary data collection methods used in quantitative studies and QI projects include self-report via survey or structured interviews, direct observation, and physiological measures (Polit and Beck, 2012, 335). It is important to select the data collection method that is suited for the DNP project goals. The data collection method should be feasible, practical, and amenable for use in the clinical setting or with the population of interest. According to Morath (2015), the Centers for Medicare and Medicaid Services (CMS) has notified hospitals participating in the inpatient quality reporting program that data collection of the severe sepsis and septic shock: Management Bundle measure will begin with discharges on or after October 2015. The measure was adopted for the fiscal year (FY) 2017 payment determination on the FY 2015 inpatient prospective payment system final rule.

DISCUSSION ON THE FINDINGS, RECOMMENDATIONS, AND CONCLUSION

Project Objective 1: To Identify the Sepsis Protocol used in the ED

The analysis findings are discussed related to the project objectives. The first objective of the project was to identify the sepsis protocol used in the ED. During the month of May 2016, the hospital sepsis task force created the ED sepsis bundle order set, the standard of work in the ED, and the ED sepsis alert management flow diagram. The process was discussed by the sepsis committee leadership during the ED huddles, and the ED nursing staff and physicians were educated about the process. According to Butcher (2016), each hospital has its own sepsis task force, and the processes used to carry out the work are determined at the department level within each facility. The use of the sepsis bundle has reduced the death toll from the condition, and the CMS is trying to standardize care for the huge population of patients who acquire it. According to Gauer (2013), surveys of medical centers instituting early goal directed therapy sepsis programs demonstrated a 45% relative risk reduction in mortality rates. Prospective studies show that the use of standardized hospital order sets hastens fluid resuscitation and appropriate antibiotic therapy, resulting in lower 28-day mortality rates.

Project Objective 2: To Explore the Effectiveness of the Sepsis Protocol Utilized in the ED.

Lactate Management

The second objective was to explore the effectiveness of the sepsis protocol utilized in the ED. The raw data were collected from the hospital data analyst before the implementation of sepsis protocol in the ED and after the implementations of the sepsis protocol in the ED by the hospital sepsis committee. The Severe sepsis measures and post protocol findings reveals that none of the implementation measures significantly changed in either direction after protocol implementation. The ED nurses reported the lactate levels are only sometimes ordered with the blood cultures and 35% of them reported that the lactate levels are always ordered with the blood culture levels, and about eight percentage of the nurses reported that the lactate is hardly ever ordered. The physicians (57%) of them stated they order the lactate levels always with the blood culture level and 42.9% of them order the lactate with the blood culture sometimes. Only 51% of the nurses were aware of the correct tube used for sending the blood for lactate level to the lab. The minimum value of lactate of concern for about 59% of the nurses were above two, and 27% of the nurses responded as the lactate level of four, and 14% of the nurses were concerned about the lactate level of 2.5.

The physicians' response showed about 57.1% of them were concerned about the lactate level of more than two, 28.6% of them were concerned about the lactate level of four, and 14.3% of them were concerned about the lactate level of 2.5. According to Rhee *et al.* (2015), serum lactate monitoring is central to risk stratification and management of sepsis and is now part of a potentially quality measure. The 11-year trends in lactate testing and predictors of failure to measure lactates in patients with severe sepsis are examined using retrospective cohort study. The two U.S. academic hospitals from 2003 to 2013 was selected for the study. Among hospitalizations with blood culture orders, rates of lactate measurement increased from 11% in 2003 to 48% in 2014 $(p < 0.001$ for linear trend). Rates of repeat lactate measurement within 6 hours after lactate levels more than or equal to 4.0 mmol/L increased from 23% to 69% $(p < 0.001)$. Patients were progressively less likely to be on vasopressors at the time of first lactate measurement (49% in 2003 vs 21% in 2013, $p < 0.001$). Despite these trends, lactates that were measured at the time of suspected sepsis in only 65% of patients with severe sepsis were significant predictors of failure to measure lactate (adjusted ORs 7.56, 95% CI: 6.31–9.06 and 2.08, 95% CI: 1.76–2.24, respectively). Elevated serum lactate levels have long been known to identify patients with severe hypoperfusion and predict death. Measuring lactate levels have been shown to stratify patients with suspected sepsis, to prompt, aggressive early treatment, and to help monitor the impact of therapy.

Implementation of bedside lactate measurement in the emergency department has also been associated with reduced time to administration of intravenous fluids with suspected sepsis and decreased rates of ICU admission and mortality. For these reasons, lactate testing in all patients with suspected severe sepsis has become increasingly emphasized and is now a key component and is now a key component of the Surviving Sepsis Campaign (SSC) Guidelines. In the most recent version of the guidelines, lactate measurement is a core component of the 3-hour bundle, while repeat lactate measurement in patients with hyperlactatemia is part of the 6-hour bundle. Onset of suspected sepsis while hospitalized and admission to a nonmedical service, were risk factors for failure to draw a lactate. The National Quality Forum's adoption of the SSC guidelines means that lactate measurement in severe sepsis could be included in future quality measures for public reporting and payment.

Broad Spectrum Antibiotic Management

The pre- and post- protocol findings in the ED did not show significant change in the antibiotic administration. The five percentage of nurses in the ED responded the delay in treating the severe sepsis is due to profiling of Zosyn by the pharmacy. Also, nine percentage of the physicians preferred the pharmacist to attend code sepsis to assist with the antibiotics of choice. Most of the physicians (71.4%) were confident in choosing the right antibiotic for the patient and 28.6% of the physicians were not confident in selecting the appropriate antibiotics in treating the sepsis patients.

According to Goer (2016), early appropriate antibiotic therapy is associated with improved clinical outcomes. Consensus guidelines recommend antibiotic therapy within one hour of suspected sepsis. In septic shock, the initiation of antibiotic therapy within one hour increases survival and with each hour antibiotic therapy is delayed, survival decreases by about 8%. Empiric antibiotic therapy should be based on the most likely source, clinical context (community-vs-hospital-acquired sepsis), recent antibiotic use, and local resistance patterns. Empiric antibiotic therapy should be narrowed or redirected when the causative organism has been identified, thereby reducing the risk of resistance or superinfection.

The Septic Shock Measures

The septic shock measures pre- and post- protocol, finds that most of the measures did not demonstrate a significant change after protocol implementation. The only measure of resuscitation with crystalloid fluids not received in three hours increased from 54% to 72% after the implementation of the protocol indicates that the protocol may have resulted in either less use of fluids or in greater delays in providing the fluids. According to Gauer (2013), the highest priority in early sepsis is establishing vascular access and initiating fluid resuscitation. Hypovolemia, myocardial depression, and hypoperfusion result in hypotension, which is the most important event leading to increased morbidity and mortality in patients with sepsis. Delaying fluid resuscitation can worsen fluid resuscitation and worsen tissue hypoxia, leading to multiple organ dysfunction. The average fluid resuscitation volume in two recognized sepsis trials was five liters in six hours and 6.3 liters in 12 hours. Response to fluid resuscitation and continued rates of administration beyond the first 12 hours should be successfully assessed by blood pressure response, tissue perfusion, and urine output. Optimal survival occurs with a positive fluid balance (i.e., intravenous fluid input minus urine output) of 3 to 4 liters at 12 hours. There were different responses from the ED nurses related to the fluid replacement varying from two liters to five liters for the sepsis patients in the ED. The physicians' responses varied from the use of three liters to five liters for the severely septic patients in the ED during the first six hours. The sepsis mortality rate pre- and post-protocol, finds a decrease from 34% to 28%, but the difference was not found to be statistically significant.

Vasopressor Therapy

The ED nurses responded that the vasopressors are given often (54%) and Levofed (54%) is given through the central line. Also, 46% of the ED nurses responded that the Dopamine was hardly ever used. The physicians' 71.4% of them responded that they hardly use Dopamine and 43% of them use other vasopressors. The ED nurses about 51% of them were familiar with the SIRS criteria and 49% of them were somewhat aware of it. According to Kleinpell, Aitken, and Christa (2013), vasopressor therapy should be initiated to target a mean arterial pressure (MAP) of 65 mm Hg. Vasopressor therapy is often required in severe sepsis/septic shock to maintain perfusion in the face of life-threatening hypotension, even when hypovolemia has not yet been resolved. Below a threshold MAP, autoregulation in critical vascular beds can be lost, and perfusion can become linearly dependent on pressure. Norepinephrine is recommended as the first-choice vasopressor. Epinephrine is recommended when an additional agent is needed to maintain adequate blood pressure. Vasopressin up to 0.03 units per minute can be added to norepinephrine with the intent of increasing MAP to the target level or decreasing the dosage of norepinephrine. Low-dose vasopressin is not recommended as the single initial vasopressor for treatment of sepsis-induced hypotension and vasopressin doses higher than 0.03 to 0.04 units per minute should be reserved for salvage therapy (failure to achieve adequate MAP with other vasopressor agents). Dopamine should be used as an alternative vasopressor agent to norepinephrine only in highly selected patients (e.g., patients with low risk of tachy-arrythmias and absolute or relative bradycardia). Phenylephrine is not recommended in the treatment of sepsis shock except in circumstances where norepinephrine is associated with serious arrhythmias. The cardiac output is known to be high and blood pressure persistently low, as salvage therapy when combined inotropic/vasopressor drugs and low-dose vasopressin have failed to achieve the MAP target. Another guideline recommendation is that low-dose dopamine should not be used for renal protection. Additionally, the guidelines recommend that all patients requiring vasopressors have an arterial catheter placed as soon as practical if resources are available.

Vital Signs Review

The physicians' response related to the cause for delay in treating sepsis patient in the ED is lack of recognition of potential sepsis in triage (28.5%). The other barriers in the early identification of sepsis is report of abnormal vital signs by the support staff (54% of the nurses responded it as reported almost always, 35% of the nurses responded it is reported only sometimes, and 11% of them responded the abnormal vital signs are hardly reported. According to Kenzaka *et al.* (2012), a prospective observational study of 206 patients with sepsis was carried out to investigate the vital relationship between signs and Sequential Failure Assessment (SOFA) score in the emergency department of the Toyooka Public Hospital. The aim of this study was to assess a possible association between vital signs and the Sequential Failure Assessment (SOFA) score in patients with sepsis. The blood pressure, respiratory rate, body temperature, and heart rate were measured on arrival at the hospital and the SOFA score was also determined on the day of admission. Bivariate correlation analysis showed that all the vital signs were correlated with the SOFA score. Increased respiratory rate and the shock index were significantly correlated with disease severity with sepsis. Evaluation of these signs may therefore improve early identification of severely ill patients at triage, allowing more aggressive and timely interventions to improve the prognosis of these patients.

Bedside Cardiovascular Ultrasound

The ED physicians (57.1%) were somewhat competent in performing an IVC ultrasound and the other 42.9% were not at all competent in performing an IVC ultrasound. According to Seif *et al.* (2012), assessment of hemodynamic status in a shock state remains a challenging issue in Emergency Medicine and Critical Care. As the use of invasive hemodynamic monitoring declines at bedside—a focused ultrasound has become a valuable tool in the evaluation and management of patients in shock. Early recognition and appropriate treatment of shock have been shown to decrease mortality. Incorporation of a bedside ultrasound in patients with undifferentiated shock allows for rapid evaluation of reversible causes in patients and improves accurate diagnosis in undifferentiated hypotension.

Leg Raises and Fluid Challenge

The leg raises and fluid challenge not in six hours pre-protocol aggregate was (82%), and post-protocol aggregate was (76%). It did not demonstrate a significant change after protocol implementation. According to Dong *et al.* (2012), in critically ill patients with hypoperfusion, intravascular volume expansion (VE) is a cornerstone of hemodynamic therapy. Early resuscitation protocols, including fluid therapy, can be lifesaving early in the course of sepsis. However, VE may induce peripheral and pulmonary edema, and worsen microvascular perfusion and oxygen delivery in patients with right or left ventricular dysfunction. Passive leg raising (PLR) was supposed to transfer venous blood from the legs toward the intrathoracic compartment, increasing the intrathoracic blood volume and the cardiac preload. PLR is a reversible maneuver that mimics rapid VE by shifting venous blood from the lower limbs toward the intrathoracic compartment. The classic lower limb raising mimics a 300 ml VE. Thus, PLR increases the cardiac and increases SVI if the heart is preloaded dependent.

Project Objective 3: To Identify the Barriers in using the Sepsis Protocol in the ED

The third objective was to identify the barriers in using the sepsis protocol in the ED. The barriers related to the implementation of a protocolized approach for severe sepsis from the ED nurses include central line insertion (89%), the time required to carry out the orders (59%), access to protocol medications (59%), and measuring lactate (54%). The physicians' responses related to the significant barriers in the resuscitation of severe sepsis patients in the ED include lack of agreement with the protocol outlies with Early Goal Directed Therapy (EGDT) (35%), the nursing staff required to perform EGDT (20%), and the central line catheter insertion is 15%. The ED nurses responded to the causes for the delay in the treatment of severe sepsis. The contributors to the delay in treatment is the diagnosis of sepsis by the physicians (35%), lack of recognition of potential sepsis in triage (16%), and the other cases is knowledge deficit, lab delays, and delay in availability of ICU beds. The physicians' response related to the cause for delay in treating sepsis patients in the ED is lack of recognition of potential sepsis in triage (28.5%) and delay in diagnosis of sepsis by physicians (14.2%). The other causes given by the physicians are knowledge deficit regarding appropriate management, nursing delays, and lack of bed space in the ED. According to Falgout (2016), the potential barriers to success are knowledge deficit of sepsis, severe sepsis or septic shock, distinguishing the difference of each, delay in recognition or diagnosis, knowledge deficit of sepsis best practices, or guidelines, the lack of knowledge of sepsis initiative, communication failures, delay in early or appropriate treatment, threat of physician autonomy, improper or lack of use of sepsis screening tool, resources or resource utilization, lack of standardized policy and procedure for treatment, attitude, support of team members, assumed costs associated with unnecessary treatment or testing, failure to see sepsis as time critical, and time is life in treating sepsis.

Project Objective 4: To Recommend Measures to Improve Sepsis Bundle Outcomes

The fourth objective was to recommend measures to improve sepsis bundle outcomes in the ED. The ED nurses who participated in the survey wanted to be educated on early identification of sepsis and set protocol (100%). The other recommendation (65%) is to add vasopressors in the Omnicell, to add more staff in triage to identify sepsis earlier (57%), to improve collaboration between MD, RN and the pharmacist (51%), and to improve the RN and nursing aide shortages (43%). Also, the other recommendations are to focus on nurse driven sepsis protocol, to improve the bed availability in the ED for the possible sepsis patients, to place a standing order for nurses to improve the sepsis bundle outcomes, and to give the privilege to the nurses to call code sepsis in the triage to facilitate early treatment for the sepsis patients. The physicians' suggested to improve the ED space and keep more beds available for the patients with sepsis, to provide the accepted antibiotic regimen for the ED physicians to treat the patients with sepsis, to educate the ED consultants and the ED intensivists related to sepsis bundles, to educate the nurses regarding the completion of timely orders, and to update the protocols with current evidence-based process. The planned education program on sepsis will bring about changes in the practice.

CONCLUSION

It was identified that the sepsis/septic shock management protocol did not lead to improved patient outcomes as evidenced by the statistical findings. As patient outcomes are not affected by the protocol, it will be beneficial to improve the factors holding back the performance. Also, it is critical to provide educational opportunities regarding the protocol itself or its implementation, as well as providing a check as to the validity of the implementation measures and identifying any barriers to a full protocol implemented that may require remediation.

According to American Association of Colleges of Nursing (2006), the Doctor of Nursing Practice (DNP) Graduate utilizes the scientific knowledge to develop and evaluate the care delivery approaches that meet the current and future needs of the patient population. Based on the scientific findings of the sepsis project, the recommendations should be utilized to improve the quality of care. The recommendation is to improve the sepsis bundle outcomes in the ED in collaboration with the organizational leadership team that can be applied in a healthcare setting by the ED physicians and the ED nurses to promote their job satisfaction and in providing quality care for the patients.

To sum up, sepsis and associated septic shock are among the serious health complications and may be associated with undesirable social, clinical, and economic outcomes. It is the responsibility of scholar-practitioners to work with supportive organizations to steer the development of guidelines which are aimed at lowering sepsis-related mortality rates and in empowering nurses and practitioners taking care of sepsis patients, improving timely and accurate sepsis recognition, and promoting the use of appropriate treatment interventions. Finally, regular evaluations of sepsis protocols should be warranted to ensure improvements in the sepsis protocol designs and overall treatment outcomes. Promoting the team collaboration between nurses, physicians, pharmacist, lab, and other personnel in the ED, will promote early identification and in treating the patient promptly within the time frame.

REFERENCES

American Association of Colleges of Nursing. (2006). The essentials of doctoral education for advanced nursing practice. Retrieved from http://www.aacn.nche.edu/dnp/Essentials.pdf

American Association of Colleges of Nursing. (2016). Vision and mission. Retrieved from http://www.aacn.nche.edu/about-aacn/vision-mission

Batchen, L. P. (2016). A policy exemplar: Policy revision regarding item development and testing, delivery methods for first and second semester BSN students. In Bemker, M. & Schreiner, B. (Eds.), The DNP Degree & Capstone Project: A Practical Guide (pp. 157–160). Lancaster, PA: DEStech Publications, Inc.

Centers for Medicare & Medicaid Services. (2013). Quality improvement projects. Retrieved from https://www.cms.gov/Medicare/Health-Plans/Medicare-Advantage-Quality-Improvement-Program/6QIP.html

Chism, L. A. (2013). *The Doctor of Nursing Practice: A Guidebook for Role Development and Professional Issues* (2nd ed.). Burlington, MA: Jones & Bartlett.

Conner, T. B. (2014). Differentiating research, evidence-based practice, and quality improvement: Understanding QI. *American Nurse Today. 9*(6). Retrieved from http://www.americannursetoday.com/differentiating-research-evidence-based-practice-and-quality-improvement/

Dellinger, R., Levy, M., Rhodes, A., Annane, D., Gerlach, H., Opal, S., . . . Moreno, R. (2013). Surviving sepsis campaign: International Guidelines for management of severe sepsis and septic shock, 2012. *Intensive Care Medicine, 39*, 165–228. doi:10.1007/s00134-012-2769-8

Dong, Z, Fang, Q, Zheng, X. and Shi, H. (2012). Passive leg raising as an indicator of fluid responsiveness in patients with severe sepsis. *World Journal of Emergency Medicine.* 3930. pp. 191–196. doi: 10.5847/wjem.j.jssn.1920-8642.2012.03.006

Falgout, N. (2016). The role of the UCLA sepsis champions & the sepsis toolbox. Retrieved from https://sepsis.mednet.ucla.edu/files/view/sepsisday/7.pdf

Gauer, L. R. (2013). Early recognition and management of sepsis in adults: The first six hours. *American family physicians. 88*(1). PP. 44–53.

Goldstein, Z. W. (2011). Quality collaborative. A partnership sponsored by the Greater New York Hospital Association and the United Hospital Fund. Retrieved from Quality_Colloborative_Winter_2010_2011.pdf.

Grove, K., S, Burns, N and Gray, R. J. (2013). *The Practice of Nursing Research. Appraisal, Synthesis, and Generation of Evidence* (7th ed.). St. Louis: Elsevier.

Joint Commission Center for Transforming Healthcare. (2016). Reducing sepsis mortality. Retrieved from http://www.centerfortransforminghealthcare.org/projects/detail.aspx?project=8

Kenzaka, T, okayama, M, Kuroki, S, Fuki, M, Yahata, S, Hayashi, H, Kitao, A, Sugiyama, D, Seif, D, Perera, P, Mailhot, T, Riley, D. and Mandavia, D. (2012). Bedside ultrasound in resuscitation and rapid ultrasound in shock protocol. Critical care research and practice. doi: 10.1155/2012/503254

Kleinpell, R, Aitken, L and Schorr, A. C. (2013). Implications of the new international sepsis guidelines for nursing care. *American Journal of Critical Care, 22*(3). pp. 212–222. doi: 10.4037/ajcc2013158

Moser, H. (2014). Early recognition and rapid intervention of sepsis: Implementation of a focused educational initiative emphasizing early goal-directed therapy in the emergency department. *Journal of Nursing Education and Practice, 4*(6). doi: 10.5430/jnep.v4n6p23

Moran, K., Burson, R. and Conrad, D. (2014). *The Doctor of Nursing Practice Scholarly Project: A Framework for Success.* Burlington, MA: Jones & Bartlett Learning.

Morath, J. (2015). CMS announces data collection for sepsis bundle measure: measure specifications will be posted to quality April 1. Retrieved from http://www.calhospital.org/cha-news-article/cms-announces-data-collection-sepsis-bundle-. . .

Polit, D. and Beck. C. (2012). *Nursing Research: Generating and Assessing Evidence for Nursing Practice* (9th ed.). Philadelphia, PA: Lippincott Williams & Wilkins.

Rhee, C, Murphy, V., M, Li, L, Platt, R and Klompas, M. (2015). Lactate testing in suspected sepsis: trends and predictors of failure to measure levels. *Critical Care Medicine, 43*(8). pp. 1669–1676. doi: 10.1097/CCM.0000000000001087.

Schetter, J. (2013). Spotlight on Success: Implementing Nurse-Driven protocols to reduce CAUTIs. *Joint Commission Resources. 11*(4). Retrieved from http://www.tnpatientsafety.com/Portals/0/Meetings/Regional%20Meetings/August%202014/joint-commission-resources.pdf

Surviving Sepsis Campaign. (2012). Obtain blood cultures prior to administration of antibiotics. Retrieved from http://www.survivingsepsis.org/SiteCollectionDocuments/Bundle-3-Hour-Sepsis-Step2-Blood-Cultures.pdf

The Advisory Board Company. (2016). Achieving Top-of-License Nursing Practice. Best practices for elevating the impact of the frontline nurse. Retrieved from https://www.advisory.com/sitecore%20modules/web/international/research/global-centre-for-nursing-executives/studies/2013/achieving-top-of-license-nursing-practice/expand-nurse-clinical-decision-making/nurse-driven-protocol-starter-list/starter-list-of-protocols

The Greater New York Hospital Association. (2016). STOP Sepsis Collaborative. Retrieved from http://www.gnyha.org/whatwedo/quality-patient-safety/building-infrastructure-for-clinical-advancement/stop-sepsis-collaborative

Tromp, M., Tjan, D. H. T., Zanten, A. R. H., Gielen-Wijffels, S. E. M., Goekoop, G. J. D., Boogaard, and M., Pickkers, P. (2011). The effects of implementation of the surviving sepsis campaign in the Netherlands. *Netherland Journal of Medicine, 69*, 292–298.

CHAPTER 9

If I Greet You at The Front Door, Will You Leave Sooner?

THERESA KATERINA HALEY, DNP, MSN-ED, MSN-FNP, NP-C

INTRODUCTION TO THE PRACTICE GAP

Emergency medicine providers know everyday patients in waiting rooms face increased mortality because they have not seen a healthcare provider (HP). In 2015, over 141 million individuals visited emergency departments (EDs) across the United States, which equates to 45.1 per 100 individuals (CDC, 2018). Nationally, a patient waits approximately 22 minutes before they see a HP and spends a total of 166 minutes in the department before discharge (CDC, 2018). Common sense dictates the sooner a patient has been seen by a provider, the sooner at risk patients are identified and immediate treatment commences.

Implementation of value-based purchase programs is tied to hospital reimbursement, and most ED providers contracted to hospitals are feeling the pressure to achieve a turnaround time to discharge (TAT-D) of less than 150 minutes from the current average which is greater than 225 minutes (Morgan *et al.*, 2015). When patients arrive at the ED and see a crowded waiting room, they often leave without being seen. Not only are these patients not receiving care, placing their health and recovery at risk, but there is also a significant loss in revenue. Evidence demonstrates that every patient who leaves the ED without being seen represents a loss in revenue equivalent to $800 (Salway *et al.*, 2017). Patients who leave without being seen also represent lost admission charges further impacting hospital revenue.

The reality is that healthcare is a growth industry; hospitals are investing in expanding their EDs in response to rapidly increasing patient census. According to Wilson and Cutler (2014), patients admitted through the ED will exceed 24% and represent a profit margin to the

181

hospital of approximately 21%, with a projected profit growth of 11.7% by the year 2023.

The practice site where this scholarly project took place was in a 425-bed acute care facility with an ED that has 44 beds and a capability of expanding to 53 hall beds and treatment chairs. This ED admits 30 to 50 patients per day with 7% to 10% of these patients admitted to the intensive care unit. Prior to the practice change project, the door-to-provider (DTP) was greater than 90 minutes and the turnaround time to discharge (TAT-D) > 249 minutes. Additionally, important to the practice site was a 5.2% left without being seen (LWBS) rate that equated to a loss in revenue over $3 million and a projected lost admission revenue exceeding $39.5 million dollars.

DEFINITION OF TERMS

Recognizing the technicality of this DNP project it is important for the reader who has not had exposure to the emergency medicine specialty to understand the various terms that were incorporated into this project.

Healthcare Provider (HP)

The term healthcare provider is, according to the Food and Drug Administration (FDA) (FDA, 2017), defined as: "a Doctor of Medicine or Osteopathy, Podiatrist, Dentist, Chiropractor, Clinical Psychologist, Optometrist, Nurse Practitioner, Nurse-Midwife, or a Clinical Social worker who is authorized to practice by the State and performing within the scope of their practice as defined by State law." The HP in this study refers to either a nurse practitioner or a physician assistant.

Door-to-Provider (DTP)

The actual time when a patient signs in and a chart is opened to the time when the provider first sees the patient.

Turnaround Time to Discharge (TAT-D)

The actual time from when the patient signs in and their chart is created in the electronic health record until they are discharged from the emergency department.

Length of Stay (LOS)

The entire length of time a patient is in the emergency department including discharge and when admitted patients transfer out of the department.

Left Without Being Seen (LWBS)

Patients who arrive into the emergency department and have an electronic chart created for their visit but leave prior to being seen by a provider.

Medical Screening Exam (MSE)

The Emergency Medical Treatment and Active Labor Act (EMTA-LA) states that any patient who comes to the emergency department requesting examination or treatment for a medical condition must be provided with an appropriate medical screening examination (MSE) by a qualified medical person to determine if he is suffering from an emergency medical condition (CMS, 2012).

Emergency Severity Index (ESI)

Is a five-level emergency department triage algorithm utilized in the United States. ESI triage is based on the acuity of a patient's presenting complaint and the number of resources their care is anticipated to require. ESI 1 is a patient requiring immediate resuscitation, typically arriving by ambulance. ESI 2 patients are considered emergent and at high risk of deterioration if they wait, often these patients arrive by ambulance but frequently walk through the front door and require multiple resources. ESI 3 patients are stable but will require 2 or more resources; ESI 4 patients are considered less urgent, stable requiring only one resource: and ESI 5 patients are nonurgent who do not require any resources (AHRQ, 2012).

PROBLEM IDENTIFICATION—ENVIRONMENT AND TARGET POPULATION

The goal was to improve the overall TAT-D by decreasing the length of time patients wait to see a provider (DTP) and determine if there would be a financial benefit. The impact on extended DTP and TAT-D set up a perfect storm for adverse events in the lobby, an increase in the LWBS metric which impacts both patient outcomes and revenue. Although there had not been a sentinel event, there had been several near misses because patients had to wait to see a provider.

Further defining the problem included evaluating organizational need, narrowing the patient population, and determining the times where patient volume surges were most frequently seen. Using a tracer methodology approach, several days of observation and dissecting where the greatest impact on patient outcomes exists was the approach used to delineate the inclusion criteria and define the scholarly question.

SCHOLARLY MODEL—LITERATURE REVIEW

Once the scholarly question was defined, the development of the PICOT question became the next important step in the DNP project design process. To facilitate developing the PICOT question, a very detailed and multi-stage review of literature was embarked upon. There is an abundance of evidence that demonstrates the extent to which hospitals and providers are going to alleviate the issues of overcrowding in the ED, increased DTP time and overall LOS.

The first stage of the literature review was broad based and aimed at improving the scholar's general knowledge of the regulatory implications for the practice problem. Current federal, state, organizational, and provider group policies and practice guidelines were the foundation for this literature review. Using the references sited in practice guidelines, the scholar expanded the literature search to expand understanding of the science of ED throughput.

Over the course of didactic study, a continuous and comprehensive review of the evidence was conducted through the databases CINAHL, MEDLINE, the Cochrane Library, and Joanna Briggs Institute, which were accessed and searched extensively. Key words utilized included provider in greet, provider in triage, ED length of stay, door to doctor time, triage, ED patient satisfaction, ED throughput goals, ED patient flow, and ED LEAN process. Thesaurus options of the databases CINAHL, MEDLINE, and the Cochrane Library were utilized to attempt to capture any additional research that related to advanced practice providers in emergency medicine. The search excluded nursing process and protocols in the ED and ED nursing triage, because the focus of this project was to evaluate the evidence as it pertained to advanced practice provider efficiency in triage and the impact on DTP and TAT-D.

THE PICOT QUESTION

Would patients with an Emergency Severity Index (ESI) Score of 3, 4, or 5 who presented to the ED and received an MSE done by an HP upon sign-in, have diagnostic orders initiated, result in a decrease DTP time less than 30 minutes and a TAT-D below 180 minutes? Concurrently, would the LWBS rate decrease, thereby improving revenue capture? This was the ideal complex multifaceted project identified that could lead to meaningful and sustainable change for patients arriving for care in the ED and was the premise for the DNP scholarly project.

THEORY IDENTIFICATION

Ray's theory as a metaparadigm speaks to what is probably the most important factor in the metaparadigm, the person (Haley, 2014). Without the person (i.e., patient) there is no need for a healthcare provider, and the bureaucracy of the complex organization is diminished in its relevance. Never has the metaparadigm of the person been more important to complex healthcare organizations than it is in today's value-based purchasing model of reimbursement (Haley, 2014). It is for this reason that the Theory of Bureaucratic Caring spoke to the DNP scholar's choice when applying the structure for the practice change that ultimately demonstrated a decrease in metrics for DTP and TAT-D and resulted in a significant decrease in the LWBS rate.

Ray's theory (Coffman, 2014) encompasses the foundations of emergency medicine that creates a cohesive operation:

- *Nursing*—Partnering with nursing, the healthcare provider provides ethical, spiritual and holistic care of the patient and forms a relationship that transforms the urgency of their health concern into the foundation of a healing process (Coffman, 2014).
- *Person*—Patients arriving at the greet window of the ED represent spiritual and cultural beings who seek to find answers to their health emergency. To build an effective relationship with the

patient, a healthcare provider must incorporate spiritual and cultural understanding into each encounter (Coffman, 2014).

*   *Health*—Recognizing the view of health is in the eye of the beholder, and each patient formulates their personal reality of their own health based in part on what their views of health are as well as the influence of those close to them (Coffman, 2014).

*   Environment—A complex and often chaotic environment, it is in the ED that the patient often does not understand the factors that go into determining when and where in the ED they will be seen; it is here that the caring, compassionate attitudes and communication frequently fail (Coffman, 2014).

Ray's theory purports that the definition of caring has a wide range of meaning depending upon the setting and the position held by the healthcare professional (Coffman, 2014). In the setting of the ED, the need to work expediently often results in a failure to communicate effectively with patients so much so that there is a perception of a lack of caring and compassion. Yet to the HP, expedient recognition of an emergent condition, coordinating care and taking comprehensive action are all examples of caring. According to Mahmoudi *et al.* (2017), by the very work that is done in the ED, the meaning of caring falls outside of the traditional understanding of what caring means. The Theory of Bureaucratic Caring speaks to the practice environment and supported the scientific legitimacy of this scholarly project.

CHANGE MODEL IDENTIFICATION

This scholar incorporated into the project John Kotter's Eight Step Process of Successful Change, a proven model for driving effective change in healthcare (Small *et al.,* 2016). Kotter's model recognizes the approach to change through the fundamental steps creating a foundation for success. It is through this model that the importance of building a strong coalition and the power of creating a sense of urgency to implement change lays the groundwork for effective change. Persuasive communication and empowering others to act creates short-term gains that reward staff who are working to bring about meaningful change. Kotter stressed the importance of maintaining a vision for change and bringing together like-minded staff who can articulate the impact of meaningful change and the organizations success.

Kotter's eight steps (Small *et al.*, 2016) include:

1. Acting with urgency
2. Developing the guiding coalition
3. Developing a change vision
4. Communicating the vision buy-in
5. Empowering broad-based action
6. Generating short-term wins
7. Don't let up
8. Make change stick

While developing this project, it was understood that change, no matter how big or small, required vigilance, effort, cooperation, and a coalition with the fortitude and the power to lead. In healthcare, when change is mandated with little input or collaboration with frontline staff, the efforts to bring meaningful change will fail. The scholar recognized early on that effective change requires a holistic approach to be successful. Utilizing an effective change model enhances the likelihood meaningful change can occur and be sustained.

STAKEHOLDER IDENTIFICATION AND COLLABORATION

As a nurse practitioner in the ED and a DNP scholar, the goal was to identify and develop a meaningful project that would produce meaningful and sustainable change. There were many competing issues all important to ED throughput which created a situation for designing a unique and innovative approach to the scholarly project.

Two of the major stakeholders, the medical director and assistant medical director for the ED provider group, were identified early on as mentors and the two preceptors who would guide the scholar to design, develop, implement, and successfully complete the scholarly project. Several meetings were held with ED and hospital leadership where the pre-intervention TAT-D and DTP times were discussed and the impact on the LWBS rate and revenue was presented.

The health care provider (HP) group was consulted, and all agreed to participate in the study providing they retained their practice independence which leadership supported. Nursing leadership was consulted and was supportive of the DNP project but did advise that there would be no support for changing nurse staffing levels, adding nursing FTE's or altering the workflow of the nurses who staffed the greet window. The manager for ED registration was consulted and is fully supportive of the project. The scribes were advised of the project and change in HP provider assignment but are limited stakeholders in that each scribe is assigned to work with each HP wherever the HP sees patients.

PROBLEM TO IDENTIFICATION

Understanding the Clinical Problem

There were many key issues impacting the increased DTP and TAT-D metrics. A lack of inpatient beds often results in admitted patients being boarded, which in turn results in a lack of core ED beds where newly arrived patients can be evaluated and treated. There is a rapid medical evaluation (RME) area where patients are supposed to be treated and dispositioned quickly; however, overcrowding has resulted in this area frequently becoming saturated with sick patients requiring large workups and extended stays.

Another barrier that lengthens the DTP and TAT-D pertains to nurse staffing and a state mandated four patients per nurse ratio and a limited number of nursing staff on duty. A state survey determined that patients who were seen by a provider then returned to the lobby pending results should fall under the nurse-to-patient ratio, creating further strain on nurse staffing.

The most significant observation was the length of time it took to have a patient complete the greet process, be evaluated by a provider, have diagnostic exams ordered, and complete the registration process. During times of high census, it was not unusual for patients to wait more than 90 minutes to see a provider after the initial greet process. This DTP time greater than 90 minutes along with other identified obstacles contributed heavily to a TAT-D which exceeded 249 minutes and a 5.2% LWBS rate.

Formulating Appropriate, Realistic Interventions

This DNP scholarly project required dedicated physical space in the greet area and preset scheduling of HPs. It was agreed upon by the provider group that the HP who arrives at 1600 will be assigned to greet from 1600 to 2000 hours and will then rotate to the triage area. The HP scheduled at 20:00 will start his/her shift assigned to greet until 23:30, at which time this HP will rotate to the RME area.

While assigned to the greet area, the HP completed the following steps for each patient interaction to ensure each component of the DNP scholarly project was adhered to. As the patients arrived through the front door of the ED, they proceeded to the greet desk where the RN was the initial point of contact for the patient. The RN performed a quick registration which included the basic patient demographics, name, date of birth and/or social security number, and arrived the patient into the system so that the chart appeared on the ED track board. The RN obtained the presenting complaint, vital signs to include height and weight, verified allergy information, and assigned the ESI level. Once the patient was arrived into the system, the HP, from the waiting room section of the tracker, clicked on the patient's name assigning him/herself as the provider. As the patient was providing information to the RN, the HP listened to the presenting complaint and initiated diagnostic and treatment orders. Once the HP assigned him/herself, the scribe clicked the RME tab in the patient chart; this action by the scribe stopped the DTP clock. This action also informed the registration department that the patient had been seen by a provider and was now eligible for full registration. The scribe then proceeded to open an RME note and document the MSE using the MSE template. When the RN finished with the patient at greeting, the HP closed the patient chart and unassigned him/herself, making sure to reassign the patient to a "waiting for room" status. The HP then reviewed the MSE and signed the note, sending it to the attending physician assigned by the scribe. The patient, in the meantime, was returned to the waiting area of the ED to await registration and complete diagnostic workup and/or treatments ordered before being called for the full provider exam and final disposition.

Launch

After receiving approval from the facility and university Internal Review Boards, the 10-week quality improvement project was implemented. The first two weeks focused on staff and provider education regarding the need for process improvement as well as the process change to be implemented. Through multiple in-services and meetings with stakeholders and staff, the DNP scholar provided evidence-based education to promote support for the project. The DNP scholar found a weaker knowledge base among nursing staff as it pertains to the detailed impact of prolonged throughput, patients waiting in the lobby and the risks associated with continuing business as usual. The DNP scholar provided focused education and mentoring for all nursing staff pertaining to the weaknesses identified and toward the end of the implementation period and observed nursing staff independently take ownership for lobby awareness and advocating to move patients more efficiently.

Challenges—Barriers and Challenges

There were a few limitations that impacted this projects outcome and possibly were the result of an increase in the TAT-D. One limitation was the variability in nursing staff working in the RME that made it difficult for patients to receive the treatments ordered by the HP in greet. Other limitations that placed a strain on the process were the unexpected traumas and alerts (stroke, myocardial infarction and sepsis) that diverted resources such as radiology and lab to these priority patients thus resulting in a delay in diagnostics for those patients whose orders were placed by the HP in greet. An increase in admissions was also observed during the implementation phase, resulting in more patients being boarded in the ED. Perhaps this phenomenon was due to the increased volume, as there were fewer LWBS patients.

DATA COLLECTION

This project incorporated a non-probability convenience sample which consisted of all patients who presented to the greet window, signed in to be seen in the ED and had an ESI score of 3, 4, or 5 assigned. This project was a quality improvement project; therefore, it was not necessary to recruit patients individually, nor was patient consent for participation required. ESI level 1 and 2 patients were excluded given the critical nature of these patients and their need for admission as opposed to discharge from the ED.

A pre- and post-implementation design was utilized for the purposes of this project. The comparison data for the pre-intervention phase utilized similar patient volume for a 10-week period in 2017. Only those patients discharged from the ED were included for evaluation. Data pertaining to patients admitted to the hospital from the ED were excluded from analysis.

Following conclusion of the 10-week period, analysis of the pre- and post-intervention arms of the scholarly project were conducted using SPSS software, version 25.0 to perform data analysis (IBM, 2017).

DATA COLLECTION TO ANALYSIS

The principal outcome measures for this scholarly project examined if improvement in DTP, TAT-D, and LWBS metrics were achieved through placing an HP in the greeting phase of the project. The paired t-test provided a scientifically acceptable level of confidence; the differences between the means of the pre- and post-intervention arms was such that the likelihood resulted in a correlation equal to the targeted result (DTP below 30 minutes and TAT-D below 180 minutes). The chi-square test of independence was chosen to measure the LWBS metric between the pre- and post-intervention arms of the study. This test of independence evaluated the relationship between the pre- and post-intervention arms to determine if there was a significant relationship between the LWBS metrics.

Statistical Analysis—Methods to Bring Meaning to the Data

It should be noted that in the pre-implementation data, most of the patients who presented to the greet window were assigned an ESI 3 score ($n = 274$). This is important because it is this acuity of patients who require more than one resource (i.e., lab, x-ray, ultrasound, CT scan) prolonging their stay in the ED, while the next lowest acuity level, ESI 4, representing 204 patients, requires only one resource (i.e. lab or x-ray). There were also patients within the pre-implementation period who presented but were not assigned an ESI score ($n = 19$). It is unclear how patients were seen and discharged from the ED without an assigned ESI score and is a phenomenon that was brought to ED leaderships attention during the data collection period.

In the post-implementation period, an ESI 3 acuity level was assigned to the largest segment of the patients ($n = 106$) and ESI 4 was the second most often seen ($n = 83$). During the implementation period, only six patients who presented to the greet window and were seen by the HP in greet were not assigned an ESI score by the greet nurse. As with the pre-implementation period, it is unknown if these patients were seen and discharged by a provider.

A total of 5,580 patient records were obtained during the pre-implementation period, with acuities of 3, 4, or 5. A total of 5,111 patient records were obtained during the post-implementation time period, with acuities of 3, 4, or 5. A two-way frequency table was used to demonstrate the counts and percentages of individuals across the pre- and post-implementation periods as it pertains to discharged disposition. Most patients in both the pre- and post-implementation periods were discharged from the ED, n = 4,456 and n = 4,070 respectively. In the pre-implementation period, patients who eloped from the ED numbered 1.1% but increased during the implementation period to 4.2% of patients. During the pre-implementation period, 5.2% of patients LWBS after triage, as opposed to 0.9% of patients in the post-implementation period.

Analysis of the distribution of arrival methods included the pre- and post-implementation periods. While the second largest percentage of patients arrives by ambulance in both the pre-and post-implementation periods, the greatest numbers of patients arrive via the front entrance of the ED by car. In the pre-implementation period, 73.5% (n = 4,100) of patients arrived by car and post-implementation, 72.6% (n = 3,712). It is noted that other modes of transportation to the ED were analyzed—all with less than a 5% impact on the number of patients who come through the front door in either the pre- or post-implementation periods.

This project only considered patients who arrived through the front entrance of the ED and were assigned an acuity ESI score of 3, 4 or 5 in both the pre- and post-implementation periods. The most common level of acuity was ESI 3 (60.3% of patient's pre-implementation and 61.5% of patient's post-implementation). Statistically, patients assigned an acuity ESI score of 5 were rare.

One of the primary goals of this project was to decrease the DTP time from the pre-implementation median of greater than 90 minutes to a DTP median time of less than 30 minutes in the post-implementation period. The median time is the metric reported to the Centers for Medicare and Medicaid Services (CMS) and utilized at this facility. In the pre-implementation period, the median DTP was 46 minutes; post-implementation the median DTP was three minutes.

Because the typical DTP times certainly appeared much lower in the post-implementation period, it was important to determine whether this indicated an underlying change in the DTP times or if this could have been due to a simple random difference in the patients who came during each time period. For this reason, a Mann-Whitney U test was conducted to compare the two independent groups of patients between the pre- and post-implementation period. While the Mann-Whitney U and the Wilcoxon W and Z statistics are equivalent to one another, the test was ultimately interpreted through the p-value. The p-value was < 0.001, meaning there had been no real change in the underlying median DTP following the implementation of the process change. There was less than a 0.1% chance that random differences in patient circumstances would have led to a change in the median DTP times.

The other phenomenon of interest in the project was the impact on TAT-D between the pre- and post-implementation periods. The same analysis used to evaluate the project's result on DTP was used to evaluate outcomes on TAT-D. The median TAT-D in the pre-implementation period was 186 minutes and increased to a median of 201 minutes in the post-implementation period. A Mann-Whitney U test was conducted comparing the median TAT-D times from pre- to post-implementation, confirming there was a statistically significant increase in the median TAT-D in the post-implementation period.

Finally, the metric concurrently studied within this project was the LWBS rate. The pre-implementation period analysis showed that pre-implementation 5.2% of patients ($n = 289$) LWBS and only 1% ($n = 49$) in the post-implementation period left before being seen by a provider. Although there is a significant difference between the pre- and post-implementation periods, a chi-square test of independence was conducted to compare the percentages across the two implementation periods. The only component of the chi-square that is interpreted is the p-value, which was less than 0.05, indicating a significant decrease in the number of LWBS patients in the post-implementation period.

What cannot be overlooked as a strength of this project is the impact on revenue captured as a result of the decreased LWBS rate. During the post-implementation period, the percentage of patients who LWBS ($n = 49$) resulted in a $39,200 loss in revenue over the 10-week period. However, it is estimated that an additional $192,000 in revenue was captured over the 10-week period because more patients ($n = 241$) remained to see a provider. In the post-implementation period, the decision to admit also increased 1.6% (to 13.8%). Perhaps this is because more patients were being seen or because of the diagnostic ordering differences among HPs ordering tests that may not have been previously ordered. This increase in admissions ($n = 706$) resulted in a revenue gain over $29 million over the course of the 10-week implementation period.

POST PROJECT CONSIDERATIONS AND SUSTAINABILITY

The findings of this project successfully demonstrated the ability to decrease the length of time it takes for a patient to see a HP upon arrival into the ED and have their diagnostic and treatment orders initiated. Those patients who are deemed too sick to wait are identified more quickly and immediately provided care, improving patient outcomes. In the past, these patients waited a minimum of 90 minutes to see a provider, increasing their risk for adverse outcomes or worse yet, leaving without being seen while not realizing the gravity of their illness. Greeting patients at the front door and making them aware they are being seen by a provider gets their attention. Patients who realize their diagnostic and treatment orders have been initiated within minutes of arrival are less likely to leave.

The results of this project have many similarities to previous studies that successfully demonstrated that getting a provider to the patient at the earliest possible point does effectively decrease DTP and the LWBS rate; however, consistent with the evidence, there were roadblocks that either extended or failed to improve TAT-D (Burstrom et al., 2016; Weston et al., 2017; Pierce et al., 2016). Therefore, it is reasonable to ascertain for those facilities who can reallocate provider staff without interrupting patient flow these results may be applicable beyond this DNP scholar's population and setting.

CONCLUSIONS AND REFLECTIONS

Developing a Doctor of Nursing Practice (DNP) scholarly project that would improve ED metrics, revenue and most importantly patient outcomes was the driving motivator for this scholar. I recognized that during times of high volume, placing a provider at the point of entry where ambulatory patients arrive into the ED provides the earliest possible identification of those at risk patients, allowing for immediate care and overall improvement in patient outcomes. Not only are patient outcomes improving as a result of this project, but the increase in revenue captured is significant. As healthcare costs rise, hospitals and providers are keenly aware that sustainability requires continuous process improvement and revenue loss of any amount is not an option.

The role of the DNP leader is to translate evidence to bring about positive change within the clinical setting. Successful DNP programs recognize that to take the DNP scholar from doctoral novice to leader requires a building block approach. For me, each didactic course served as the foundation for successfully designing, implementing and completing a meaningful change project. Throughout each course, an ongoing systematic review of evidence elevated my understanding of and ability to translate meaning for evidence-based research. Gaining an appreciation for literature reviews allowed me to successfully translate existing evidence and develop a project that resulted in improved patient outcomes, increased revenue and, most importantly, demonstrated sustainability. There are many learning curves throughout doctoral study; however, the result is a confident, articulate DNP leader who stands ready to assume greater leadership roles and promote evidence-based practice change.

REFERENCES

Agency for Healthcare Research and Quality (AHRQ) (2012). Overview of the Emergency Severity Index. In *Emergency Severity Index (ESI): A Triage Tool for Emergency Department Care. Version 4. 2012 Edition*. Ch 2. Retrieved from https://www.ahrq.gov/sites/default/files/wysiwyg/professionals/systems/hospital/esi/esi-handbk.pdf

Burström, L., Engström, M. L., Castrén, M., Wiklund, T. and Enlund, M. (2016). Improved quality and efficiency after the introduction of physician-led team triage in an emergency department. *Upsala Journal of Medical Sciences, 121*(1), 38–44. Retrieved from: https://doi.org/10.3109/03009734.2015.1100223

Centers for Medicare & Medicaid Services (CMS). (2012). Emergency Medical Treatment and Labor Act (EMTALA). Retrieved from: https://www.cms.gov/Regulations-and-Guidance/Legislation/EMTALA/

Centers for Medicare & Medicaid Services (CMS). Hospital Results. In Hospital Consumer Assessment of Healthcare Providers and Systems (HCAHPS). 2018. Retrieved from: https://www.medicare.gov/hospitalcompare/compare.html

Coffman, S. (2014). Theory of bureaucratic caring. In M. R. Alligood (Ed.), *Nursing Theorists and Their Work*, 8th ed. Ch 8, 98–119. St. Louis, MO: Elsevier Mosby.

Food and Drug Administration (FDA). (2017) Code of Federal Regulations, Title 21. Retrieved from: https://www.accessdata.fda.gov/scripts/cdrh/cfdocs/cfcfr/CFRSearch.cfm?fr=810.2

Haley, T. (2014). Scientific underpinnings: Theory of bureaucratic caring. *NR700 Scientific Underpinnings*. Chamberlain College of Nursing. March 27, 2014.

Mahmoudi, H., Mohmmadi, E. and Ebadi, A. (2017). The meaning of emergency care in the Iranian nursing profession. *Journal of Critical Care Nursing, 10*(1). doi: 10.5812/ccn.10073

Morgan, M. W., Salzman, J. G., LeFevere, R. C., Thomas, A. J. and Isenberger, K. M. Demographic, Operational, and Healthcare Utilization Factors Associated with Emergency Department Patient Satisfaction. *Western Journal of Emergency Medicine, 16*, no. 4 (2015): 516, doi: 10.5811/westjem.2015.4.25074

Pierce, B. A. and Gormley, D. (2016). Practice improvement: Are split flow and provider in triage models in the emergency department effective in reducing discharge length of stay? *Journal of Emergency Nursing, 4*(2), 487–491. doi:10.1016/j.jen.2016.01.005

Salway, R. J., Valenzuela, R., Shoenberger, J. M., Mallon, W. K. and Viccellio, A. (2017). Emergency department (ED) overcrowding: Evidence-based answers to frequently asked questions. *Revista Medica Clinica Las Condes, 28*(2), 213–219. Retrieved from: https://doi.org/10.1016/j.rmclc.2017.04.008

Small, A., Gist, D., Souza, D., Dalton, J., Magny-Normilus, C. and David, D. (2016). Using Kotter's change model for implementing bedside handoff: A quality improvement project. *Journal of Nursing Care Quality, 31*(4), 304–309. doi: 10.1097/NCQ.0000000000000212

Weston, V., Aldeen, A., Gravenor, S., Jain, S., Schmidt, M. and Malik, S. (2014). 213 Effectiveness of resident physicians as triage liaison providers in an academic emergency department. *Annals of Emergency Medicine, 64*(4). doi: 10.5811/westjem.2017.1.33243

Wilson, M. and Cutler, D. (2014). Emergency department profits are likely to continue as The Affordable Care Act expands coverage. *Health Affairs, 33*(5), 792–799. doi: https://doi.org/10.1377/hlthaff.2013.0754

The Development and Implementation of Admissions Criteria for a Clinical Decision Unit

COLLEEN CROSBY, DNP, MSN, RN BC-NE

PROBLEM STATEMENT

Increased Emergency Department (ED) wait times and patients leaving EDs without being seen are serious issues nationwide. Both problems arise, in part, from patients increasingly seeking primary care at EDs rather than with their primary care physicians (Scrofine, 2014). This trend necessitates reconsidering the way patients are directed at point of first contact; consequently, clinical decision units (CDUs) have become a vital component of strategies to optimize hospital metrics.

At the author's practice site, a 150-bed New York hospital, observation patients have conventionally been placed throughout the hospital wherever there is a vacant bed, rather than in a dedicated CDU with well-defined admissions criteria. Due in part to this practice, the hospital's length of stay (LOS) for observation patients exceeded national guidelines of 26 hours. My doctor of nursing practice (DNP) project culminated in the opening of a CDU, after developing and implementing inclusion/exclusion criteria for CDU admissions, with the goal of decreasing CDU patients' mean LOS to less than 18 hours. In addition, the project was designed to address elevated numbers of patients leaving the ED without being seen by a provider (approximately 6%) and above average times from arrival to being seen in an ED treatment room. This is a critical concern for this hospital.

It was anticipated that opening of a CDU, with established admission criteria from the ED, would free up ED beds. This revision in policy and practice was anticipated to reduce ED left-without-being-seen (LWBS) numbers below 3%, while decreasing arrival-to-treatment times for ED patients.

The protocol was developed by a project leader (the author) and approved by a multidisciplinary team. Appropriate training was delivered to staff, which included education in inclusion/exclusion criteria for admission to the CDU and use of an audit form to measure if admissions criteria were being followed.

The design of the protocol took into account other factors: the multifactorial and reciprocal relationship between reduction in wait times (and LOS) and maintaining maximum occupancy for the CDU's 11 beds and fine-tuning communication between units. It was acknowledged from the outset that the efficacy of the CDU could not be fully judged, nor its value to the hospital fully realized, without consideration of the unit's function as a system component. Specifically, the CDU's efficacy needed to be weighed in balance with its role in the fiscal and staffing landscape of the ED and the hospital as a whole to understand whether its "positives"—fiscal or operational—would outweigh its possible "negatives."

PURPOSE STATEMENT

The purpose of this project was to improve efficiency and treatment times of ED patients through the implementation of a CDU for admitted patients. Research supports the usefulness of CDUs in alleviating overcrowding by judiciously moving patients deemed appropriate candidates out of the ED to the CDU at the first opportunity (Gabele *et al.,* 2016).

PROJECT OBJECTIVES

The efficacy of any project can be judged only by placing its stated objectives in juxtaposition with measurable data arising from its implementation. Firmly rooted in evidence based practice, the CDU sets its project objectives accordingly:

1. Develop a CDU protocol that exactingly establishes inclusion-exclusion criteria for CDU admission, then follow it consistently and without to decrease incidence of inappropriate admissions.
2. Educate staff prior to opening of the CDU to ensure each consistently identifies appropriate patients according to protocol-based admissions criteria.

3. Decrease average ED door-to-treatment time to 60 minutes or less.
4. Decrease ED decision-to-admit times to a bed to 2.5 hours.
5. Decrease the number of patients leaving the ED prior to receiving care from the provider to 3% or less.
6. Decrease the LOS of CDU patients to 18 hours or less.

People who present to EDs request treatment for a variety of ailments. Any individual seeking medical attention in the ED must be seen regardless of race, origin, ethnicity, sexual orientation, or type of medical insurance. Frequently, the ED is overflowing with people requiring treatment. Consequently, patients may experience delays in treatment. Some may become frustrated and leave the ED without being seen by a provider (Hamrock, 2014).

Another factor contributing to extended wait times and delays in treatment is occupation of ED beds by patients awaiting test results or admissions decisions. Both practices indicate inefficient use of ED resources (Teets *et al.,* 2014). The author's practice site, acknowledging the seriousness of these problems, resolved to establish a dedicated CDU to address ED overflow. The CDU would admit short-stay (less than 24 hours) patients meeting admissions criteria to await test results and receive treatment.

Before the CDU's opening, nurses and providers received focused training in criteria for inclusion in, or exclusion from, the unit. To ensure appropriate admissions standards, a comprehensive protocol defining criteria, and a plan for preparing nurses and providers to implement the practice change, had been formulated. Often, ED patients seek treatment for issues not requiring prolonged hospitalization. Research suggests that absent of life-threatening diagnoses, and when patients have anticipated hospitalizations less than 24 hours, CDUs may be the best option (Hamrock, 2014). It seemed reasonable that transfer of short-stay patients would free up ED beds for more critically ill patients and ease the bottleneck of ED patients waiting to be treated. Patients would be brought into the triage area by the triage nurse to be assessed; an ESI number defining the priority of treatment would be assigned to the patient. Frequently, the provider sees the patient in triage and places orders to start the workup and treatment. Consequently, the CDU has the potential to decrease door-to-treatment times for ED patients.

Because CDU admissions affect overall hospital flow, care would need to be taken in the design and implementation of a protocol on which the daily functioning of the unit is based. Since identifying the target population for the unit's services—patients requiring observation less than 24 hours in duration—is central to its effectiveness, attention to detail in design of inclusion/exclusion criteria, training of staff in those criteria, and testing effectiveness of that training, formed important links in design of the CDU.

BACKGROUND

A dedicated CDU or short-stay unit located outside of the ED is a proven strategy for increasing patient throughput (Carpenter, 2015). Patients in CDUs are typically monitored for 6 to 24 hours until they are medically cleared or discharged home. Ideally, CDUs cohort short-stay patients in one physical location. Such units have been shown to decrease LOS, enhance ED access, foster patient and staff satisfaction, reduce mortality, and improve ED efficiency (Jibrin, 2008).

CDUs are specialized and serve as an alternative to inpatient admission. The success of a unit in achieving its intended purpose depends on precisely defined operational protocols and strict adherence to them, with a fixed time limit for patients who are admitted. The unit is managed by medical experts, and patients who are determined to require longer hospitals stays would not be admitted to the unit. Patients presenting with chest pain, asthma or COPD exacerbation, syncope, gastroenteritis, or community-acquired pneumonia are typically seen in CDUs (Baugh, 2011). To make informed decisions about admission to the CDU based on best-practice standards, a multidisciplinary, collaborative team was assembled to formulate inclusion/exclusion criteria.

IMPACT OF THE PROBLEM

Overcrowded EDs result in longer wait times, patient dissatisfaction, and patients leaving the ED without being treated (Ross *et al.,* 2013). Many patients seeking ED treatment are not sick enough to warrant hospital admission, yet not well enough to go home. These patients may occupy ED beds for up to 48 hours, causing a bottleneck of patients waiting to be seen by a provider, in the ED waiting room (Gabele, 2016). These "boarders" or "holds" consume a lot of resources and labor. They prevent ED staff from bringing in the next patient to be seen, causing a backup. The Institute of Medicine (IOM) has recognized ED boarding and ambulance diversion as unacceptable consequences of ED overcrowding needing to be addressed (IOM, 2006). Surprisingly, two-thirds of United States (U.S.) hospitals do not have a dedicated CDU. Most place clinical decision patients in any bed, typically in-patient beds, without reference to protocols. Such patients experience longer lengths of stay and utilize more resources than CDU patients in a unit with clearly defined protocols and dedicated staff. U.S. hospitals slowly are establishing dedicated CDUs to maximize ED throughput, decompress the ED, and decrease lengths of stay for clinical decision patients (Ross *et al.,* 2013).

POPULATION OF INTEREST

The population of interest included formal ED and CDU leadership teams and ED and CDU frontline staff in a 150-bed, upstate-New-York community hospital. Formal leadership teams consisted of 2 nurse managers, 9 charge nurses and 2 nurse educators for the ED and CDU, 55 RNs, 8 patient care techs, and 5 secretaries in both the CDU and ED.

STAKEHOLDERS

For the unit to be successful, all key stakeholders needed to share the mission and vision of the unit and the organization. Key stakeholders were hospitalists and ED providers, the medical director of the hospitalist group, the medical director of the ED, CDU and ED staff and managers, and senior leadership. Observation patients admitted to the CDU are also key stakeholders: it would be important to do patient rounds daily once the unit opened to get their feedback as well. Hospitalist and ED providers included MDs, physician assistants, and nurse practitioners. These stakeholders determined who would be admitted to the CDU and whether admissions criteria were being followed. Senior leadership was supportive and involved in the opening of the CDU, as well as in developing admissions criteria.

Early engagement and continued involvement of all stakeholders was key to the success of this project. As the project leader, I was present on site and established rapport with all stakeholders (including hospital transporters and emergency medical personnel), answered questions, and scheduled meetings with staff and stakeholders.

Rapport with stakeholders was established by involving them in developing admissions criteria, as well as answering questions or concerns about the protocol. As the project lead, I attended weekly CDU meetings and monthly ED staff meetings to review CDU metrics: LOS for clinical decision patients admitted to the dedicated, 11-bed CDU and LOS of all other clinical decision patients in the ED.

INTERVENTION/PROJECT TIMELINE

The intervention began with the project lead's introduction of the new guideline to CDU staff and ED staff through unit meetings for each group and during daily huddles organized by charge nurses at the change of shifts. The project rollout was planned for a six-week period; however, there were several delays (mostly construction) in implementing the project. The project was delineated for ED and prospective CDU staff, including education in inclusion/exclusion criteria; pre-and post-surveys were completed by participants to measure understanding of mandated education. Privacy for participants was strictly maintained: no identifying information was collected. The project leader developed an audit tool concerning CDU admissions criteria and educated CDU RNs on use of the new audit form. The project rollout was six weeks, beginning April 2018, and included staff education and 50 retrospective chart reviews before the implementation of the new protocol and 50 chart reviews after implementation.

Planning for this project had begun in August 2017 at the request of the VP of Nursing. After discussion with management, assessment and analysis of the hospital's established practice of placing clinical decision patients throughout the hospital (rather than in a dedicated CDU) was reviewed. Literature review and gap analysis were performed, and a PDCA cycle was planned.

The rollout for the project was established after IRB approvals from my university and the practice site. Because the success of the project also hinged upon its timely completion, a detailed rollout plan was developed and, once construction delays were resolved, closely followed.

- *Week 1*: Kickoff meeting to introduce project to key stakeholders.

The project lead attended unit meetings for ED, CDU, and providers to communicate with and educate staff and providers on project details. All staff and providers at the ED and CDU unit meetings were educated about the CDU protocol and data collection tool. An initial survey was completed by staff to measure effectiveness of education provided on the CDU protocol.

- *Week 2*: The project lead presented revisions of protocol based on input from staff, providers, and management and led weekly meetings of the project team. The project lead directed the use of the data collection tool upon opening of the CDU.
- *Week 3*: The project lead monitored the use of the admissions/exclusion criteria and led weekly meetings of the project team. The project lead also facilitated ongoing communication with staff and providers regarding inclusion/exclusion criteria and oversaw revisions to the criteria based on input from stakeholders.
- *Week 4*: The project leads organized weekly team meetings and the continued study of the effectiveness of the implementation of the admission/exclusion criteria.
- *Week 5*: The project lead continued to modify admission/exclusion criteria as necessary and lead the weekly team meeting.
- *Week 6*: The project lead completed the project and chart reviews, worked with the project statistician in data analysis and interpretation, offered a final evaluation of effectiveness of the protocol, and disseminated results.

CDU Protocol

The project lead developed the inclusion/exclusion (admissions) protocol for the CDU with input from stakeholders and educated the nursing staff (approximately 60) in the ED and CDU. Educational materials included the protocol and a PowerPoint presentation addressing each area of it.

CDU Knowledge Level

The project lead developed a questionnaire to evaluate whether learners' knowledge regarding inclusion/exclusion criteria increased after education in the protocol. It is important to determine the validity and reliability of a tool. Validity expresses the degree to which a measurement measures what is says it is measuring, whereas reliability refers to the degree to which results obtained by a measurement or a procedure can be replicated (Bolarinwa, 2016). The pre- and post-questionnaire developed by the project leader utilized a Likert scale, with possible answers being strongly agree, agree, disagree, strongly disagree, or true or false. A statistician was consulted early in the project to help audit proper data collection and to assist with analysis of data for the project.

THEORETICAL FRAMEWORKS AND LITERATURE REVIEW

This DNP project was informed by two theoretical frameworks: the Donabedian Model (Donabedian, 1966), and Rogers's Diffusion of Innovation Theory (Rogers, 1995). The Donabedian Model was chosen because of its focus on quality care and outcomes. The Donabedian Model necessitated a thorough review of the CDU admissions criteria and education of the CDU and ED staff, providers, and key stakeholders. The Donabedian conceptual framework uses structure, process, and outcome as standards to guide a project and monitor progress, making its evidence-based orientation ideal for this DNP project.

Everett Rogers's Diffusion of Innovation Theory (Rogers, 1995) offers insight into behavioral changes typical among adopters, classifying them into useful categories: innovators, early adopters, early majority, late majority, and laggards. Early adopters were instrumental in making implementation of the new CDU admission criteria successful. During the confirmation stage, nursing staff continuously utilized CDU admissions criteria and communicated to colleagues (especially laggards and the providers) why those criteria needed to be followed. I reviewed many theories and frameworks before concluding that the Donabedian Model and Rogers's Theory were congruent with this project's aims; they in turn helped the author identify and better comprehend relationships between phenomena. It is critical to have the right theoretical framework to guide and support your project. A thorough literature search going back seven years was completed using CINAL, PubMed, and Medline. The use of the university library to research differences between observation units, short-stay units, and clinical decision units was invaluable. Several articles underlined the importance of clearly delineated admissions criteria for governing CDU decision-making.

DATA COLLECTION PROCEDURES

MOU Knowledge Level

A thorough explanation of the new protocol and inclusion-exclusion criteria was presented to staff in the CDU and ED in April 2018. The staff completed pre-and post-education tests to determine the effectiveness of mandated education in CDU admissions criteria. The project lead developed a codebook, and results from pre-and post-education tests were entered in SPSS spreadsheets and analyzed.

ED Metrics

The project leader completed a retrospective audit of 50 patients admitted as clinical decision patients throughout the hospital for the three weeks preceding opening of the CDU. For the three weeks immediately after its opening, 50 CDU-patient charts were audited to measure admit-to-CDU times. In addition, the project leader used aggregate data to track ED door-to-treatment-room times and LWBS for three weeks prior to opening of the CDU and for the first three weeks post-implementation.

The Meditech electronic medical records system tracks LOS for clinical decision patients through MIDAS, a program that supplies the hospital with aggregate data monthly. The project lead compared LOS of clinical decision patients in a bed for three weeks directly prior to opening of the CDU, with LOS of clinical decision patients in the new CDU for the first three weeks after opening. All data was analyzed using SPSS software.

Emergency room core metrics for patient length of stay and left-without-being-seen data are reported monthly from the Centers for Medicare & Medicaid Services (CMS). Data supplied by both Midas Health Analytics and CMS is "aggregate"; consequently, patient identification information is not linked to metrics and confidentiality is strictly maintained.

PLAN FOR ANALYSIS/EVALUATION

Upon completion of the DNP project, results from pre- and post-education staff questionnaires were entered in an SPSS spreadsheet and prepared for analysis. Normality was assessed using the Kolmogorov-Smirnov test and confirmed; linearity and homoscedasticity were confirmed by using SPSS to analyze scatterplots and residuals. A paired samples t-test was performed to compare participants' survey responses pre- and post-education regarding CDU admissions criteria (*time 1* and *time 2*, respectively). The significance of differences in survey scores pre- and post-education was analyzed for both CDU staff and ED staff.

ED door-to-treatment time by a provider and admission time-bed time was analyzed using retrospective chart audits of 50 clinical decision patients; specifically, admission to bed time was compared for clinical decision patients admitted from the ED hospital-wide three weeks before opening of the CDU with the same metrics for patients admitted to the CDU during the three weeks after its opening. LWBS data for the ED was collected for the first three weeks prior to opening of the CDU and compared to the same metric for the first three weeks after opening of the CDU. Correlation analysis revealed the direction and strength of the correlation between these two LWBS variables (Pallant 2016).

ANALYSIS OF RESULTS

The DNP project included three major components: development of, and education in, admissions criteria for a CDU; opening of a CDU; and collection and analysis of four metrics related to CDU effectiveness. To assess the efficacy of educational intervention, a ten-question, multiple-choice test was administered to 52 participants. Each participant received two same numbered copies of the ten questions, one marked pre-test and the other post-test. Confidentiality of all participants was maintained throughout. Test questions were designed to measure participants' understanding of CDU admissions criteria prior to training in the CDU admissions criteria protocol. Developing pre- and post-education surveys proved difficult. The advice of experts helped me to develop perspective in what was an unfamiliar task. Finally, with the evaluation instrument approved, each participant completed pre- and post-education tests. An SPSS spreadsheet, educdu.sav, was created from uploaded data.

The difference in means of two *educdu.sav* variables—*pretotal* and *posttotal* (measuring pre- and post-education total scores, respectively)—was analyzed using a paired samples t-test. The difference in means (-0.442), t-value (-3.976), and two-tailed p value of 0.000 confirmed a difference in pre- and post-test means significant at the $p = 0.01$ level. In addition, the effect size statistic $\eta^2 = 0.2366$ demonstrated unequivocally the efficacy of CDU admissions education in improving the working knowledge and decision-making of participants.

Paired-samples t tests for individual questions on the pre- and post-education revealed a difference of means for question 4 that was very significant ($p = 0.005$ and $\eta^2 = 0.142$), but none of the other questions was significant even at a $p = 0.05$ level. For three questions—numbers 2, 5, and 8—all 52 participants answered correctly on both pre- and post-education evaluations. Many of the prospective participants had engaged in informal discussions of CDU admissions policy over time prior to the education component, and the exceptional mean total scores pre- and post-education—19.50 and 19.94, respectively—demonstrated the effectiveness of informal communication in imparting the essentials of short-stay units.

The efficacy of educational intervention was mirrored in significant improvements in four metrics central to the purpose of the CDU: percent of left-without-being-seen CDU patients; CDU length of stay; door-to-treatment times for ED patients; and ED admit-to-bed times. Specifically, the DNP project was designed to reduce ED patient door-to-treatment times from a pre-implementation mean of 76.40 minutes to 60 minutes or less, percent LWBS ED patients from a pre-implementation weighted mean of 3.55% to less than 3.00%, and ED decision-to-admit times from a pre-implementation mean of 565.22 minutes to less than 150 minutes. Simple descriptive statistics using SPSS were adequate to analyze the extent to which these goals were met.

The post-implementation LWBS goal of less than 3.00% was met: LWBS post implementation plummeted to 2.21%. Mean ED door-to-treatment time also showed improvement: post-implementation, time to being seen by a provider had dropped to 17.02 minutes. Emphatically, the goal of 60 minutes or less was met. Mean ED admit-to-bed time post-implementation decreased from a pre-implementation mean of 565.22 minutes to 142.82 minutes. In addition, LOS dropped from a pre-implementation mean of 35.38 hours to a much-improved 12.12 hours under new CDU admissions guidelines and to 26 hours hospital wide. All metrics, pre- and post-, were normally distributed; for each, both mean and standard deviation decreased post-implementation.

DISCUSSION OF THE FINDINGS

Traditionally, patients who require further evaluation and testing beyond the first few hours in the ED have been admitted to an inpatient hospital bed. CDUs or short-stay units are becoming common in hospitals because they provide an alternative to admission or discharge (Stang et al., 2015). The ultimate goal of a CDU is to improve the quality of medical care for patients through extended evaluation and treatment, up to 24 hours, while reducing inappropriate admissions and length of stay, thereby improving ED throughput and reducing healthcare costs.

In total, 52 staff and providers were educated, pre- and post-test admissions operational knowledge was measured, and test data were analyzed using a paired samples t-test. The difference in pre- and post-test means was significant, demonstrating the effectiveness of CDU admissions education in improving the functional knowledge of CDU and ED team members. Baugh et al. (2015) emphasize that it is essential ED and CDU staff and providers are educated regarding CDU admissions criteria, further stressing the importance of subsequent adherence to those criteria.

Project results revealed a decrease of mean door-to-provider time from 76.40 minutes before to 17.02 minutes after CDU admissions criteria were in place. Without doubt, the CDU opening had a significant impact on this metric, but an additional measure put in place by the ED's medical director and nurse manager also played a role: assigning a provider to triage allowed patients to be seen sooner and to start treatment earlier. This also helped to decrease door-to-treatment time for ED patients. The ED nurse manager took four additional agency nurses to supplement staffing, helping patients receive treatment sooner. Silverman and Choppa (2016) described the benefits of opening a CDU as follows: decreased inpatient admissions, lower costs for patients and hospitals, decreased wait times for ED patients, decreased ED LWBS by a provider, and improved ED throughput.

DNP project results saw mean ED admit-to-bed time post-implementation drop to 142.82 minutes from a pre-implementation mean of 565.22 minutes. Although this was a significant improvement, PDCA analysis suggested further improvement could be realized if the admitting hospitalist wrote admission orders and the history and physical were performed in the CDU (rather than the ED). Hamrock (2014) confirms that quickly transferring patients to the CDU will decrease ED overcrowding, ED patient wait-times, and percent of patients leaving the ED without being seen by a provider.

A pre-implementation LWBS mean of 3.55% improved to 2.21% under the CDU protocol. Several factors contributed to this improvement: the CDU opened 11 additional beds; CDU staff actively pulled patients from the ED to the CDU, decreasing time patients were in the ED and freeing up ED beds for other patients; the ED medical director assigned a provider to triage to see patients sooner and to begin treatment. The last intervention also helped decrease ED LWBS patients. The ED nurse manager took four additional agency nurses to help supplement staffing; this resulted in patients being triaged expeditiously, further decreasing percent LWBS.

Post-implementation, LOS dropped from a mean of 35.38 hours to a much-improved 12.12 hours for the dedicated-CDU patients. Baugh *et al.* (2015) concluded, in their Monte Carlo simulation reflecting current clinical practice, that both observation status and where observation patients are managed are critical to clinical outcomes and overall costs for patients and hospitals. Silverman and Chopra (2016) and Gabele (2016) determined that clinical decision services provided in CDUs decrease short-stay inpatient admissions, LOS, and costs.

The outcomes element of the Donabedian framework consisted of the effect the CDU opening had on patients' overall status and represents the combined effect of structure and process (Gabele, 2016). The Donabedian Model has been used in studies treating conditions specified in the project's CDU admissions criteria and has been shown to improve quality of care provided in management of these diseases (Naranjo and Viswantha, 2011). The Donabedian Model emphasizes that focus on metrics is essential. Four operational metrics discussed previously all demonstrated significant improvement. Several researchers have suggested that LOS, ED throughput, wait times, patient outcomes, and patient satisfaction all improve when CDU patients are cohorted in one area and clear criteria specify which ones are appropriate for CDU admission (Hamrock, 2014; Barrett, Ford, and Smith, 2012; Stang *et al.*, 2015; Ross *et al.*, 2013; Baugh, 2011; Scrofine, 2014; and Hess and Nestler, 2012).

Project statistics confirmed an overwhelming majority of admitted patients—90%—were found to have met the CDU criteria. When a patient was deemed no longer appropriate for CDU—the patient no longer met CDU admissions criteria—the charge nurse notified the provider to transfer the patient to another unit. This was not always easy: at times, no beds were available elsewhere. The results showed that all metrics, pre-and post implementation, were normally distributed (Kolmogorov-Smirnov statistic > 0.05), and for each metric both mean and standard deviation decreased, suggestive of both an increase in effectiveness and a decrease in process variation. It is essential to continue to collect and analyze data, evaluate processes, and appraise the impact of CDU admissions criteria; the PDCA cycle supports iterative planning, implementation, and study. Taylor *et al.* (2013) described the importance of collecting and analyzing data monthly and the importance of cycle iteration to improve outcomes.

CONCLUSIONS

A dedicated CDU with clearly defined criteria is a proven strategy to decrease ED wait times and improve ED throughput (Carpenter, 2015); this outcome was confirmed by the present DNP project. The goals and objectives of this project were achieved. The opening of the CDU was a sharp departure hospital-wide in how observation patients were admitted and positively influenced the care provided to those patients. Implementation of an evidence-based intervention at the practice site had a positive impact on all patient outcomes. The DNP project will be sustained by nurse managers of the CDU and ED and by the senior leadership team. CDU admissions criteria continue to be reviewed and revised to meet changing patient and organization needs. The CDU continues to have a positive impact on length of stay for observation patients while improving ED patient throughput.

REFERENCES

Barrett, L., Ford, S. and Smith, P.W. (2012). A bed management strategy for overcrowding in the emergency department. *Nursing Economics*, 82–85.

Baugh, C. V. (2011). Emergency departments observation units: a clinical and financial benefit for hospitals. *Health Care Management Review, 36*(1), 28–37.

Baugh, C., Liang, L., Probst and Sun, B. (2015). National cost savings from observation unit management of syncope. *Academic Emergency Medicine*, 934–941.

Bolarinwa, O. A. (2015). Principles and methods of validity and reliability testing of questionnaires used in social and health science researchers. *Nigerian Postgraduate Medical Journal, 22*(4), 193–201.

Carpenter, J. S. (2015). Improving congestive heart failure care with a clinical decision unit. *Nursing Economics, 33*(5), 255–262.

Donabedian, A. (1966). Evaluating the quality of medical care. *Milbank Q., 44*, 166–203.

Gabele, D. B. (2016). Medical observation units and emergency department collaboration. Improving patient throughput. *The Journal of Nursing Administration*, 360–365.

Hamrock, E. P. (2014). Relieving emergency department crowding: simulating the effects of improving patient flow over time. *Hospital Administration*, 43–47.

Hess, E. and Nestler, D. (2012). Transforming the emergency department observation unit. *Cardiology Clinics, 30*(4), 501–521.

Jibrin, I. Y. (2008). Maryland's first inpatient chest pain short stay unit as an alternative to emergency room-based observation unit. Critical Pathways in Cardiology, 35–42.

Naranjo, L. S. & Viswanatha, P (2011). Applying Donabedian's theory as a framework for bariatric surgery accreditation. *Bariatric Nursing and Surgical Patient Care, 6* (1), 33–37.

Pallant, J. 2013. SPSS Survival Manual: A Step by Step Guide to Data Analysis. New York: McGraw-Hill.

Ross, M., J. Hockenberry, R. Mutter, M. Barrett, M. Wheatley, and S. Pitts. 2013. Protocol-driven emergency department observation units offer savings, shorter stays, and reduced admissions. *Health Affairs, 32*(12), 2149–2156.

Scrofine, S. F. (2014). Emergency department throughput. *The Journal of Nursing Administration*, 375–377.

Silverman, M. & Chopra, P. (2016). How to develop a successful observation unit. *Emergency Physicians Monthly.*

Stang, A.S., Crotts J., Johnson, D.W. Hartling, L. & Guttmann, A. (2015). Crowding measures associated with the quality of emergency department care: a systematic review. *Academy of Emergency Med.*, 643–56.

Taylor MJ, McNicholas C, Nicolay C, *et al.* (2013). Systematic review of the application of the Plan–do–study–act method to improve quality in healthcare. *BMJ Qual Saf* Published Online First: 11 September 2013. doi:10.1136/bmjqs-2013001862

Teets, C., Roth, L., Boderman, C., Hoch, E. (2014, Winter). Observation Status: Getting it Right the First Time. *Pennsylvania Nurse, 69*(4) pp. 20–27.

CHAPTER 11

Patient Safety Policies in an Acute Psychiatric Setting

OBED ASIF, DNP, RN

PROBLEM IDENTIFICATION/STATEMENT

The problem statement identified for this Doctor of Nursing Practice (DNP) project was focused on ways in which nurses can be instrumental in reducing the incidence of aggression and violence in the inpatient, psychiatric healthcare setting. It is important for nurses to both recognize and address signs that potential violence may occur. Part of that process lies in the nurses being away of the patient thoughts and actions that may generate from them.

According to Ridenour *et al.* (2015), patients with a psychiatric diagnosis may feel isolated. Daily routines of medication and treatment enforcement can make psychiatric inpatients more anxious, and the result could be violent actions directed toward the treatment team.

Psychiatric inpatients exhibit some of the highest rates of violence towards healthcare professionals, especially during forensic hospital treatment. This can be noted by the types of diagnoses patients in a forensic psychiatric facility often have. For example, there was an increased risk of violent behavior by schizophrenic patients in the practice setting (Kivimies *et al.*, 2014). Complex diagnoses, often with violent predispositions, force healthcare workers to focus on preventing violent acts that may be intended for them or others in their care. This need often keeps healthcare workers from focusing on other aspects of patient care.

Patients' inability to cope with rejection, disappointment, or other undesired feelings were associated with a higher likelihood of becoming violent while being mandated to an inpatient treatment setting (Bousardt *et al.*, 2016). The rise in patient aggression and violent incidents

213

reported through staff feedback has demonstrated a need for a quality improvement project to change safety policies and develop a protocol to help reduce the risk of aggression and violence towards staff and other patients. According to Morrison *et al.* (2002), exposure to violence in the forensic psychiatric inpatient sector affects employees and has implications for the quality of care provided.

DEVELOPING PROJECT FOCUS AND OBJECTIVES

According to Bemker and Schreiner (2016), developing an implementation plan that would be cost efficient and improved quality of outcome in the areas of patient satisfaction can reduce harm. An accurate risk prediction would facilitate the development of a violence prevention protocol that reflects policy based on current evidence preventative measures (Stevenson *et al.*, 2015). The focus of the DNP project was to develop safety policies and create a safety plan that was designed to help nurses recognize common predictors related to potential aggression and violence among psychiatric patients.

The goal of this project was to implement safe practice policies and protocols within a forensic psychiatric inpatient practice setting. Objectives are measurable actions that result in goal achievement (Moran *et al.*, 2017). The following objectives are proposed in this DNP project to support this goal.

1. Develop a patient violence policy and protocol for implementation
2. Implement a safety training program for staff that addresses changes in policies and procedures for the management of patient violence
3. Evaluate the effectiveness of the policy, protocol, and program through chart review, surveys, and randomized observation for appropriate application of the policy and protocol over the following three weeks post policy implementation

The overall outcome of this DNP project was met. This project helped the nursing staff and other healthcare providers become familiar with current and evidenced-based practice related safety policies and protocols. The DNP project was an effective source for healthcare worker safety, risk of violence, injury reduction, and better patient outcomes.

In addition, the DNP project benefited the staff who used the safety findings to obtain effective strategies for gaining insight into safety. The safety methods and techniques helped nursing staff and other healthcare workers to better prepare and handle violent incidents safely. The DNP project may also be helpful for future researchers in relation to differing situations and safety approaches.

DESCRIPTION OF PROBLEM/TARGET POPULATION

The focus of the literature search was to find scholarly documentation that provides evidence related to safety and the risk of violence and injury to the staff members when providing care for psychiatric inpatients. The literature review, directed toward the project topic, was helpful in developing safety policies and protocols for the nursing staff and other healthcare workers at the practice setting. To reach this goal, systematic reviews and previous research studies were evaluated for their content and appropriateness to this project. A comprehensive literature review provides evidence to defend a logical argument supporting the need for the value of the proposed scholarly project (Moran *et al.*, 2017).

Research by Stevenson *et al.* (2015) described the experience of registered nurses with violent patients on acute care, psychiatric, and inpatient units. Data taken from a 12-month period demonstrated that almost one-third (29%) of the nurses in the study were physically assaulted, nearly half (44%–55%) were emotionally and verbally abused, whereas others (19.5%) experienced sexual abuse. Gross (2016), when citing the work of Seager, reviewed statistical information through state public records related to aggressive incidents, violence, and assaults that were reported in five state hospitals in California. Over 42% of the assaults reported, 11,000, were documented to be directed toward hospital staff.

According to Iozzino *et al.* (2015), there was a significant potential for violence within the psychiatric inpatient setting. Exposure to a violent environment can directly affect physical and mental health of nurses and other healthcare workers. Due to the nature of the problem, the safety of health care workers was a priority.

In a study conducted by Short *et al.* (2008), a team of clinicians at the Ohio Department of Mental Health developed guidelines for injury-free management of psychiatric inpatients in pre-crisis and crisis situations.

The guidelines focus on best practices of effective communication. The healthcare workers are not to use the word "no" when talking to patients; all responses needed to be framed in a positive way and needed to be utilized while patients appear calm and controlled.

These healthcare workers were interviewed and surveyed frequently (at least weekly) for their input regarding effectiveness to update the guidelines. This descriptive methodology for investigation of the information and the criteria was established and needed for the safety guidelines used in the psychiatric facilities with aggressive patients. The safety guidelines were based on eight elements of care associated with positive communication practice by all nursing staff and other healthcare workers over a four-year period, in a psychiatric patient setting. The outcomes of the safety guidelines resulted in a paradigm shift in which the staff no longer found getting hurt on the job acceptable.

The evidence from this investigation indicated that overall violence and aggression decreased and reduced incidents by 90% (from 91 to 9; Short *et al.*, 2008). The incidents recorded by the Occupational Safety and Health Administration (OSHA) decreased by 70% (from 40 to 9 incidents); loss of workdays decreased by 77% (from 22 to 5 incidents); use of restraint and seclusions decreased by 36% (from 301 to 191 incidents); patient complaints decreased by 37% (from 291 to 181 incidents); and psychiatric codes decreased by 25% (from 346 to 259 incidents). The findings noted here support that safety guidelines reduced a rate of violence and aggression of psychiatric patients toward healthcare workers. The review and synthesis of scholarly literature, methods, and techniques discussed above support and are clearly relevant to the project topic after the new practices were initiated (Short *et al.*, 2008).

Safe care has always been a concern within the profession of nursing. Safety for both staff and patient remain a priority in relation to the work environment. As previously noted, this was especially true when addressing safety needs in a psychiatric facility (Stevenson *et al.*, 2015). The literature clearly identifies the prevalence of aggression of psychiatric inpatients and that the need for prevention was clearly indicated.

The population of interest in the DNP project was the nursing staff, which includes registered nurses (RNs), licensed vocational nurses (LVNs), and psychiatric technicians (PTs) who provide direct patient care on the units for over six to seven hours a day. Incidents of patient aggression and violence are higher among nursing staff. Psychiatric nurses report the highest violence victimization rates of all types of nurses (Jonker *et al.*, 2008).

According to The Joint Commission's publication, National Patient Safety Goals for Hospitals Standards (2008), sound treatment design and intrinsic delivery of safe high-quality inpatient services support the goals to decrease and eliminate staff injuries. By offering specific insights into policy and protocol related to violence noted in the healthcare environment, this review of scholarly literature identifies methods and techniques in supporting the project topic and its aim (Moran *et al.*, 2017).

DNP PROJECT INTERVENTIONS

Theoretical frameworks help in understanding forces that maintain current behavior and identify those that need to be modified to bring about change (Smith, 2001). The theoretical foundation that supported this project was that of Kurt Lewin (Lewin, 1992). The use of a change model may become an important tool for continuing education for evaluators or organizations as the beginning of a journey toward evidenced-based practice (EBP) demonstrated through projects in clinical settings.

Lewin's Theory of Change was a classic or fundamental approach to managing change in a healthcare setting (Cummings, Bridgman, and Brown, 2016). Manchester *et al.* (2014) discusses the mechanism for EBP planners to anticipate the contextual effect as programs unfreeze their host settings, create movement, and become refrozen. Therefore, planning for contextual change appears equally important as planning for the actual practice outcomes among providers and patients. Lewin's theory was a positive impact directed toward nurses at the practice site, via policy change and educating nurses.

The systematic quantitative review by Tölli *et al.* (2017) identified current knowledge and effects of training interventions for managing patients' challenging behavior. According to Young *et al.* (2017), the process evaluation results provided contextual information about intervention implementation and delivery with which to interpret other aspects of the program. The evidence-based training interventions that focus on safely managing the challenging behavior of patients were observed and evaluated.

The significance of the DNP project intervention was assessed for the participants' attentiveness to education and training on the safety policy and safety plan. The nursing staff from the pilot units were followed through with in-services and completion of safety policy training. The participants also self-reported on instances of improvement in patient care as a function of their training and experience. The findings on the incidental reports included changes in the number/types of patients' interpersonal interactions during care and counseling practices.

The project leader observed significant results of nursing staffs' frequent and safer involvement in patient education, team collaboration, documentation, and other service changes. The delivery of staff training to address current patient-related violence and aggression identified needs for additional training for the nursing staff. According to Tölli *et al.* (2017), the individuals need to evaluate staff competence in managing challenging patients' behavior.

In relevance to clinical practice, the nursing staff who received adequate training would consider the training relevant to their working situations. The nursing staff who frequently care for assaultive patients were addressing the lack of staff safety to the organization and management and suggested safety policy review and training needs (West, Galloway, and Niemeier, 2014). The review of updated safety policies promoted safety awareness, staff confidence, and staff support during care and incidents of aggressive, assaultive acts directed by psychiatric inpatients.

During the project implementation and evaluation phase, the data gathered for such events was considered highly personal and sensitive. Careless handling can cause a loss of privacy and affect personal data (Costa, Andrade, and Novais 2013). The project leader met with the project mentor, stakeholders, course instructor, and academic mentor to seek guidance when conducting activities, while maintaining privacy and confidentiality of participants' data information and technology procedures. Responsible methods were exercised to protect the confidentiality and privacy of the participants (Smith *et al.,* 2017).

The following individuals are considered to have an interest in this DNP project, are stakeholders of this project, and helped with advertisement of the safety plan using inter-hospital intranet, email, and standard mail: administrative departments such as the Psychiatric Nursing Director, Standards Compliance Manager, Project Mentor, Safety Manager, and Information Technology Director. The safety policy was distributed by the assistance of the managers and mentors on the units. The project leader was conscientious of appropriate incentives, when indicated. According to Taylor-Piliae and Froelicher (2007), providing incentives creates excellent communication, personal attention, encouragement, and attendance of the audience.

Nurses on the pilot units were given a pre-knowledge survey regarding their baseline understanding regarding management of the combative patient. The safety plan was distributed on the units through a safety policy handout. The safety policy was reviewed through 20 to 30 minutes of formal in-services to the RN, LVN, and PT on the pilot units. The synopsis of safety policy was extracted into a safety plan and wall posters were created and displayed for easy access of safety tips to promote and maintain safe environment for the staff on the pilot units. The safety policy review, training, and education were also implemented through formal in services during new employee orientation and annual mandatory education.

The primary goal of the safety plan was to establish and maintain an optimum level of safety in the workplace. The following safety plan was included in the safety policy. The project lead provided the updated safety policy to the unit managers and nursing mentors; the policy was reviewed with unit staff. The unit staff signed an attendance sheet upon completion of the safety policy review and 20 to 30 minutes of formal training. A laminated copy of the safety plan was also distributed in the units. Upon completion of review of safety policy and plan, the data on patient aggression and violence through incident reports were reviewed again in four to six weeks to determine the safety plan effectiveness.

This safety plan implementation helped unit nursing staff by providing them with a uniform approach to assessment, intervention, and treatment when handling violent psychiatric inpatients. The project lead provided in-services training on the safety policy and safety plan. The project leader met with an auditor to collect data from the incidental reports for the number of incidental episodes of patient aggression and violence towards staff on the units. Additional data were reviewed by the project leader in the patient charts, in which a patient's current progress was documented as an ongoing treatment and evaluation. The course instructor, academic mentor, and project mentor continued to guide the project lead and support project development. The Touro University statistician assisted with statistical techniques and actual outcomes.

Managing a DNP project includes the guiding of the participants and stakeholders, processes, time necessary to complete the project, and answering the project question (Bemker and Schreiner, 2016). The DNP project conducted at a psychiatric hospital with a focus on implementing safety measures to staff members that provide patient care. The project timeline activities include building close working relationships with key stakeholders, obtaining Institutional Review Board (IRB) approval, weekly project team meetings, implementation of new safety program, and continual evaluation and a staff communication plan. The anticipated project timeline was approximately four to six weeks. The week by week plan was as follows.

Week 1

The project leader set up a meeting with the key stakeholders to introduce the DNP project and plans for the intervention implementation. The project leader arranged meeting with key stakeholders, including the administrative director, and explained the details of the project. During this week, the project lead began initial preparations on data gathering tools. The safety plan was distributed to the stakeholders for review; confidentiality and protection of the personal and private information of the participants was maintained.

Week 2

The project leader reviewed feedback provided by stakeholders and completed a final revision of the safety plan. A weekly update was coordinated to discuss the project status with the project team, which included the project mentor, content expert, academic mentor, and project instructor. Emphasis was placed on incorporating input and feedback from the project team and stakeholders, as well as discussing the importance of inclusions and exclusions of elements in the safety plan.

Week 3

The project leader set up a meeting with the managers of pilot units, nurse mentor, nurse educator, and information technology director to discuss safety plan details and in-services. The project leader conducted a pre-knowledge survey on the safety plan with the nursing staff. During this week, the project lead finalized the safety plan PowerPoint presentation, prepared handout materials, displayed wall posters, and began providing 20 to 30 minute in-services of the safety plan to the nursing staff of the pilot units.

Weeks 4 to 5

The project leader observed interaction with nursing staff to determine if training provided was being practiced. The project leader also monitored incidental reports involving patient violence to determine factors leading to violence and actions taken by staff members. Reports of unit observations and incident reports were presented to the project team for analysis and recommended actions or modifications to safety program. The project leader continued to conduct unit observations and incident report audits and report findings during project team meetings for recommended actions or modifications. The project leader conducted a post knowledge survey on the safety plan for the nursing staff.

Week 6

The final evaluation of the safety plan dissemination, intervention outcome, and results determined the effectiveness of the intervention through reviewing charts, post knowledge surveys, and data analysis interpretations. The safety policy was reviewed through in-services on the pilot units to promote awareness of safety for nursing staff during patient care.

The DNP project promoted the safety plan through the safety policy, which was designed to help nurses recognize common predictors related to potential aggression and violence, be aware of a patients' history of trauma, and enhance effective communication (what, when, when, how, who, and why) with patients. The project also helped nurses communicate with the clinical staff, locate psychiatric emergency equipment, and collaborate with the treatment team. An empirical knowledge of the safety plan provided staff with tools to prevent violence and minimize its consequences.

DATA COLLECTION, MEASUREMENT TOOLS, ANALYSIS

The statistical analysis selected was used to evaluate the impact of the interventions on safety of the nurses with high scores and the statistical significance of safety awareness and safety preparation, where practitioners commonly see this particular behavior in (1) those patients who became violent and (2) those who did not become violent. A nonparametric t-test, such as the Mann-Whitney test, comparing those who became violent from those who did not. The behaviors were evaluated with a high significant difference ($P < 0.05$). The intended outcomes would indicate a decrease in reduced assaultive incidents and improved confidence and job satisfaction among psychiatric nursing staff, promoting positive and effective patient care as a response to the interventions.

During the evaluation phase, the project lead maintained privacy of information by de-identifying names of participants, date of birth, and other personal information when collaborating with the training department, standards of compliance departments, and electronic services using an intranet for updated data from incident reports at the practice setting. Ongoing progress and the positive impact of the safety plan were reviewed, and any pertinent information was collected from the stakeholders by meeting with them weekly and as needed. Gathering research data following these methodologies often requires preparing situations, tasks, or activities that engage participants to interact with a specific theme or to mobilize specific communication skills (Canals, 2017).

Various studies suggest that it was beneficial to develop instruments and protocols that are tailored to the unique needs/experiences of collecting data (Simons, 2011). A variety of tools and instruments were used for implementation and evaluation of the following project. The updated safety policy was distributed through inter-hospital mail and intranet.

The pre-and post-knowledge survey scores within the individual to control for the variations among individuals. This was analyzed using a Mann-Whitney test, which also refers to repeated measures used when groups of independent and dependent variables indicate data output on two different occasions or under two different conditions (Pallant, 2016). Using statistical analysis, the project leader for the DNP project was implementing interventions to support the nursing staff in reducing patient related aggressive and assaultive incidents, and promoting safety improvement during patient care.

During training, the nurse educator provided a handout on the safety plan to each member of the nursing staff. The safety plan inservices were conducted using handouts and a PowerPoint presentation. During the DNP project development, various databases were been used to collect pertinent data related to incidences of violence. The pre- and post knowledge questionnaires were conducted with unit nursing staff.

In discussion with Peek-Asa et al. (2009) through email, the validity and reliability of the tool were assessed to ensure accuracy and training staff until less than a 5% error rate was accomplished before using the tool. The site assessors were trained on the tool until they had a consistent and replicable interpretation of the items. The final evaluation of the safety plan dissemination, intervention, and outcome and the results determined the effectiveness of the intervention through reviewing charts, post knowledge surveys, and data analysis interpretations. The safety policy was reviewed through in-services on the pilot units to promote awareness of safety for nursing staff during patient care.

Based on the findings in Table 11.1, there was a total of 17 incidents of patient violence directed toward other individuals, with 11 of those incidents reported on Unit A and six incidents reported on Unit B. A pre-and post-questionnaire was used to measure the understanding of safety plan policy. The analysis of variables used a Wilcoxon signed rank test to evaluate the effect of the training intervention. The results of the pre-and post-questionnaires linked the pre-test scores with the post-test scores to control for variation among individuals.

There was a total of 15 reported incidents of violence directed toward other individuals, in which 10 of those incidents are reported on Unit A and five reported on Unit B. The reported incidents of violent behavior reduced from 22% to 20% following an educational intervention. This was a decrease by 2%. The pre-and post-questionnaire was completed by 12 participants.

The results from the questionnaires indicated that there was an increase of knowledge, awareness, and training among 10 participants on the safety policy and safety plan from 66% to 83%, with one participant scheduled off work and unable to attend and one participant a no show. The results of the pre- and post- questionnaires showed an increase of 17% following implementation of the safety policy and safety plan. Based on the pre- and post-chart reviews, the above table showed that there was an increase of the nurses' knowledge and awareness of safety following the education intervention.

TABLE 11.1. Safety Improvement.

Pre- and Post-Intervention Over 3 Months	Behavioral Incidents of Among 75 Patients	Behavioral Incidents of Among 75 Patients Safety Policy Updates	Knowledge & Awareness of Among 12 Nurses
Pre-Intervention	17 (22%)	2014	8 (66%)
Post-Intervention	15 (20%)	2018	10 (83%)
Improvement	2 (2%)		2 (17%)

CONCLUSION

The rising trend in patient aggression and violent incidents reported through staff feedback demonstrated a need for a quality improvement project. Therefore, a change in safety policies and the development a protocol helped reduce the risk of aggression and violence toward nursing staff. The strong evidence-based results of the review of synthesis indicated this model could be used in similar healthcare settings and could provide a positive impact.

The QI project was expected to promote safety and awareness at a practice site by implementing a safety policy and a training in-service to staff. The data analyzed included knowledge questionnaires and electronic health records. Both parametric (t-test, Pearson) and nonparametric (Mann-Whitney U, Chi Square) statistical tests were used to analyze the data. According to Bemker and Schreiner (2016) descriptive statistics consisted of raw proportions for each of the variables pre- and post-interventions. Questionnaires were stratified by individual categories. The post questionnaires were used to assess the data. which was consistent with changes in behavior, knowledge, and attitude of the participants (Fernández-Morano et al., 2015). Evaluation of the intervention used qualitative and quantitative data to analyze the findings.

Results from the questionnaires indicated that there was an increase of knowledge, awareness, and training among 10 participants on the safety policy and safety plan from 66% to 83%, with one participant scheduled off work and unable to attend and one participant a no show. The results of the pre- and post- questionnaires showed an increase of 17% following implementation of the safety policy and safety plan. Based on the pre- and post-chart reviews, the data showed that there was an increase of the nurses' knowledge and awareness of safety following the education intervention.

The comparison of results from pre- and post-chart reviews following the education intervention showed an increase of the nurses' knowledge and awareness of safety procedures and overall improvement care, including a reduction in violent incidents by patients toward the nurses. This project illustrates the direct relationship between knowledge and performance. When staff members were knowledgeable regarding policies and expectations are clearly outlined, their performances were enhanced, leading to favorable outcomes.

REFERENCES

Bemker, M., & Schreiner, B. (2016). *The DNP degree & capstone project: A practical guide.*

Bousardt, A. C., Hoogendoorn, A. W., Noorthoorn, E. O., Hummelen, J. W., and Nijman, H. I. (2016). Predicting inpatient aggression by self-reported impulsivity in forensic psychiatric patients. *Criminal Behaviour & Mental Health, 26*(3), 161–173. doi:10.1002/cbm.1955

Canals, L. (2017). Instruments for Gathering Data. Available from: http://web.a.ebscohost.com.lbproxy2.touro.edu/ehost/detail/detail?vid=11&sid=c99a99e8-39dd-4935-9eb86426ad4614e8%40sessionmgr4006&bdata=JnNpdGU9ZWhvc3QtbGl2ZQ%3d%3d #AN=ED573582&db=eric

Costa, Â., Andrade, F., & Novais, P. (2013). Privacy and data protection towards elderly healthcare. In M. M. Cruz-Cunha, I. M. Miranda, P. Gonçalves, M. M. Cruz-Cunha, I. M. Miranda, P. Gonçalves (Eds.), Handbook of research on ICTs for human-centered healthcare and social care services, Vols. I & II (pp. 330–346). Hershey, PA, US: Medical Information Science Reference/IGI Global. doi:10.4018/xxx-x-xxxx-xxxx-x.ch017

Cummings, S. S., Bridgman, T. T. and Brown, K. K. (2016). Unfreezing change as three steps: Rethinking Kurt Lewin's legacy for change management. *Human Relations, 69*(1), 33–60.

Fernández-Morano, T., de Troya-Martín, M., Rivas-Ruiz, F., Blázquez-Sánchez, N. and Buendía-Eisman, A. (2015). Sensitivity to change of the beach questionnaire to behaviour, attitudes and knowledge related to sun exposure: quasi-experimental before-after study. BMC public health, 1560. doi:10.1186/s12889-015-1415-0

Iozzino, L., Ferrari, C., Large, M., Nielssen, O. and de Girolamo, G. (2015). Prevalence and risk factors of violence by psychiatric acute inpatients: A systematic review and meta-analysis. *Plus one, 10*(6), e0128536. doi:10.1371/journal.pone.0128536

Gross, L., (2016, October 3). State of health at California psychiatric hospitals, epidemic of patients' assaults on staff goes untreated. Public Media for Northern California. Retrieved from psychiatric-hospitals-epidemic-of-patients-assaults-on-staff-goes-untreated/

Jonker, E., Goossens, P., Steenhuis, I. and Oud, N. (2008). Patient aggression in clinical psychiatry: Perceptions of mental health nurses. *J Psychiatric Mental Health Nursing, 15,* 492–9.

Kivimies, K., Repo-Tiihonen, E., Kautiainen, H. and Tiihonen, J. (2014). Previous forensic mental examination is a useful marker indicating effective violence relapse prevention among psychotic patients. *Nordic Journal of Psychiatry, 68*(5), 311–315. doi:10.3109/08039488.2013.8

Lewin, M. (1992). The impact of Kurt Lewin's life on the place of social issues in his work. *Journal of Social Issues, 48,* 2, 15–29.

Manchester, J., Gray-Miceli, D. L., Metcalf, J. A., Paolini, C. A., Napier, A. H., Coogle, C. L. and Owens, M. G. (2014). Facilitating Lewin's change model with collaborative evaluation in promoting evidence-based practices of health professionals. *Evaluation and Program Planning, (47)* 82–90. doi:10.1016/j.evalprogplan.2014.08.007

Moran, K., Burson, R and Conrad, D., (2017). The doctor of nursing practice scholarly project. (2nd ed.)., Jones and Bartlett Learning. Burlington, MA.30770

Morrison E1., Morman G., Bonner G., Taylor C., Abraham I., Lathan L. (2002) Reducing staff injuries and violence in a forensic psychiatric setting. *Arch Psychiatr Nurs.*

Jun;16(3):108-17. Retrieved from http://psychology.wikia.com/wiki/Client_violence

Pallant, J. (2016). A step by step guide to data analysis using IBM SPSS. (6th ed.) Berkshire, England: McGraw-Hill Education.

Peek-Asa, C., Casteel, C., Allareddy, V., Nocera, M., Goldmacher, S., Ohagan, E. and Harrison, R. (2009). Workplace violence prevention programs in psychiatric units and facilities. *Archives of Psychiatric Nursing, 23*(2), 166–176. doi:10.1016/j. apnu.2008.05.008

Ridenour, M., Lanza, M., Hendricks, S., Hartley, D., Rierdan, J., Zeiss, R. and Amandus, H. (2015). Incidence and risk factors of workplace violence on psychiatric staff. Work, 51(1), 19–28. Available from: https://doi.org/10.3233/WOR-141894

Short, R., Sherman, M. E., Raia, J., Bumgardner, C., Chambers, A. and Lofton, V. (2008). Safety guidelines for injury-free management of psychiatric inpatients in pre-crisis and crisis situations. *Psychiatric Services (Washington, D.C.), 59*(12), 1376-1378. doi:10.1176/appi.ps.59.12.1376

Simon, R. I. (2011). Patient violence against health care professionals. *Psychiatric Times, 28*(2), 16–21.

Smith, C. T., Nevitt, S., Appelbe, D., Appleton, R., Dixon, P., Harrison, J. and Tudur Smith, C. (2017). Resource implications of preparing individual participant data from a clinical trial to share with external researchers. *Trials*, 181-8. doi:10.1186/ s13063-017-2067-4.

Smith, M. K. (2001). Kurt Lewin: groups, experiential learning and action research. The Encyclopedia of Informal Education. http://www.infed.org/thinkers/et-lewin. htm, 1–15.

Stevenson, K. N., Jack, S.M., O'Mara, L. and Legris, J. (2015). Registered nurses' experiences of patient violence on acute care psychiatric inpatients units: an interpretive description study. *BMC Nursing, 14*(1), 1–13. Doi: 10.1186/s12912-ow5-0079-5

Taylor-Piliae, R. and Froelicher, E. (2007). Methods. Methods to optimize recruitment and retention to an exercise study in Chinese immigrants. *Nursing Research, 56*(2), 132–136.

The Joint Commission, (2008). National patient safety goals: Behavioral healthcare program. Oakbrook Terrace Ill. Retrieved from www.jointcommission.org/patient-safety

Tölli, S., Partanen, P., Kontio, R. and Häggman-Laitila, A. (2017). A quantitative systematic review of the effects of training interventions on enhancing the competence of nursing staff in managing challenging patient behaviour. *Journal of Advanced Nursing, 73*(12), 2817–2831. doi:10.1111/jan.13351

West, C. A., Galloway, E. and Niemeier, M. T. (2014). Resident aggression toward staff at a center for the developmentally disabled. Workplace Health & Safety, 62(1), 19–26.

Young, G. J., Lewis, A. L., Lane, J. A., Winton, H. L., Drake, M. J. and Blair, P. S. (2017). Statistical analysis plan for the urodynamics for prostate surgery Trial; Randomized evaluation of assessment methods (UPSTREAM). *Trials*, 181-7. doi:10.1186/s13063-017-2206-y

Assessment of Knowledge Regarding Obesity Preventative Methods Among African American Children Ages 9 to 11

SELENA A. GILLES, DNP, ANP-BC, CNECL, CCRN

PROBLEM IDENTIFICATION/STATEMENT

In the United States (U.S.), childhood obesity has become a significant healthcare concern. Obesity has reached epidemic proportions affecting 17% of all children and adolescents in the U.S. In 2009–2010, non-Hispanic black girls were significantly more likely to be obese than non-Hispanic white girls (Centers for Disease Control and Prevention [CDC], 2012). Results from the 2007–2008 National Health and Nutrition Examination Survey (NHANES) showed that among New York City (NYC) children ages 6 to 11, 21.3% were obese versus 19.6% nationally (CDC, 2011; New York City Obesity Task Force, 2012). In addition, two out of five NYC elementary school children remain overweight and obese (New York City Obesity Task Force, 2012).

Not only is it a problem in high-income countries like the U.S., but also overweight and obesity are now dramatically on the rise in low and middle-income countries, especially in urban settings. According to the World Health Organization (WHO) (2013), more than 10% of the world's adult population is obese. Worldwide, obesity has nearly doubled since 1980. More than 40 million children under age five were overweight in 2011 globally. In addition, there are more than 30 million overweight children living in developing countries and 10 million in developed countries (WHO, 2013a). The prevalence of overweight and obesity are highest in the WHO Regions of the Americas, where 62% of the population are overweight and 26% are obese (WHO, 2013b).

227

DEVELOPING PROJECT FOCUS AND OBJECTIVES

The purpose of this study was to assess the knowledge of obesity preventative methods among African American children ages 9 to 11 in a community center in Brooklyn, New York. The study answers the clinical question, "Among African American children ages 9 to 11, what percentage of children have knowledge of obesity preventative methods?" The effectiveness of an implemented education program on obesity preventative measures was also determined. One of the objectives of this study was to help these children shape a positive behavioral history for the future by focusing on the benefits of healthy eating and teaching them how to overcome the hurdles to making healthy choices. It was of top priority to get children to commit to a plan of action to engage in health promoting behaviors to attain positive health outcomes.

DESCRIPTION OF PROBLEM/TARGET POPULATION

For children, overweight is defined as a body mass index (BMI) at or above the 85th percentile and lower than the 95th percentile, when compared to children of the same age and sex. Obesity is defined as a BMI at or above the 95th percentile (CDC, 2012). Studies have shown a correlation between socioeconomic status and obesity. Wang and Zhen (2006) examined these trends using national representative data collected in the NHANES between 1971 and 2002 for 30,417 U.S. children ages 2 to 18. Researchers concluded that there were considerable race, sex, and age differences observed in association with overweight and socioeconomic status. Not only was the prevalence of overweight and obesity higher in blacks than in whites consistently across all socioeconomic groups, but also African American children with a high socioeconomic status were at increased risk for overweight and obesity. Researchers concluded that it is vital to tailor prevention and management efforts to each particular ethnic group to ensure efficiency and effectiveness (Wang and Zheng, 2006). Gamble *et al.* (2012) examined obesity and health risk of children in the Mississippi Delta. Among 1136 children in first through fifth grade studied, 47.1% were overweight and 28.8% obese. Researchers suggested that the obesity epidemic is continuing to manifest in minority children of low socioeconomic status at an increasingly younger age (Gamble *et al.,* 2012). In a study by Slusser *et al.* (2005) that examined nutritional problems among low-income children of elementary school age in Los Angeles, researchers found that more than 35% of the 913 students grades K through 12 were classified as being at risk for being overweight or were overweight. The prevalence of overweight children was the highest among the African American and Hispanic children (Slusser *et al.*, 2005). Slusser *et al.* (2005) concluded that development of multiple school-based intervention programs is crucial.

Cultural Attitudes and Behaviors

In the African American culture, food is used to celebrate special events, holidays, and birthdays and can be seen as a symbol of health and wealth (Purnell and Paulanka, 2008; Purnell, 2012). Their diet is frequently high in fat, cholesterol, and sodium, but low in fiber, fruits, and vegetables (Purnell and Paulanka, 2008). Commonly preparing foods by frying, barbequing, and using gravy or sauces, African Americans tend to eat more animal fat and prefer vegetables cooked as opposed to raw (Purnell and Paulanka, 2008; Purnell, 2012). Being overweight is often seen as positive or a sign of good health, with carrying additional weight affording them the ability to lose weight in times of sickness (Purnell and Paulanka, 2008; Purnell, 2012).

Researchers have uncovered that obese children are more likely to consume diets high in fat and low in fruit and vegetables than their normal-weight counterparts (Chen and Wang, 2011; Wang *et al.*, 2006; Wang *et al.*, 2007; Williams *et al.*, 2008). In examining obesity prevalence and associated risk factors among fifth to seventh grade African American adolescents participating in the HEALTHY-KIDS study, researchers discovered that over a seven-day period, 55% of adolescents consumed fried and/or high fat foods two or more times a day. In addition, 70% drank two or more sodas a day. Most adolescents did not eat the recommended servings of fruits and vegetables (Wang *et al.*, 2006; Wang *et al.*, 2007). Williams *et al.* (2008) examined breakfast consumption patterns in association with weight status and nutrient adequacy in African American children and concluded that children ages 6 to 12 are more likely to skip breakfast. Chen and Wang (2011) discovered that overweight or obese African American boys and girls had better food self-efficacy and healthier food choice intentions than their non-overweight peers, indicating that heavier adolescents may have a stronger desire to choose foods lower in fat and sugar (Chen and Wang, 2011). In a study that examined obesity among minority parents and children in relation to parents' food choices and eating habits, researchers discovered that food choices for parents and children are closely connected with culturally determined eating habits, foods that can be easily accessed, and foods that require minimal time for preparation (Sealy, 2010).

Perceptions

Researchers have uncovered that parents' perceptions and attitudes about their child's weight influence behaviors that will affect the child's health. Payas, Budd, and Polansky (2010) examined the relationship between parental concern for child's weight and childhood obesity (Payas, Budd, and Polansky, 2010). Almost half of the participants were considered obese, with a BMI greater than 30. In addition, mothers with a higher BMI were more likely to perceive their children as weighing more and were more concerned about their children's weight. According to the study, urban mothers were realistically aware that their children are either at risk or actually overweight (Payas, Budd, and Polansky, 2010). In looking at a child's perception of ideal body image (IBI) in relation to obesity and lifestyle behaviors in African American adolescents, Chen and Wang (2011) discovered that IBI was related to weight status in African American girls. The researchers found that girls with larger IBIs were more likely to be overweight or obese. In their study, 54% of overweight or obese boys and 78% of girls reported considering themselves being overweight or obese (Chen and Wang, 2011).

In a study that compared African American girls' and their parents' perceptions of girls' weight concerns and weight control behaviors, researchers discovered that girls reported engaging in weight control behaviors more frequently than parents perceived their daughters' behaviors (Dalton *et al.,* 2007). Parents consistently underreported girls' weight control behaviors, such as binging, purging, and skipping meals (Dalton *et al.,* 2007). The study concluded that increases in girls' endorsements of overconcern with weight, shape, and weight control behaviors were associated with increases in parent's perceptions of girls' endorsements. The majority of parents underreported girls' frequency of unhealthy behaviors (Dalton *et al.,* 2007).

Health Implications

Obese children are more likely to have high blood pressure and high cholesterol, which are risk factors for heart disease. According to the CDC (2012), 70% of obese children had at least one cardiovascular disease (CVD) risk factor, and 39% had two or more (CDC, 2012). Obesity has a strong correlation with atherosclerosis, with risk factors that accelerate the development of atherosclerosis beginning in childhood (National Heart, Lung, and Blood Institute [NHLBI], 2012). There is also evidence that there is an increase in the prevalence of overweight and hypertension, notably among ethnic minority children (Sorof *et al.* 2004). Obesity tracks most strongly from childhood into adulthood, among all the risk factors associated with CVD (NHLBI, 2012). According to the NHLBI (2012), the presence of obesity in childhood and adolescence is associated with increased evidence of atherosclerosis at autopsy. It is predicted that adolescent obesity will likely increase adult CHD by 5% to 16% over the next 25 years, with more than 10,000 excess cases of CHD predicted to be attributed to increased obesity in childhood (NHLBI, 2012).

Obese children also have an increased risk of impaired glucose tolerance, insulin resistance, and Type 2 diabetes mellitus (T2DM). According to the American Diabetes Association (ADA) (2013), about 1 in every 400 children and adolescence have TT2DM (ADA, 2013). The risk for T2DM rises with increases in BMI. In addition, approximately 85% of children with T2DM are overweight or obese at the time of diagnosis (ADA, 2013). In a study that examined the prevalence of risk for T2DM in 1076 school children ages 8 to 13, researchers discovered that nearly one third of children were overweight, with a higher prevalence among males and among African Americans and Hispanics (Urrutia-Rojas and Menchaca, 2006). In addition, nearly one fourth of the children in the study were found to be at risk for T2DM (Urrutia-Rojas and Menchaca, 2006).

Other health risks associated with childhood obesity include increased risk for fatty liver disease, gallstones, joint problems, musculoskeletal discomfort, and breathing problems, such as sleep apnea and asthma (CDC, 2012). Obese children and adolescents have a greater risk of social and psychological problems, such as discrimination or poor self-esteem, which can continue into adulthood. Obese children are more likely to become obese adults (CDC, 2012; Mayo Clinic, 2012). If children are overweight, obesity in adulthood is likely to be more severe. Adult obesity is associated with a number of serious health conditions, including heart disease, diabetes, and some cancers (CDC, 2012; Mayo Clinic, 2012).

PROJECT INTERVENTIONS

With increased recognition of the role of behavior in health promotion, the theoretical framework utilized for this study was Pender's Health Promotion Model (HPM) (Pender, 1996). The HPM is based on theories of human behavior and is an elaborate model that promotes healthy behaviors. The HPM offers a guide to explore the complex biopsychosocial processes that motivate individuals to engage in behaviors directed toward enhancing health, including prior related behavior influencing beliefs, affects, and enactment of health promoting behavior (Pender, Murdaugh, and Parsons, 2011). Application of the model to behavioral risks, such as poor nutrition, which can lead to obesity, necessitates the importance of assessing individual understanding of obesity, its long-term health effects, and preventative methods. According to Pender *et al.* (2011), individuals tend to invest time and resources in activities that have a high likelihood of positive outcomes. In addition, behaviors associated with positive effects are likely to be repeated, whereas those associated with negative effects are likely to be avoided. In Pender's model, the greater a commitment to a specific plan of action, the more likely health promoting behaviors are maintained over time (Pender, Murdaugh, and Parsons, 2011). With the use of the HPM in this study, the emphasis was placed on healthy eating and exercise in its relation to weight loss. The end goal of this study was to encourage these children to engage in health promoting behaviors to attain positive health outcomes.

Setting

The neighborhood selected for the study was in the southeastern portion of Brooklyn, NY, with over 200,000 residents, including a 60% African American population with a childhood obesity rate of 20.4% (The City of New York, 2011; NYU Furman Center, 2012). According to the New York City Department of Health and Mental Hygiene (NYCDOH, 2006) community health profile, more than one third of its residents were overweight and one fourth were obese (NYCDOH, 2006). In this neighborhood, overweight and obese adults were twice as likely to report having diabetes than their normal or underweight counterparts. In addition, residents who were born in the U.S. were more likely to be obese than those born elsewhere (NYCDOH, 2006). A windshield survey of the neighborhood revealed well-kept public places at which residents can gather to engage in physical activity, very few bike lanes, plenty of franchise fast food restaurants, and very little supermarkets that offer a variety of fresh fruit and vegetables.

Because the research supports developing obesity education programs for African American children, including school community-based programs, the study took place in a community center that serves more than 1,200 people daily (Fletcher *et al.*, 2009; Moyers, Bugle, and Jackson, 2005; Stines, Perman, and Sudharshan, 2011; Perman *et al.*, 2008). The center is a major source of educational, recreational, cultural, fitness, sports, and social-service programs for its residents, serving the diverse populations living in Southeast Brooklyn, including Jewish and African American families and a large population of immigrant families from the Caribbean, Asia, and Israel. As a primary source of support for working parents and their children, the center has social services, childcare, and recreational activities, including a day care program, after-school care, special needs programs, and youth and adult programs.

DATA COLLECTION, MEASUREMENT TOOLS, ANALYSIS

A quasi-experimental research design was utilized for this pilot study. This descriptive single sample study used a prospective design to answer the research questions. African American children ages 9 to 11 were assessed for their awareness of obesity preventative methods. The effectiveness of an educational intervention related to these subjects using a pre test and post-test design was determined. The study was used to understand if there is a need for further research or the development of further educational programs in this area based on the findings.

Sample

The sample population was recruited from the after-school program at the community center. The inclusion criteria for the study was African American ethnicity, age range of 9 to 11 years old, and able to speak, read, and write in English. The age range was determined based on the NHLBI Guidelines for Cardiovascular Health and Risk Reduction in Children and Adolescents. According to their recommendations, at ages 9 to 11, children should undergo universal lipid screening, a determinant of cardiovascular disease (NHLBI, 2012). After obtaining institutional IRB approval, potential participants for the study were initially identified by the community center director based on the inclusion criteria. The principal investigator (PI) visited the center during child pick up hours to speak with parents and recruit children for the study. The consents and assents were distributed to the 40 parents at the community center whose children met the inclusion criteria. Of these, nine were returned. There were no exclusions, so all nine took part in the study. The parents of the participants were provided full disclosure of the intent of the study and the research questions. The final sample was comprised of five girls and four boys. The final sample of participants ($n = 9$) ranged in ages from 9 to 11, with a mean age of 9.6 years. The sample was comprised of nine-year olds (33.33%, $n = 3$) and 10-year olds (66.67%, $n = 6$), with all participants being fourth graders.

Instrument

The instrument (Appendix A) utilized, The Children's Healthy Lifestyle Knowledge Assessment Tool, assessed children's knowledge regarding daily servings of food groups, healthy food choices, and time spent for daily physical activity and screen time. Utilized as both a pre test and a post-test, this tool contains 12 multiple-choice questions. The questions on the tool were developed by the PI based on information about obesity preventative measures as referenced by from the CDC, NHLBI, AHA, and the United States Department of Agriculture (USDA) (CDC, 2013: NHLBI, 2012; AHA, 2013b, USDA, n.d.).

Procedure

The study was conducted in a section of the community center's gymnasium that was utilized for group learning, with only the students who returned the parental consent and assent. On the day of the study, the PI was introduced to the children by the community center director. The PI began by explaining the purpose of the study and obtaining demographic information that included sex, age, and grade level. The PI explained and administered the pre-test (Appendix A) to all of the children. The children were allowed 10 minutes to complete it before it was collected and placed in an envelope labeled "Pre-test." The pre-test was confidential and did not contain any identifying information. No identifying demographic data was linked to any of the participants' pre tests.

Following the pre-tests, the children participated in a forty-minute educational intervention on obesity preventative methods. This included two interactive activities derived from the AHA and the *Let's Move* campaign. The children participated in activities that educated them about nutrition and exercise. Similar to the questions on the pre-test, the first activity involved identifying "everyday," "sometimes," and "never" foods adapted from AHA's *Food is Fuel* activity. The PI explained the difference between "everyday," "sometimes," and "never" foods to the children. "Everyday" foods are more nutritious and provide better fuel for the body. They also have vitamins and nutrients that the body can use every day. "Sometimes" foods do not have as much nutritional value and they can have a lot of calories, sugar, or unhealthy fats. "Never" foods are very unhealthy and should never be consumed (AHA, 2013b). Utilizing the surface of a desk and index cards with pictures of various foods, the children placed their cards under the "everyday," "sometimes," or "never" column. Each child was given eight cards. Once all of the children placed their cards, the PI reviewed the card placements and made necessary corrections. Subsequently, the PI continued to educate the children by informing them that one way to prevent obesity is to keep a diet balanced by picking foods from both the "everyday" and "sometimes" categories (AHA, 2013b). The children were then educated about the importance of having at least five servings of fruits and vegetables each day. In addition, participating in at least 60 minutes of physical activity each day, which balances energy in and energy out, was also stressed (AHA, 2013a; CDC, 2013). The second activity involved strategies to break up television time, derived from *Let's Move's Kids Take Action Plan*. The PI initiated a discussion related to how much time the children spend in front of a screen, including television, video games, and computer screens. The PI informed the children of the importance of limiting screen time to 2 hours a day (*Let's Move*, n.d.). The PI also discussed with the children ways to break up screen time with physical activity such as active house chores, jumping jacks, and dancing (*Let's Move*, n.d.). The PI then led the children in a brief physical activity that involved dancing to an up-tempo song to emphasize the importance of physical activity and gave them creative ways to stay active.

Immediately following the educational intervention, the PI administered the post-test, a replica of the pre-test. The children had 10 minutes to complete it before it was collected and placed in an enveloped labeled "Post-test." The post-test was confidential and did not contain any identifying information. No identifying demographic data were linked to any of the participants' post-tests. The children were sent home with AHA's Balance It Out handout that gave them information on daily serving requirements in the different food groups. In addition, they were given *Let's Move's Kids Take Action Plan* (AHA, 2013a; *Let's Move,* n.d.). The parents were sent home with *Let's Move African American Fact Sheet* and the *Let's Move* Pledge (*Let's Move,* n.d.).

Data Analysis

Data analysis began with descriptive statistics. SPSS was utilized for the analysis of all statistics for the research study. The frequency distributions and percentages of mean pre-test and post-test scores of The Children's Healthy Lifestyle Knowledge Assessment Tool were examined. The clinical question involved determining what percentage of children had knowledge of obesity preventative measures. To determine this, each pre-test was given an overall percentage score based on the number of correct responses out of the 12 questions, rounded to the nearest whole number. Based on the score, they were placed in one of four categories. Category 1 consisted of a score that ranged from 0 to 25, identifying the participant as "Not Knowledgeable." Category 2 consisted of a score that ranged from 26 to 50, labeling the participant as "Has Very Little Knowledge." Category 3 consisted of a score that ranged from 51 to 75, identifying the participant as "Somewhat Knowledgeable." Lastly, Category 4 consisted of a score that ranged from 76 to 100, identifying the participant as "Knowledgeable." Comparing the percentage of correct answers, as well as the participant category placements, on a pre-test and post-test was utilized to determine the effectiveness of the education intervention on healthy eating and physical activity.

Project Outcome

Pre and post intervention data were examined for the group as a whole, not by individual participant results. In looking at the pre-test item analysis (Table 12.1), when asked *How many servings of fruits and vegetables should I eat each day?*, only 44.4% of the group chose the correct answer of 5 servings. The majority of the group selected limiting screen time to less than or equal to 2 hours, with 44.4% selecting 2 hours and 33.3% selecting 1 hour of screen time. Time spent for physi-

TABLE 12.1. The Children's Healthy Lifestyle Knowledge Assessment Pre-test Item Analysis.

Item #	Question	Percentage Correct
1	How many servings of fruits and vegetables should I eat each day?	44.4% ($n = 4$)
2	How many hours should I limit my screen time to each day?	44.4% ($n = 4$)
3	How many minutes of activity should I get each day?	44.4% ($n = 4$)
4	"Everyday, Sometimes, or Never"—Chicken	44.4% ($n = 4$)
5	"Everyday, Sometimes, or Never"—Cookies	77.8% ($n = 7$)
6	"Everyday, Sometimes, or Never"—Strawberries	100% ($n = 9$)
7	"Everyday, Sometimes, or Never"—Donuts	22.2% ($n = 2$)
8	"Everyday, Sometimes, or Never"—Juice	88.9% ($n = 8$)
9	"Everyday, Sometimes, or Never"—Macaroni and Cheese	55.6% ($n = 5$)
10	"Everyday, Sometimes, or Never"—Milk	88.9% ($n = 8$)
11	"Everyday, Sometimes, or Never"—Soda	44.4% ($n = 4$)
12	"Everyday, Sometimes, or Never"—Yogurt	55.6% ($n = 5$)

cal activity was evenly distributed between 60 minutes (44.4%) and 90 minutes (44.4%). When labeling foods "everyday," "sometimes," or "never" foods, the items most frequently labeled correctly included cookies, strawberries, juice, and milk. Chicken was equally labeled "everyday" (44.4%) and "sometimes" (44.4%). Donuts were labeled "never" by 77.8% ($n = 7$) of the group. In addition, 55.6 % ($n = 5$) of the group selected soda as a "never" food.

Based on the pre-test overall percentage score, participants were then put into 1 of 4 categories (Category 1 score of 0–25; Category 2 score of 26–50; Category 3 score of 51–75; Category 4 score of 76–100). Eleven

TABLE 12.2. Group Analysis: Percentage of Children Knowledgeable of Obesity Preventative Measures.

Item #	Pre-test Category	Percentage
1	"Not knowledgeable"	0% ($n = 0$)
2	"Has very little knowledge"	33.3% ($n = 3$)
3	"Somewhat knowledgeable"	55.6% ($n = 5$)
4	"Knowledgeable"	11.1% ($n = 1$)

TABLE 12.3. *Group Analysis: Education Intervention*
Effectiveness Evaluation.

Category	Pre-test Mean = 56.44	Post-test Mean = 85.22
1	0 (n = 0)	0 (n = 0)
2	33.3 (n = 3)	0 (n = 0)
3	55.6 (n = 5)	0 (n = 0)
4	11.1 (n=1)	100 (n = 9)

percent of the group was categorized as "knowledgeable" of obesity preventative measures through healthy eating, limiting screen time, and physical activity (Table 12.2).

The scores pre intervention revealed a minimum score of 42% and maximum of 75%, with a mean of 56.44%. According to the pre test, only 11.1% (n = 1) of the children were categorized as "knowledgeable" of obesity preventative measures. In contrast, 55.6% (n = 5) were "somewhat knowledgeable." The scores post intervention revealed a minimum score of 75% and maximum of 100%, with a mean of 85.22%. The mean difference pre and post intervention (Table 12.3) showed an increase of 28.78 and an increase of frequency the group categorized as "knowledgeable" of 88.9%. This is statistically significant, $p < 0.05$ (Table 12.4).

TABLE 12.4. *Significance. Paired Samples Test.*

	Paired Differences							
				95% Confidence Interval of the Difference				
	Mean	Std. Deviation	Std. Error Mean	Lower	Upper	t	df	Sig. (2-tailed)
Pair 1, PRETEST SCORE– POSTTEST SCORE	−28.778	15.254	5.085	−40.503	−17.052	−5.660	8	

DISCUSSION

The results from this project show that the sample population was not knowledgeable of obesity preventative measures and that an educational intervention on healthy living would increase participant knowledge, giving them the information they need to lead a healthy lifestyle.

The biggest barrier in conducting and implementing this research project occurred in the recruitment phase. In addition, this small sample size was not a true representation of the community center's or the neighborhood's population. Another barrier was participant attentiveness. The children were motivated to learn and retain the proposed educational information but often had to be redirected and refocused. This small sample size, along with the one group pre-test and post-test design, weakens the results and does not allow for generalizability. In addition, subgroup differences, such as gender and age, could not be analyzed because pre and post intervention data were not analyzed individually but were done for the group as a whole. In addition, demographic data weres not linked to the pre-test and post test.

Recommendations for the Future

Shaping children's positive behaviors for the future by reinforcing the importance of healthy food choices and regular physical activity is of top priority. As previous studies have suggested, interventions conducted by community agencies are promising. Placing an emphasis on healthy eating and exercise can help children to develop and make a commitment to a plan of action of healthy eating and daily physical activity. In utilization of Pender's HPM, a major area of focus for future study will be how interpersonal influences determine an individual's predisposition to engage in health promoting behavior. Such interpersonal influences include expectations of significant others, social support, and modeling. In addition, utilizing these initiatives cannot only further aide children in being successful at combating childhood obesity, but also can also help get their parents involved. This study can be replicated in other communities and have the potential for greater impact with a larger sample size and a continuous education intervention that is spread out over time. In addition, to assess the impact of knowledge on overall health, pre and post BMI and food diaries can be utilized.

Nurses can play an intricate role in developing interventions that guide children toward adopting healthy lifestyles. As the studies have shown, educating our children is essential in eradicating childhood obesity, especially in the African American community. We need to utilize screening tools to identify children at risk. By addressing the learning needs of the children in our community and focusing on health promotion, practitioners can aide in eliminating health related knowledge deficits in the community. It is critical to improve healthcare outcomes by focusing on quality improvement strategies. Results from this and prior studies shows that school and community-based programs work. As nurses, it is important to teach children and adults about prevention of obesity and potential long-term health consequences of obesity going untreated.

We have to improve patient and population health outcomes by partnering with healthcare professionals in the community, in addition to supporting health promotion and illness prevention for these children and their families. This can be done by developing programs to educate children about the multifaceted risk factors of obesity, especially nutrition and physical activity. Forming partnerships with public health agencies, educational institutions, community and faith-based organizations, and governmental units to develop family nutritional and activity based programs should be a priority. These therapeutic relationships that are developed with professionals can facilitate optimal care and patient outcomes. More research needs to be done regarding the cultural aspects of food choices and viewpoints on physical activity.

CONCLUSION

In the U.S., childhood obesity has become a significant healthcare concern. With the rise in the prevalence of obesity in the U.S. over the past 30 years, parents are essential in eradicating childhood obesity. Obesity is more prevalent among African American children. They are at risk of developing several chronic diseases like Type 2 diabetes mellitus and cardiovascular disease. Health professionals in the community can play an intricate role in developing interventions that guide children toward adopting healthy lifestyles that can reduce childhood obesity and the health risks associated with it.

APPENDIX A: PRE-/POST-TEST: "CHILDREN'S HEALTHY LIFESTYLE ASSESSMENT TOOL"

Directions: Circle the best answer

How many servings of fruits and vegetables should I eat each day?

a. 0
b. 2
c. 5
d. 10

How many hours should I limit my screen time to each day?

a. 1
b. 2
c. 4
d. 6

How many minutes of activity should I get each day?

a. 10
b. 60
c. 90
d. 120

"**Everyday**" foods are more nutritious and provide better fuel for your body. They also have vitamins and nutrients that our body can use every day.

"**Sometimes**" foods do not have as much nutritional value and they can have a lot of calories, sugar or unhealthy fats.

"**Never**" foods are not nutritious and we should never eat them.

Look at the foods listed below and decide if they are "**everyday**," "**sometimes**," or "**never**" foods. Circle the best answer

Chicken

a. Everyday
b. Sometimes
c. Never

Cookies

a. Everyday
b. Sometimes
c. Never

Strawberries

a. Everyday
b. Sometimes
c. Never

Donuts

a. Everyday
b. Sometimes
c. Never

Juice

a. Everyday
b. Sometimes
c. Never

Macaroni & Cheese

a. Everyday
b. Sometimes
c. Never

Milk

a. Everyday
b. Sometimes
c. Never

Soda

a. Everyday
b. Sometimes
c. Never

Yogurt

a. Everyday
b. Sometimes
c. Never

REFERENCES

American Diabetes Association (2013a). *Diabetes basics* Retrieved September 28, 2013 from http://www.diabetes.org/diabetes-basics/diabetes-statistics/

American Diabetes Association (2013b). *Diabetes basics healthy eating* Retrieved September 28, 2013 from http://www.diabetes.org/diabetes-basics/prevention/checkup-america/healthy-eating.html

American Heart Association (2013a). *Balance it out food categories poster*. Retrieved February 10, 2014 from http://www.heart.org/idc/groups/heart-public/@wcm/@ global/documents/downloadable/ucm_305577.pdf

American Heart Association (2013b). *Food is fuel*. Retrieved February 10, 2014 from http://www.heart.org/idc/groups/heart-public/@wcm/@global/documents/down-loadable/ucm_305557.pdf

Centers for Disease Control and Prevention. (2011). *Prevalence of overweight, obesity, and extreme obesity among adults: united states, trends 1960–1962 through 2007–2008*. Retrieved September 28, 2013, from http://www.cdc.gov/nchs/data/ hestat/obesity_adult_07_08/obesity_adult_07_08.htm

Centers for Disease Control and Prevention. (2012). *Basics about Childhood Obesity*. Retrieved September 28, 2013, from http://www.cdc.gov/obesity/childhood/basics. html

Centers for Disease Control and Prevention. (2013). *Combatting childhood obesity*. Retrieved September 28, 2013 from http://www.cdc.gov/features/PreventChild-hoodObesity/

Chen, X.X., & Wang, Y.Y. (2012). Is ideal body image related to obesity and lifestyle behaviours in African American adolescents? *Child: Care, Health & Development, 38*(2), 219–228. doi:10.1111/j.1365-2214.2011.01227.x

The City of New York (2011). *Community snapshot 2011 CD18: canarsie, Brooklyn*. Retrieved April 30, 2014 from http://www.nyc.gov/html/acs/downloads/pdf/ cd_snapshots/brooklyn_cd18.pdf

Dalton, W., Klesges, L., Beech, B., Kitzmann, K., Kent, A. and Morris, K. (2007). Comparisons between African American girls' and parents' perceptions of girls' weight concerns and weight control behaviors. *Eating Disorders, 15*(3), 231–246.

Executive Office of the President of the United States (2010). *Solving the problem of childhood obesity within a generation*. Retrieved September 25, 2013 from http:// www.letsmove.gov/sites/letsmove.gov/files/TaskForce_on_Childhood_Obesity_ May2010_FullReport.pdf

Fletcher, A., Cooper, J.R., Helms, P., Northington, L. and Winters, K. (2009). Stemming the tide of childhood obesity in an underserved urban African American population: A pilot study. *The ABNF Journal, 20*(2), 44.

Gamble, A., Waddell, D., Allison Ford, M., Bentley, J. P., Woodyard, C. D., & Hallam, J. S. (2012). Obesity and health risk of children in the Mississippi delta. *Journal of School Health, 82*(10), 478–483. doi:10.1111/j.1746-1561.2012.00725.x

Horodynski, M.A., Arndt, M. J. (2004). "Eating-together" mealtimes with African-American fathers and their toddlers. *Applied Nursing Research, 18* (2005) 106–109.

Let's Move (n.d.). *Kids take action*. Retrieved February 10, 2014 from http://www. letsmove.gov/sites/letsmove.gov/files/pdfs/TAKE_ACTION_KIDS.pdf

Let's Move (n.d.). *Our pledge*. Retrieved February 15, 2014 from http://www.lets-move.gov/sites/letsmove.gov/files/pdfs/OurPledgeAccessible.pdf

Let's Move (n.d.). *The Facts for African Americans*. Retrieved February 15, 2014 from http://www.letsmove.gov/sites/letsmove.gov/files/Let%27s_Move_Fact_Sheet_ for_African%20Americans.pdf

Mayo Clinic. (2012). *Childhood obesity risk factors*. Retrieved October 24, 2013, from http://www.mayoclinic.com/health/childhood-obesity/ds00698/dsection=risk-factors

Moyers, P., Bugle, L. and Jackson, E. (2005). Perceptions of school nurses regarding obesity in school-age children. *Journal of School Nursing* (Allen Press Publishing Services Inc.), *21*(2), 86–93. doi:10.1177/10598405050210020501

National Heart, Lung, and Blood Institute (2012). *Expert panel on integrated guidelines for cardiovascular health and risk reduction in children and adolescents*. Retrieved September 12, 2013 from http://www.nhlbi.nih.gov/guidelines/cvd_ped/ peds_guidelines_sum.pdf

New York City Department of Education (2012). *Progress Report 2011-12*. Retrieved October 8, 2013 from http://schools.nyc.gov/OA/SchoolReports/2011-12/Progress_ Report_2012_EMS_K276.pdf

New York City Department of Education (2013). *School Wellness Programs*. Retrieved October 20, 2013 from http://schools.nyc.gov/Academics/FitnessandHealth/default. htm

New York City Department of Health and Mental Hygiene (2006). *Community health profiles take care canarsie and flatlands*. Retrieved April 30, 2014 from http://www. nyc.gov/html/doh/downloads/pdf/data/2006chp-208.pdf

NYU Furman Center (2012). *Brooklyn community district profiles BK18 flatlands canarsie*. Retrieved April 30, 2014 from http://furmancenter.org/files/sotc/SOC2012_ BK18.pdf

Office of the Press Secretary (2010). *Presidential memorandum—establishing a task force on childhood obesity*. Retrieved September 29, 2013 from http://www.whitehouse.gov/the-press-office/presidential-memorandum-establishing-a-task-force-childhood-obesity

Office of the Press Secretary (2011). Presidential proclamation—national childhood obesity awareness month. Retrieved September 29, 2013 from http://www.whitehouse.gov/the-press-office/2011/08/31/presidential-proclamation-national-childhood-obesity-awareness-month

Ogden, C L, Carroll, M, Curtin, L, Lamb, M, Flegal, K (2010) Prevalence of high body mass index in US children and adolescents 2007–2008. *Journal of American Medical Association, 303*(3), 242–249.

Payas, N., Budd, G. M., & Polansky, M. (2010). Exploring Relationships Among Maternal BMI, Family Factors, and Concern for Child's Weight. *Journal of Child & Adolescent Psychiatric Nursing, 23*(4), 223–230. doi:10.1111/j.1744-6171.2010.00248.x

Pender, N. (1996). *Health promotion in nursing practice* (3rd ed.) Stanford, CT: Appleton & Lange.

Pender, N., Murdaugh, C., Parsons, M. (2011). *Health Promotion in Nursing Practice* (6th ed.). Upper Saddle River, NJ: Pearson Education, Inc.

Perman, J.A., Young, T.A., Stines, E., Hamon, J., Turner, L.M. and Rowe, M.G. (2008). A community-driven obesity prevention and intervention in an elementary school. *Journal of the Kentucky Medical Association. 106*(3):104–8.

Purnell, L.D. & Paulanka, B. (2008). *Guide to culturally competent health care.* (2nd ed). Philadelphia, PA: F.A. Davis Company.

Purnell, L.D. (2012). *Transcultural health care: a culturally competent approach.* (4th ed). Philadelphia, PA: F.A. Davis Company.

Sealy, Y. (2010). Parents' food choices: obesity among minority parents and children. *Journal of Community Health Nursing, 27*(1), 1–11. doi:10.1080/07370010903466072

Slusser, W., Cumberland, W., Browdy, B., Winham, D. and Neumann, C. (2005). Overweight in urban, low-income, African American and Hispanic children attending Los Angeles elementary schools: research stimulating action. *Public Health Nutrition, 8*(2), 141–148.

Sorof, J., Lai, D., Turner, J., Poffenbarger, T. and Portman, R. (2004). Overweight, ethnicity, and the prevalence of hypertension in school-aged children. *Pediatrics, 113*(3 Part 1), 475–482.

Stines, E., Perman, S. and Sudharshan, S. (2011). Nurse Practitioner-Coordinated Childhood Obesity Early Intervention and Prevention Program. *Bariatric Nursing & Surgical Patient Care, 6*(3), 111–114. doi:10.1089/bar.2011.9960

Urrutia-Rojas, X. and Menchaca, J. (2006). Prevalence of risk for type 2 diabetes in school children. *Journal of School Health, 76*(5), 189–194. doi:10.1111/j.1746-1561.2006.00093.x

United States Department of Labor (2013). Occupational employment and wages, May 2012 Nurse Practitioner. Retrieved November 23, 2013 from http://www.bls.gov/oes/current/oes291171.htm

Williams, B., O'Neil, C., Keast, D., Cho, S. and Nicklas, T. (2008). Are breakfast consumption patterns associated with weight status and nutrient adequacy in African-American children? *Public Health Nutrition, 12*(4), 489–496. doi:10.1017/S1368980008002760

World Health Organization (2013a). Obesity and overweight. Retrieved September 26, 2013 from http://www.who.int/mediacentre/factsheets/fs311/en/index.html

World Health Organization (2013b). Obesity. Retrieved September 26, 2013 from http://www.who.int/gho/ncd/risk_factors/bmi_text/en/index.html

Part 4: Health Policy and Education Application

Implementing a Clinical Nurse Leader Shared Governance to Raise Nursing-Reported Empowerment

VERONICA RANKIN, DNP, RN-BC, NP-C, CNL

PROBLEM IDENTIFICATION/STATEMENT

My fulltime job prior to and during my Doctor of Nursing Practice (DNP) program journey was Clinical Nurse Leader (CNL) coordinator at my organization. As the CNL coordinator, my main responsibility was to ensure that CNL practice continued to advance and improve quality patient-related outcomes and that it also aligned with the American Association of Colleges of Nursing (AACN) white paper definition of the role. I identified, in this role as CNL Coordinator, the need to continue to raise empowerment within the practice of the CNL role to ensure that CNLs successfully act as change agents at the bedside. As a result, I employed many tactics over the years to raise empowerment and strengthen CNL credibility and practice quality. Unfortunately, some tactics failed to achieve the outcomes that I anticipated. The tactics I employed included more structured monthly workgroup meetings, robust annual retreats, meaningful annual requirements that reflected CNL training, and the institution of a CNL professional binder. Within the monthly workgroup meetings, I added a section on the agenda to allow CNL representatives to share important key points from their respective shared governance council meetings with the group. I felt the need to incorporate shared governance into the meetings, because it was well supported in the literature as a conduit for strengthening nursing empowerment. Although well supported at the medical center with CNLs embedded in unit based councils (UBCs), service lines, and organizational practice councils, there was no CNL shared governance structure (CNL Council). There was an Advanced Practice Council in place at the medical center, but because CNLs are not recognized as

247

advanced care practitioners, they could not serve on this council. Implementing a shared governance report out seemed beneficial at first, but it soon proved to be insufficient in impacting CNL empowerment.

Upon entering my DNP program, I realized that my project should focus on raising CNL empowerment and should therefore incorporate shared governance and some method of measuring empowerment. But before I can further expound upon my project, I must provide a high-level understanding of the CNL role.

CNLs are masters prepared advanced generalists trained to oversee the lateral integration and quality of clinical care provided to a cohort of patients (American Association of Colleges of Nursing [AACN], 2013; L'Ecuyer *et al.*, 2016). As the newest masters prepared role added to the profession of nursing in more than 40 years (Harris, Roussel, and Thomas, 2014), this role complements, instead of competes with, other clinically based graduate level nursing roles with a primary focus on patient outcomes (Rankin, 2015). CNLs serve as change agents, promoting practice transformation through the implementation of evidence-based practice at the point of care (AACN, 2007). This is done to improve processes of care that influence quality and patient safety to optimize patient outcomes (Bender *et al.*, 2016; L'Ecuyer *et al.*, 2016). This role is not an advanced practice nursing role such as the nurse practitioner, midwife, clinical nurse specialist, or nurse anesthetist, in which prescriptive authority and/or diagnosing capability is a responsibility. Nevertheless, it requires advanced clinician and nursing leadership skills to help drive positive outcomes at the bedside, where care is delivered.

In response to healthcare related challenges, the CNL role was implemented in the fall of 2009, where this DNP project took place. The program grew from 4 certified graduates in 2010 to more than 30 certified graduates in 2017. The medical center is the only facility that employs the CNL role throughout the diverse system's network of more than 40 facilities and 100 clinics. Furthermore, the medical center employs the largest number of certified practicing CNLs within one setting throughout the entire nation. Despite administrative oversight ensuring that practice aligns with the AACN CNL White Paper (AACN, 2007) and system goals, opportunities exist in self-governance and empowerment of this new role.

My initial idea was to create a leadership council within the CNL group to help vet ideas, drive timely decision-making, and effect change cohesively throughout my workplace. Although I wanted to ensure that all CNLs had an active voice, oftentimes it was difficult to make progress on change because of ineffective planning due to an excessive amount of opposing ideas or opinions, as well as the undertaking of too many initiatives simultaneously. My faculty advisor decided that this project idea was too close to research, which did not fit the criteria for a quality improvement scholarly project. Although this news was very disturbing, it helped me begin the process of formulating my quality improvement project idea using the concepts of importance that I identified early on.

LITERATURE SEARCH

To formulate my quality improvement DNP project idea, I searched the literature to explore the concept and purpose of nursing shared governance and its relation to nursing empowerment. A thorough electronic search of four databases included the following: The Cumulative Index to Nursing and Allied Health (CINAHL), Education Resources Information Center (ERIC), PubMed, and OVID. The search terms used were as follows: shared governance, nursing shared governance, governance council, structural empowerment, empowerment, empowerment survey, nursing council, nursing leadership, and unit-based council. Citations from selected articles were tracked and searched for more evidence within the literature. The searches were limited to full text peer-reviewed articles published in academic journals in less than five years and written in English. These limitations excluded many articles, but of those remaining, many more articles were excluded due to lack of appropriateness to the project's focus and subject matter. A total of 24 articles were relevant to this project and were therefore included in this literature review.

Numerous tools that measured empowerment, shared governance, autonomy, and job satisfaction were identified in the literature. These tools included the following: Conditions for Workplace Effectiveness Questionnaire-II (CWEQ-II), the Index of Professional Nursing Governance, the shared governance survey, the caring nurse-patient interactions scale, the safety climate survey, and the organizational culture inventory. The findings of the literature review were organized into overarching themes, including nursing engagement, autonomy, nursing satisfaction, nursing retention, and shared governance. Lastly, an evidence matrix was constructed to organize the evidence found in the literature.

Nursing Engagement

Shared governance is supported and described in the literature as an effective method to enhance nurse engagement because of its ability to promote professional nursing practice and shared decision-making among nursing staff that practice at the point of care (Jordan, 2016; Meline and Brehm, 2015; Sullivan, Warshawsky, and Vasey, 2013). McDonald *et al.* 2010 assessed the relationship of nursing participation in formalized work structures such as nursing councils and their perception of work empowerment. These authors used the same CWEQ-II tool to measure this relationship among registered nurses employed at a Veterans Affairs teaching hospital in an urban region of the United States (U.S). Of the 423 nurses within the target population, 138 (33%) nurses responded but only 122 (29%) surveys were completely filled out. The survey results revealed that the nurses felt a moderate amount of structural empowerment. Results of the survey also revealed that of the four CWEQ-II subscales, opportunity rated moderately high, resources and support both rated moderately high, and information rated moderately low. Organizational informal power rated moderately high and organizational formal power rated moderately low. McDonald *et al.* (2010) found significant correlational differences in the relationship of meeting attendance and support, as well as informal power and communication of information from meetings to nursing peers. This study supports the concept of empowered nurse engagement in pertinent professional matters to promote healthy productive work environments.

A study conducted by Wang and Liu (2013) supports the concept of nursing engagement by concluding that nurses who feel valued by their organization are engaged and more inspired to positively influence colleagues to achieve work goals in an efficient manner. This study used a predictive, non-experimental approach that included a random sample of 300 nurses working in two tertiary hospitals in China. Wang and Liu (2013) used three tools, including the Utrecht Work Engagement Scale, the Practice Environment Scale of the Nursing Work Index, and the Psychological Empowerment Scale, to evaluate the influence of the nursing environment and empowerment on nursing engagement. Study findings revealed a significant relationship between the practice environment and nursing empowerment that positively and directly influences engagement. Additionally, this study found that the practice environment could indirectly influence nursing engagement through the use of nursing empowerment. This essentially supports the notion that empowered CNLs will be more effective and engaged in their jobs.

Autonomy

A study by Bish, Kenny, and Nay (2012) revealed that nurses who feel supported and empowered to act autonomously lead change through their own decision-making abilities and therefore perform higher quality work and show higher levels of retention. Clavelle *et al.* 2016 stressed the importance of a shared governance structure transitioning into a professional governance structure that provides four foundational attributes to include "accountability, professional obligation, collateral relationships and decision-making" (Clavelle *et al.*, 2016, 310). Within the decision-making attribute, the authors note the need for an organized formal governance structure that demonstrates ownership for practice related decisions, identifies evidence-based opportunities and problems, and then creates, implements and evaluates the impact of made decisions (Clavelle *et al.*, 2016). These recommendations encourage governance by experts of the profession. Experts are called to serve as the accountable, autonomous members of the group that are obligated to advance outcomes through effective collaboration and effective decision-making (Clavelle *et al.*, 2016).

Nurse Satisfaction

Work by Choi *et al.* (2016) supported the premise that nursing empowerment significantly influences nursing job satisfaction. Choi *et al.* (2016) surveyed 200 nursing staff members at both a large private hospital and a public hospital in Malaysia. Using a Likert scale, employees answered questions assessing transformational leadership, empowerment, and job satisfaction at the workplace. Statistical analysis was conducted to determine the relationship between empowerment and job satisfaction. Results revealed a positive effect of transformational leadership on job satisfaction and empowerments, as well as a positive effect of empowerment on job satisfaction (Choi *et al.*, 2016).

Burkman *et al.* (2012) found that nursing job satisfaction was enhanced by activities such as expanding succession planning efforts, enhancing growth opportunities within leadership areas, promoting interprofessional collaboration activities, and continued professional development of mentors. These findings greatly support nurses aspiring to advance within their work area and specifically how these actions can positively affect job satisfaction.

Boswell *et al.* (2017) conducted a literature review on 27 articles using the terms job satisfaction, empowerment, work engagement, and shared governance. This review identified job satisfaction as a continued important outcome of shared governance, but it also noted that job satisfaction alone does not exclusively make up a healthy work environment. Boswell *et al.* (2017) noted that empowerment was a significant key factor in the attainment of job satisfaction for nurses.

A search of the literature found that the CWEQ-II was used frequently in studies throughout the world. One such study conducted by Teixeira *et al.* (2016) validated the CWEQ-II scale for use in the Portuguese population. These authors found that nursing empowerment produces positive personal and professional outcomes specifically in the areas of job satisfaction, autonomy, and care quality, as well as organizational and professional commitment.

A systematic review of the literature to synthesize studies that evaluated the relationship between nursing empowerment and job satisfaction was conducted by Cicolini *et al.* (2014). Of the 596 articles originally found, 12 articles were included in the analysis. The review revealed that although structural empowerment and psychological empowerment both affect job satisfaction; they each affect job satisfaction differently. Structural empowerment significantly affects job satisfaction and commitment to the organization. Psychological empowerment significantly affects feelings of burnout within nursing. Cicolini *et al.* (2014) recommended the finding to be used by nursing leaders to create and maintain empowering work environments that will improve nurse retention as well as organizational and patient outcomes.

Nurse Retention

It is well supported in the literature that nurses who feel empowered through well-ordered organizational structure experience higher levels of job satisfaction and lower levels of work related stress, which therefore leads to high retention rates (Hyrkas and Morton, 2013). The concept of retention is especially important in today's healthcare environment when nursing shortages are a common issue and expected to worsen in the upcoming years (Meng *et al.*, 2014). A report from the 2016 National Healthcare & RN Retention Report identified that the national turnover rate in nursing was 17.1%, which is higher than the

2014 report of 16.4%, averaging $37,000 to $58,400 per nurse for orientation and training costs (NSI Nursing Solutions, Inc., 2016). Nurse leaders must seek out opportunities to retain experienced, trained staff to promote top quality care provision and ensure an adequate surplus of trainers for less experienced staff (DiNapoli, *et al.* 2016; Hayes, Douglas, and Bonner, 2014). Based on the literature review, empowering high performing CNLs to self-govern and serve as leaders will help advance and progress a CNL program.

Meng *et al.* (2014) found that the lack of structural empowerment leads to nursing burnout, which negatively influences the quality of care provision and professional outcomes. The authors conducted a qualitative study using an anonymous questionnaire administered to 219 nurses in mainland China. The purpose of the study was to explore relationships among perceived structural empowerment, psychological empowerment, nursing burnout, and the intent to stay using the structural equation modeling tool. Results revealed that structural and psychological empowerment both positively affect nurses' intent to stay in their current jobs. Results also revealed that both structural and psychological empowerment negatively affect burnout and burnout in-turn negatively effects the intent to stay in the current job. Nurses who feel loyal, self-determining, important, and enthusiastic about their jobs prefer to stay in their roles and contribute more effectively to their organizations (Meng *et al.,* 2014).

Furthermore, Bish *et al.* (2012) noted in their study that nurses' abilities to perform well and respond to challenges may depend upon their perceived levels of power, job satisfaction, and ability to serve as effective change agents. They also noted the importance of structurally empowered nurse leaders in driving change, demonstrating an open responsive culture that supports top quality care, interprofessional collaboration, equitable resource allocation, and the retention of skilled professionals within the workforce (Bish *et al.,* 2012). These authors suggested that structural empowerment should be used as a tool for nurse leaders to use to selectively equip nurses to aim for excellence and advocate for resources (Bish *et al.,* 2012).

Shared Governance

Joseph and Bogue (2016) conducted six studies over the course of six years to evaluate nursing shared governance to provide a structured theoretical approach. The first five studies were conducted within eight hospitals in the southern region of the U.S.. Each of the five studies were organized using the general theory for the effective multilevel shared governance model created by the authors to identify the inputs, processes and outputs of each study.

The first study conducted from 2006 to 2007 assessed the effects of the implementation of a nurse practice council (NPC) at a health system that consisted of eight hospitals and 2,400 beds in the southern region of the U.S. The NPCs were implemented with the goal of improving engagement in shared governance within the system. After an extensive literature review of 115 articles and staff interviews, the authors operationalized nine competency-based measures of unit-based councils, identified three major concepts that describe empowerment, and unexpectedly found that nurses rated themselves higher in empowerment than management personnel.

The second study, conducted between 2007 and 2008, examined leadership empowerment levels and competencies, as well as potentially impacting personality factors. This study was conducted with 248 administrators that included managers, assistant managers, directors. and other administrative personnel that led units with NPCs. Numerous tools were used to assess empowerment and helped to identify five of the eight nursing leader competencies. This study concluded that nursing leader competencies are critical to the success of shared governance as well as vertical alignments between unit nursing leadership and NPCs. The third study conducted in 2008 included only system executives and evaluated executive level philosophy concerning nursing shared governance. The results of this study revealed understanding and the value of empowerment of the executives and also identified that executives did not feel the need to act on employee empowerment. The fourth study conducted from 2009 to 2010 included nurses, assistant managers, managers, directors, and NPCs. This study tested the way in which the assets of the work environment predicts NPC effectiveness. In 2011, the fifth study included nurse managers and NPC members and chairpersons with a purpose to develop and field test a tool kit to improve the practice of NPCs. The sixth study conducted in 2012 formalized the nursing theory for shared governance called the General Effectiveness Model (GEM). The GEM approach assesses the competency levels and perceptions of both leadership staff and unit-level council members while requiring six-month self-assessment cycles to evaluate the progress of the council.

Results of these studies identified that NPCs as work teams and their effectiveness can be defined, measured, and thereby improved upon. The results also found that successful teams progress up the nine steps of the staged competencies created by the authors, resulting in the development of empowerment at various levels (Joseph and Bogue, 2016). During the six month assessment cycles, the authors recommended identifying competency focuses for improvement that are measured at all levels, such as the individual, unit, division, and organizational level (Joseph and Bogue, 2016). This article provides the first theory-focused approach to evaluating nursing shared governance. Joseph and Bogue (2016) stressed the importance of systematically studying shared governance using leadership strategies inclusive of all levels of nursing to improve outcomes for both the nurse and the patient. This study supports the concept of continued evaluation and structured planning of the shared governance council to ensure effectiveness and progress towards system goals.

The concept of continued evaluation is also supported by Porter-O'Grady (2001), who noted that successful implementation of shared governance was dependent upon tireless planning, hard work, and high-level commitment to building an empowered workplace.

Advisory Council

The literature supports implementing a small portion of a group to help guide and evaluate the progress of a council. Harris *et al.* (2014) noted the importance of an advisory council when implementing a CNL shared governance council, in particular, to ensure standardization within the system's current shared governance structure along with selecting strong influential members to serve as leaders. Altbach and Salmi (2016) noted that advisory councils are situated to offer advice concerning the strategic direction of an institution and to identify challenges to success.

Woten (2014) describes the characteristics of strong leaders as highly trusted, clear with a purpose, identified as members of the team, respected, positive-minded, creative, disciplined, excellent communicators, committed, talented, and stable. Watkins (2003) provides criteria of critically influential people within an organization, which includes expertise in the area of practice, access to information, status within the team, control, and loyalty. These criteria complement the characteristics provided by Woten without contradiction. Furthermore, McNamara (n.d.) provides guidelines for ensuring effective group performance.

The author urges a structured process for recruiting leaders that utilizes a standard form for selecting prospective candidates, meeting with candidates in advance, and providing information regarding the role. The commonality found within the literature denotes the importance of having established criteria for selecting leaders and members to support the council structure.

DEVELOPING PROJECT FOCUS AND OBJECTIVES

To properly develop a project focus and objectives, a theoretical framework had to be actualized. Kanter's Structural Theory of Organizational Empowerment asserts that the level of support applied to the structure of the work environment directly correlates to employee engagement and attitudes regarding their workplace (Nedd, 2006). This framework supported both concepts of shared governance and empowerment. Nedd (2006) cited Kanter's original work from 1977 that noted Kanter's belief that two components greatly affect perceptions of empowerment within the workplace. These dynamics are opportunity and structure of power. Opportunity refers to the chance for advancement, mobility, and increased knowledge and skills, whereas structure of power refers to the organization's authority arrangement or hierarchy.

Bish *et al.* (2012) cited Kanter's work from 1993 by categorizing three separate forces of empowerment to include formal power, informal power, and organizational empowerment structures. Formal power is described as the visible positional power, such as a job role within an organization, whereas informal power is described as the social aspects exchanged between people (Kanter, 1993). The organizational empowerment structures refer to one's ability to access data, information, and resources while securing support for one's position within the organization to successfully complete a particular task and explore opportunities for growth and continued education (Kanter, 1993; Nedd, 2006). Kanter describes power as an ability to disperse resources to accomplish goals. McDonald *et al.* (2010) noted that all forms of power influences the abilities and resourcefulness of individuals in the areas of "opportunity, power, resources, information, and support" (McDonald *et al.,* 2010, 150). A lack in these areas reflects the severity of an individual's unempowered state within their workplace, which is often times greatly influenced by the work environment (McDonald *et al.,* 2010).

According to Laschinger (2012a), the work environment also significantly influences staff engagement. Laschinger (2012a) cited Kanter's earlier work from 1977 to 1993, which noted that the Structural Empowerment Theory offers a methodology to help explain how work environments negatively or positively influence employee attitude and behavior outcomes. Factors such as job stress, satisfaction, and burnout. Kanter (1993) also noted that workplace characteristics influence employee behaviors and attitudes more than the employee's own personality. Work environments that create a culture of empowerment through effective communication and feedback will directly affect workplace productivity and teammate moral (Laschinger, 2012a).

It is well supported in the literature that nurses who feel empowered through well-ordered organizational structure experience higher levels of job satisfaction and lower levels of work related stress, which ultimately leads to high retention rates (Hyrkas and Morton, 2013; Laschinger, 2012a). The concept of retention is especially important in today's healthcare environment, in which nursing shortages are a common issue and expected to worsen in the upcoming years (Meng *et al.*, 2014). Nurse leaders must seek out opportunities to retain experienced, trained staff to promote top quality care provision and ensure adequate trainers for less experienced staff (DiNapoli *et al.*, 2016; Hayes, Douglas, and Bonner, 2014). This notion is also supported by the Institute of Medicine (IOM) (2011), stressing the need for higher education level attainment to retain a supply of educated and skilled nurses to train next generation nurses. Despite the complexity of this theory and for the purposes of this project, a schematic model has been adapted (Laschinger *et al.*, 2001) to depict and simplify the theoretical framework and concepts used to guide this project.

Clinical Setting

Based on unpublished data from the medical center (2017), the shared governance structure consisted of a coordinating council, an education council, a transformational leadership council, an exemplary professional practice council, a professional empowerment council, a new knowledge and innovation/research council, a nursing peer review council, a nursing at night council, an informatics council, service line councils, and unit-based councils (Medical Center unpublished data, 2017). Council leaders are recruited by council members and nursing leaders to serve terms delineated in the bylaws. An orientation process and tools exist to prepare new council leaders for office. Information is disseminated through all councils to nursing staff regularly. Prior to this project, a CNL representative was included in the membership of each of these councils to ensure information was also disseminated to the CNL group.

Focus and Objectives

Findings from the literature repeatedly support the implementation of shared governance to create or strengthen the perception of empowerment within nursing (Porter-O'Grady, 2001; Porter-O'Grady and Finnegan, 1984). These findings, coupled with Kanter's Structural Theory of Organizational Empowerment, were used to focus the project's objectives on assessing the current perception of empowerment, implementing a shared governance council, and then reassessing the impact of this intervention. The clinical question for this project was: "will the establishment of a shared governance council within the CNL program at the medical center improve nurse-reported empowerment using the validated Conditions for Workplace Effectiveness Questionnaire-II (CWEQ-II) tool two months of implementation?"

PROJECT INTERVENTIONS

Approval from the medical center's Institutional Review Board (IRB) and the University's IRB was obtained prior to project implementation. In January 2018, I met with my project manager to complete the medical center's shared governance checklist and choose potential CNL Advisory Council (CAC) board members using established evidence-based criteria. Following this meeting, the CWEQ-II survey was distributed electronically via SurveyMonkey to all eligible CNL members to complete over a two-week period. After the two week survey period, I recruited the selected CNLs to serve on the CAC board. Within a week, the CAC board met to brainstorm ideas for the charter and council goals and to begin planning for the first CNL shared governance council meeting. The Plan-Do-Study-Act tool (PDSA) was used to evaluate the implementation of the council process (Institute of Healthcare Improvement [IHI], 2017).

At the end of January 2018, the first CNL shared governance council monthly meeting occurred and the charter, goals, and any other decisions offered by the CAC board were discussed and voted on by the entire CNL council. Shared governance reference tools used at the medical center were used to provide structure and organization to the council meetings. At the completion of each council meeting, an evaluation of the process occurred using the PDSA. Throughout the implementation period, after the first council meeting, and prior to every monthly CNL council meeting, the CAC board met to review the charter and the PDSA tool and to discuss and plan for any additional issues as needed. Two months after the implementation of the CNL shared governance council, the CWEQ-II survey was electronically distributed to eligible CNLs for completion. A timeline of the project was created to ensure efficient implementation of the project.

DATA COLLECTION, MEASUREMENT TOOLS, ANALYSIS

Sample Demographics

A total of 25 out of 27 (93%) completed pre surveys were received prior to implementation of the CNL shared governance council. A total of 18 out of 22 (82%) completed post surveys were received at the conclusion of the project. Participants were masters prepared, CNL certified nurses working within medical-surgical areas, including high-risk obstetrics, oncology, surgical, trauma, orthopedics, and the emergency department (ED). CNL students were excluded from participating in the survey; however, they were invited to attend and participate in the CNL shared governance council meetings. Four CNL members volunteered to serve as CAC board members. Participation was encouraged but was not mandatory.

Instruments

Measurement tools included the PDSA and the CWEQ-II tool. According to the Institute for Healthcare Improvement (2017), a PDSA is a useful tool for evaluating and documenting a quick test of change. The PDSA cycle review process was used to guide and evaluate the ongoing progress of the council. The CWEQ-II survey is a modified shortened version of the original CWEQ-I and intended for use within large nursing populations (Laschinger, 2012b). The CWEQ-II consists of 21 items and is designed for use for research studies and quality improvement initiatives. The survey consists of 19 items, which assess six domains and an additional two questions related to global empowerment. The six domains include the following: (1) participant's level of opportunity in the present job, (2) access to resources, (3) access to information, (4) access to support, (5) formal power related to job activities, and (6) informal power related to organizational relationships. All items are rated using a five point Likert scale with a rating of one reflecting a response of "none" or "strongly disagree" and five reflecting a response of "a lot" or "strongly agree."

An overall empowerment score is calculated by totaling scores from the six domains. The scoring rubric provided by Laschinger (2012b) denotes that scores will range from 6 to 30. Higher scores ranging from 23 to 30 reflects strong levels of self-reported structural empowerment. Lower scores ranging from 6 to 13 indicate weak levels of empowerment, whereas scores ranging from 14 to 22 indicate moderate levels of empowerment. A global empowerment score serves as a validation index separate from the overall empowerment score. This score can be calculated by summing and averaging the scores from the two global empowerment questions. This total will range between 1 and 5. Higher scores in this range reflects stronger perceptions of workplace empowerment (Laschinger, 2012b). Laschinger *et al.* (2000) reports Cronbach's alpha reliability coefficients for the CWEQ-II on the six domains to be the following: opportunity 0.81, information 0.80, support 0.89, resources 0.84, formal power 0.69, and informal power 0.67. The authors also included a Cronbach's alpha reliability coefficient score for overall empowerment 0.89 and global empowerment 0.87.

Protecting the participants using de-identified data was collected from responses received from the pre and post–CWEQ-II survey. The CWEQ-II tool was administered using SurveyMonkey software (SurveyMonkey, 2017), which is common practice for the practice site. Data analysis was performed on the aggregate electronic report provided by SurveyMonkey.

Data Analysis

Descriptive analysis was conducted on the responses received from the pre and post–CWEQ-II surveys, at the completion of the project period, to compare if an improvement in nurse-reported empowerment had been actualized. A two-sample t-test assuming unequal variances analysis was used to compare the difference between the variables, which included the results of the pre and post survey (Moran, Burson, and Conrad, 2017). Comparable analysis provided insight concerning the impact on CNL self-reported empowerment as a result of implementing shared governance.

Findings

The results of the t-test revealed no statistical significance between the pre and post survey results. Despite the lack of statistical significance, a positive increase was demonstrated in comparing the pre and post survey score results in five of the six subscale domains. Essentially, this equates to an increase in nurse-reported access to opportunity (3.77 to 3.89), information (3.31 to 3.37), support (3.17 to 3.61), formal power (3.32 to 3.39), and informal power (4.38 to 4.40) (see Table 13.1 and Table 13.2). Although no domain subscale results revealed statistical significance, increases were noted that indicate the positive impact of empowerment within two months of implementing shared governance. The only domain subscale that revealed a decrease was the resource domain (2.60 to 2.56).

Many changes occurred during the PDSA review process that included goals to improve attendance rates at the monthly meetings, facilitate access of the communication platform, and standardize a method of CNL self-review. These changes included the completion of a CNL Shared Governance Council Charter, establishment of an official communication platform using OneNote, and an initiative to create a CNL

TABLE 13.1. CWEQ-II Pre and Post Survey Data Analysis.

Item	Pre Survey Means	Post Survey Means	Difference in Means	One-tail P-Values
Opportunity	3.77	3.89	0.12	0.343
Resources	2.60	2.56	−0.04	0.497
Information	3.31	3.37	0.06	0.399
Support	3.17	3.61	0.44	0.063
Formal Power	3.32	3.39	0.07	0.358
Informal Power	4.38	4.40	0.02	0.330
Global Empowerment	3.36	3.56	0.20	0.247
Total Structural Empowerment	20.55	21.22	0.67	0.322

TABLE 13.2. Domain Score Interpretation.

1	2	3	4	5
Weaker		→		Stronger

TSE Score Range	TSE Score Interpretation
6–13	Low levels of empowerment
14–22	Moderate levels of empowerment
23–30	High levels of empowerment

Self-Review tool. The Charter was brainstormed by the CAC and then shared with the group at the monthly meeting. Recommendations for changes were accepted and used to revise the charter until it was finalized. OneNote was unanimously agreed upon to serve as the communication platform for the group, because it is user-friendly. Scavenger hunt surveys were created and administered monthly to help the group navigate the OneNote platform. Completed surveys were tracked monthly and reported to the group at the monthly meeting. The group is currently working on creating a CNL Self-Review tool. Continued work is planned and required to complete this goal.

SUMMARY

An increase was noted in comparing the pre and post–CWEQ-II survey results reflecting a potential impact in self-reported empowerment as a result of the implementation of CNL shared governance. Although no statistical significance was noted, a positive increase noted in five of six domain subscales and both empowerment questions provides additional support concerning the positive impact of shared governance on nursing empowerment. Furthermore, post survey results in both the global empowerment question (3.56) and the total structural empowerment question (21.22) that rests on the high end of both scales reflects an overall perception rating better than average within this population.

CONCLUSIONS

The underlying theme for the project centered on nursing empowerment through the use of shared governance. Shared governance is well supported in the literature as a method of improving empowerment, autonomy and work satisfaction within the profession of nursing (Porter-O'Grady, 2001; Porter-O'Grady and Finnigan, 1984). This project used evidence to implement shared governance within a new nursing leadership role while evaluating the before and after self-reported empowerment perceptions of the participants.

Project limitations include the short implementation timeframe of four months, the significant amount of turnover experienced on all levels at the project site during and before the implementation period, and the newness of the CNL role. Project benefits include useful tools for assessing nursing empowerment and more support regarding the positive impact of shared governance on nursing empowerment. Additionally, this project can be replicated with any groups of nurses.

This project is pertinent to the CNL role because CNLs oversee the clinical care of groups of patients. The CNL role, similarly to any other nursing leadership role, requires that the nurse possess exceptional skills in critical thinking, professionalism, and clinical competence (Harris, Roussel, and Thomas, 2014). Additionally, these skills must be rooted in confidence, autonomy, and empowerment (Cook and Holt, 2000). Stanley (2006) actually defines a CNL as a "clinician who is an expert in their field, and who, because they are approachable, effective communicators and empowered, are able to act as a role model, motivating others by matching their values and beliefs about nursing and care to their practice" (Stanley, 2006, 111). The purpose of this project was built upon this premise and proved useful in evaluating CNL empowerment at the medical center.

Kanter's Structural Empowerment Theory centers on the concept of empowering staff to effect change and be productive healthcare providers. This theoretical framework was used for this project, because it provides the foundation of understanding that the level of support applied to the work environment fosters positive attitudes of autonomy, empowerment, and job satisfaction for nurses. This recommendation is especially important as these elements help to promote the IHI Triple Aim (IHI, 2018). which focuses on improving the experience of the patient, health of the population, and cost of care. The primary goal of the masters prepared CNL role is to improve patient outcomes, but empowered autonomous nursing cultures are necessary to achieve this goal. Furthermore, this project provided insight for CNL administrators in future planning purposes for the CNL program.

DISSEMINATION

At the conclusion of this project, I made great effort to present my work wherever I found an opportunity. I presented my DNP project externally at the East Carolina University DNP Poster Day and the 2018 DNP Nursing Education Symposium. I also shared my DNP project internally at the medical center with the CNL group and other colleagues. This project will also be submitted for presentation at the project site's poster symposiums that are held twice a year, along with other research and evidence-based practice events.

REFERENCES

Altbach, P., & Salmi, J. (2016). International advisory councils and internationalization of governance: A qualitative analysis. *European Journal of Higher Education, 6*(4), 328–342.

American Association of Colleges of Nursing. (2007). *White paper on the role of the clinical nurse leader*. Retrieved from http://www.aacn.nche.edu/publications/white-papers/ClinicalNurseLeader.pdf.

American Association of Colleges of Nursing (AACN). (2013). *Competencies and curricular expectations for clinical nurse leader's education and practice*. Retrieved from http://www.aacn.nche.edu/publications/white-papers/cnl.

Bender, M., Williams, M., Su, W. and Hites, L. (2016). Clinical nurse leader integrated care delivery to improve care quality: Factors influencing perceived success. *Journal of Nursing Scholarship, 48*(4), 414–422.

Bish, M., Kenny, A. and Nay, R. (2012). Perceptions of structural empowerment: Nurse leaders in rural health services. *Journal of Nursing Management, 22*, 29–37.

Boswell, C., Opton, L. and Owen, D. (2017). Exploring shared governance for an academic nursing setting. *Journal of Nursing Education, 56*(4), 197–201.

Burkman, K., Sellers, D., Rowder, C. and Batcheller, J. (2012). An integrated system's nursing shared governance model: A system chief nursing officer's synergistic vehicle for leading a complex health care system. *Nursing Administration Quarterly, 36*, 353–361. doi: 10.1097/NAQ.0b013e31826692ea

Choi, S., Goh, C., Adam, M. and Tan, O. (2016). Transformational leadership empowerment, and job satisfaction: The mediating role of employee empowerment. *Human Resources for Health, 14*(73). doi: 10.1186/s12960-016-0171-2

Cicolini, G., Comparcini, D. and Simonetti, V. (2014). Workplace empowerment and nurses' job satisfaction: A systematic literature review. *Journal of Nursing Management, 22*, 855–871.

Clavelle, J., O'Grady, T., Weston, M. and Verran, J. (2016). Evolution of structural empowerment. *The Journal of Nursing Administration, 46*(6), 308–312.

Cook, A., & Holt, L. (2000). *Clinical leadership and supervision*. In B. Dolan & L. Holt (Eds.), Accident and Emergency Theory into Practice (pp. 497–503). London: Bailliere Tindall.

DiNapoli, J., O'Flaherty, D., Musil, C., Clavelle, J. and Fitzpatrick, J. (2016). The relationship of clinical nurses' perceptions of structural and psychological empowerment and engagement on their unit. *The Journal of Nursing Administration, 46*(2), 95–100.

Harris, J., Roussel, L. and Thomas, P. (2014). *Initiating and sustaining the clinical nurse leader role: A practical guide.* (2nd ed.). Burlington, MA: Jones & Bartlett.

Hayes, B., Douglas, C. and Bonner, A. (2014). Predicting emotional exhaustion among haemodialysis nurses: A structural equation model using kanter's structural empowerment theory. *Journal of Advanced Nursing, 70*(12), 2897–2909. doi: 10.1111/jan.12452

Hyrkas, K. and Morton, J. (2013). International perspectives on retention, stress and burnout. *Journal of Nursing Management, 21*, 603–604.

Institute of Healthcare Improvement. (2017). *Plan-Do-Study-Act (pdsa) worksheet.* Retrieved from http://www.ihi.org/resources/Pages/Tools/PlanDoStudyActWorksheet.aspx

Institute of Healthcare Improvement. (2018). *The ihi triple aim.* Retrieved from http://www.ihi.org/Engage/Initiatives/TripleAim/Pages/default.aspx

Jordan, B. (2016). Designing a unit practice council structure. *Nursing Management, 47*(1), 15–18. doi: 10.1097/01.NUMA.0000475633.98128.4d

Joseph, M. and Bogue, R. (2016). A theory-based approach to nursing shared governance. *Nursing Outlook, 64*(4), 339–351.

Kanter, R. (1993). *Men and women of the corporation.* (2nd ed.). New York, NY: Basic Books.

Laschinger, H. (2012a). Organizational and health effects of workplace empowerment in health care settings. In P. Spurgeon, C. Cooper and R. Burke (Eds.), *The Innovation Imperative in Health Care Organization* (pp. 221–238). Cheltenham, England: Edward Elgar Publishing.

Laschinger, H. (2012b). *Conditions for work effectiveness questionnaire I and II: User manual.* Western University, Canada.

Laschinger, H., Finegan, J., Shamian, J. and Casier, S. (2000). Organizational trust and empowerment in restructured healthcare setting: Effects on staff nurse commitment. *Journal of Nursing Administration, 30*(9), 413–425.

Laschinger, H., Finegan, J., Shamian, J. and Wilk, P. (2001). Impact of structural and psychological empowerment on job strain in nursing work settings: Expanding kanter's model. *Journal of Nursing Administration, 31*, 260–272.

L'Ecuyer, K., Shatto, B., Hoffmann, R. and Crecelius, M. (2016). The certified clinical nurse leader in critical care. *Dimensions of Critical Care Nursing, 35*(5), 248–254.

McDonald, S., Tullai-McGuinness, S., Madigan, E. and Shively, M. (2010). Relationship between staff nurse involvement in organizational structures and perception of empowerment. *Critical Care Nursing Quarterly, 33*(2), 148–162.

McNamara, C. (n.d.). *All about facilitation, group skills and group performance management.* Retrieved from http://managementhelp.org/grp_skll/facltate/facltate.htm.

Meline, D. and Brehm, S. (2015). Sustained shared decision-making: A biennial task force process. *American Nurse Today, 10*(3), 52–54.

Meng, L., Liu, Y., Liu, H., Hu, Y., Yang, J. and Liu, J. (2014). Relationships among structural empowerment, psychological empowerment, intent to stay and burnout in nursing field in mainland china—based on a cross-sectional questionnaire research. *International Journal of Nursing Practice, 21*, 303–312.

Moran, K., Burson, R. and Conrad, D. (2017). *The doctor of nursing practice scholarly project: A framework for success*. Burlington, MA: Jones & Bartlett Learning.

Nedd, N. (2006). Perceptions of empowerment and intent to stay. *Nursing Economics, 24*(1), 13–18.

NSI Nursing Solutions, Inc. (2016). *2016 national healthcare & RN retention report*. Retrieved from www.nsinursingsolutions.com/Files/assets/library/retention-institute/NationalHealthcareRNRetentionReport2016.pdf.

Porter-O'Grady, T. (2001). Is shared governance still relevant? *Journal of Nursing Administration, 31*(10), 468–473.

Porter-O'Grady, T. and Finnigan, S. (1984). *Shared governance for nursing: A creative approach to accountability*. Rockville, MD: Aspen.

Rankin, V. (2015). Clinical nurse leader: A role for the 21st century. *MedSURG Nursing, 24*(3), 199–201.

Stanley, D. (2006). Recognizing and defining clinical nurse leaders. *British Journal of Nursing, 15*(2), 108–111.

Sullivan, H., Warshawsky, N. and Vasey, J. (2013). RN work engagement in generational cohorts: The view from rural us hospitals. *Journal of Nursing Management, 21*(7), 927–940. doi: 10.1111/jonm.12171

SurveyMonkey® Inc. (2017). SurveyMonkey. Retrieved from www.surveymonkey.com

Teixeira, A., Nogueira, M. and Alves, P. (2016). Structural empowerment in nursing: Translation, adaptation and validation of the conditions of work effectiveness questionnaire II. *Journal of Nursing Referencia, 4*(10), 39–46.

Wang, S. and Liu, Y. (2013). Impact of professional nursing practice environment and psychological empowerment on nurses' work engagement: Test of structural equation modelling. *Journal of Nursing Management, 23*, 287–296. doi: 10.1111/jonm.12124

Watkins, M. (2003). *Critical success strategies for new leaders at all levels: The first 90 days*. Boston, MA: Harvard Business School Publishing.

Woten, M. (2014). *Team building in nursing care: Implementing*. CINAHL Information Systems.

CHAPTER 14

Identify and Employ a Best Practice in Engaging Frontline Staff and Improve Overall Satisfaction

FRED CANTOR, DNP

INTRODUCTION

Improving the engagement and overall satisfaction of frontline staff is something that leadership is always striving to accomplish. In a recent study, Bhuvanaiah and Raya (2015) state that engaged employees lead to a much healthier organization, because they are satisfied, committed, innovative, and high performing. Although this concept is not foreign to most leaders, the practical application can prove to be much more difficult. The ability to truly engage staff is often one of the most daunting, yet overly rewarding, tasks that an organization is likely to face. The purpose of this DNP degree project was to identify and employ a best practice in engaging frontline staff and to improve overall satisfaction.

REVIEW OF LITERATURE

Improving overall job satisfaction and engagement has been directly linked to an increase in retention rates (Hairr *et al.*, 2014). Employees who feel that they are treated at or above their expectations are more productive and also attract more applicants than their disengaged counterparts (Toller, 2016). Zhang *et al.* (2014) showed that whenever possible, supervisors should utilize a visionary or organic approach to increase employee engagement. They went on to say that the utilization of a transactional or classical style of leadership would, in general, have a negative effect on engagement (Zhang *et al.*, 2014). The American Association of Critical Care Nurses (AACN) believes that a strong link exists between what is defined as a healthy work environment (HWE) and improvements in patient safety and overall staff engagement (AACN, 2010). Such great importance has been placed on setting a high standard of a healthy work environment that the AACN has continued to study and improve their literature and guidance on this issue.

Definition of Engagement

There are many definitions of engagement, but commonly an engaged employee is defined as someone who believes he or she is appreciated, feels involved, is committed and passionate, and feels empowered through work and working relationships (Baudler, 2011). Engagement can lead to increased retention rates, decreased overall absenteeism, increases in productivity, and an increase in the return on overall investment into staff (Gallup, 2013). Regardless of the definition utilized and engaged employee translates to one that has a high satisfaction level with both the employer and the employment. Holistically, engagement can be seen as an important indicator of overall business success (Bhuvanaiah and Raya, 2015).

Effects of Engagement

Employee engagement should be thought of as an asset to a company or a source of power to help drive overall performance (Shuck, Reio, and Rocco, 2011). The top business and corporations throughout the world understand that engagement drives outcomes and growth (Lather and Jain, 2015). A recent study found that a distinguishing feature of companies with strong financial results was the high engagement level of senior managers and their ability to engage others around them (Aon Hewitt, 2012). Overall, it is well documented that increasing the engagement level of staff throughout an organization, from the c-suite down to the frontline staff, improves outcomes, secures a better financial standing, and provides for a healthier overall work environment.

Conclusion

Although a vast amount of research and evidence are available around the idea of improving employee engagement, the idea is still very subjective. Many of the tactics, leadership styles, and best practice should be utilized in a model that is best suited for the environment that it is being applied. Leaders need to recognize that behavior is the single most important factor when discussing engagement outcomes. They must also recognize that along with behavior, their intentions must be genuine and supportive. Staff should be given tools of success, and communication lines should be established that are safe and provide for a two-way interaction. The leadership team must embrace all ideas around engagement so that their behaviors do not come off as forced and staff see and believe in the genuine approach to overall improvement. Lastly, the organization as a whole must embrace engagement, seeing this as an opportunity to change the culture for the better and improving not only core outcomes but also the attitudes of staff and the environment in which they choose to work.

THE DNP DEGREE PROJECT

Instituting a process improvement project required many steps to ensure a positive outcome. The project needed a strong design that focused on the desired outcome, well defined stakeholders and participants, robust tools, and proper methodology. Transparency was also a key piece to the success of the project. Implementation of the project was closely aligned to the Plan Do Study Act (PDSA) model, and any variation from the original plan was discussed with all team members.

Project Design

This project was designed around the implementation of a rounding system for frontline staff. The purpose of this was to gather feedback from frontline clinical staff on all aspects of their respective positions and look for opportunities for improvement. This project design was based on an extensive literature review around improving staff engagement, the outcome of which was the recommendation of utilizing stay interviews as a best practice. Stay interviews are defined as an opportunity for an employee to sit down with a leader and discuss the current position, share wants and needs, and devise a plan that helps to foster engagement (Tips to Tackle the Employee Engagement Crisis, 2016, 3–5). Along with the stay interviews, a system of continuous feedback was instituted utilizing the CASE model, which is an acronym for instilling a sense of community, being authentic and trustworthy, recognizing the significance of each person's contributions, and providing for an environment in which the staff is excited to achieve outcomes (BlessingWhite, 2013).

The project was completely voluntary for both management and staff. All managers had the opportunity to participate; however, a maximum of four were chosen for the initial pilot project. Once chosen, each manager shared the implementation plan with staff and arranged available times for the rounding process. Managers were also required to provide continuous feedback to all staff via a report utilizing the CASE model.

Population of Interest & Stakeholders

The population of interest was the front-line staff of a clinical unit within the selected agency. The specific units were chosen based on first-level manger volunteers. Once the specific units were chosen, the staff of the units had the opportunity to choose not to participate. The reason that this population is of interest links to numerous studies to support that increasing staff engagement can lead to many desirable benefits. In a recent study, Bhuvanaiah and Raya (2015) state that engaged employees lead to a much healthier organization, because they are satisfied, committed, innovative, and high performing.

They key stakeholders of this project were both the frontline staff and the many layers of leadership. The staff is the single most important asset to most companies, and the success of an organization can be heavily affected by the engagement of its employees. The leadership team can greatly benefit from increased engagement in such ways as increased staff performance and improved patient outcomes. The staff can also recognize a benefit in such ways as improved teamwork, more joy in daily activities, and improved relationships with leaders.

RESULTS

At the completion of the project implementation, a total of 58 employees completed a first rounding meeting with their direct manager. This represented a total of 60.42% of all available staff. The Intake and Telehealth/Coaching departments recognized a higher participation rate than the clinical or therapy departments. This was contributed to the fact that these staff are in the agency on a daily basis, whereas the clinical and therapy staff are in the field on a more regular basis, limiting their access to leadership. All staff who volunteered to participate were able to attend one rounding meeting. All participants who volunteered completed the entire implementation. All 58 meetings resulted in a completed rounding report, and 4 separate stop light reports were created, one for each department. The stop light reports displayed the summary of the results of the meetings.

All four managers held two separate staff meetings to share the stoplight reports. The reports were also made available to all staff via email for those who were unable to attend an in-person meeting. After discussion in a manager debriefing meeting, it was also decided to share the stop light reports with managers of other departments, because many of the identified issues transcended all units. These managers were asked to share with their staff as they saw fit.

Discussion of the Findings

All identified issues were placed on the stoplight reports and a status was applied. Staff was made aware of the initial status and a tentative timeline for an update was also communicated. Management staff found the format to be very efficient for frequent communication and agreed to continue utilization of the form going forward. Overall, the initial roll out was met with high engagement from both management and frontline staff.

There were several identified trends in the rounding meetings. The most common issue noted by staff was a recent change to a patient consent document. Staff believed the new process was laborious and inefficient. The leadership took this identified issue as an opportunity to reexamine the process and make adjustments. Another common theme was the on-call scheduling process. Many staff were unhappy with how this process was handled and requested that it was revisited. Management agreed to take this to the senior leadership meeting to discuss.

TABLE 14.1.

Department	Participated	Total	Percentage
Intake	9	9	100.00%
Clinical	20	42	47.62%
Therapy	19	33	57.58%
Coaching	10	12	83.33%
Totals	58	96	60.42%

At the conclusion of the initial four-week trial period, all managers were brought together for a debriefing. This meeting also included members of the senior management team. The results were mostly positive. The management staff felt that the tools provided helped them to be better engaged with the needs of their respective staff members. One concern for continuing the project was the amount of time necessary. It was decided by senior leadership that the monthly rounding should be done with each employee, but the managers could share the responsibility with their supervisors to help ease the work load. This was well received. A committee was formed to draft a formal rounding policy for review.

Significance and Implications for Nursing

The importance of retention has been a focus for nursing for many years. In 2002, after a considerable amount of lobbying from the American Nurses Association (ANA), President George W. Bush signed the Nurse Reinvestment Act, which authorized important recruitment and retention initiatives (Nurse Reinvestment Act Background, n.d.). This act helped to shift focus to many initiatives for nursing retention, including loan repayment programs, training grants, and faculty advancement programs. Although great benefits have been achieved, the ANA has continued to lobby for improvement and to release updated best practices.

Nursing has long been thought of as a job with a high job satisfaction rate. Unfortunately, as the census of patients continues to rise and the cost of education grows, the number of nurses entering the workforce has not kept pace. It has been projected that the shortage of available nurses will significantly rise over the next 10 to 20 years. This has put an increased emphasis on retention, engagement, and satisfaction of qualified staff (Cottingham *et al.,* 2011). Onboarding new staff is also one of the highest costs to a healthcare provider: therefore, any opportunity to reduce turnover has great financial benefits as well. Adverse patient outcomes have also been linked to increased turnover amongst clinical staff (Adams, 2016).

Understanding what drives staff to succeed can aid leadership in creating a healthy work environment, which can also translate into improved patient outcomes and satisfaction levels. The engagement of staff is a process that needs to be addressed at all times and on all levels. Nursing, as well as all staff, are finding it much easier to transition to new places of employment and new roles, which can make the job of retention even more difficult. It is vital to nursing leadership to comprehend what staff are struggling with, as well as where they are succeeding. Often leadership is focused on achieving outcomes, which can be perceived negatively by frontline staff. The purpose of this specific project was to shift the focus back on the needs and expectations of the frontline clinician.

Areas for Further Dissemination

Like a research project, the final phase for an evidence-based practice project is dissemination of the findings and outcomes. It is vital to the growth of care delivery to continually share new and proven information and process change. There are many forums for which information can be exchanged including written articles, poster presentations, oral presentations and training seminars. It is also important to integrate new knowledge gained from a project into official practice.

As the project came to fruition and positive results were recognized, senior leadership was brought together to discuss how this could translate to a more holistic culture change. The chosen practice site is part of a large healthcare corporation, which provides a lot of opportunity to share process change. It was decided that a formal rounding policy would be created for the practice site. Once this is completed, it will be shared with the corporate process improvement committee to be shared throughout the corporation.

During this process, it was also decided that going forward, monthly rounding would now be an expectation of all management staff at the practice site. Managers who were not included in the original project were in attendance at the post project debriefing, and a training session was scheduled to provide needed information for those individuals. The practice site educator was instrumental to this process, because she became the owner and principal trainer for the ongoing project.

Lastly, opportunities for more widespread dissemination were sought out. The healthcare corporation has several yearly forums to showcase the success of local projects and share information amongst clinical settings. The findings of this project were transferred to a poster presentation and presented at the yearly nursing showcase event. The poster was then converted to digital media and made available to all members of leadership throughout the corporations.

CONCLUSION

Providing a means of allowing frontline staff the opportunity to openly share concerns and information with management has been shown to improve engagement, retention, and overall satisfaction. Throughout the completion of this project, positive results were achieved by instituting a formal process for which staff could share information, as well as how they would be kept apprised of the outcomes of any raised concerns. This process was instituted with a trial group and found to be overwhelmingly successful.

The project was designed around numerous research projects identifying the best in practice for employee rounding. This lent itself well to translation into policy to achieve permanent practice change. As the project came to completion, the change in practice continued moving forward so that the outcomes could be sustained.

REFERENCES

American Association of Colleges of Nursing. (2010). AACN launches free online HWE team assessment tool. *Critical Care Nurse*, 30-30 1p.

American Association of Colleges of Nursing. (2016). AACN Releases New Edition of HWE Standards. *AACN Bold Voices, 8*(4), 7-7 1/2p.

Adams, S. L. (2016). Influences of turnover, retention, and job embeddedness in the nursing workforce literature. *Online Journal of Rural Nursing and Health Care, 16*(2), 168–195. doi:10.14574/ojrnhc.v16i2.405.

Aon Hewitt (2012). The multiplier effect-insights into how senior leaders drive employee engagement higher, retrieved from http://www.aon.com/attachments/thought-leadership/Aon-Hewitt-White-paper_Engagement.pdf

Baudler, C. R. (2011). Employee engagement: Through effective performance management by Edward M. Mone and Manuel London. *Personnel Psychology, 64*(3), 813–816. doi:10.1111/j.1744-6570.2011.01226_5.x

Bhuvanaiah, T., & Raya, R. P. (2015). Mechanism of improved performance: Intrinsic motivation and employee engagement. *SCMS Journal of Indian Management, 12*(4), 92–97.

BlessingWhite (2013). Leadership development vs employee engagement retrieved from http://blessingwhite.com/article/2013/06/20/leadership-development-vs-employee-engagement/

Bouffard, W. L. (2012). Ten leadership qualities that fuel employee engagement retrieved from http://hiring.monster.com/hr/hr-best-practices/workforce-management/improving-employee-relations/employee-engagement.aspx

Cabral, L., & Johnson, C. (2015). Generating staff buy-in for the patient-centered medical home. *Physician Leadership Journal, 2*(5), 64–67.

Cottingham S., DiBartolo M.C., Battistoni S. and Brown T. (2011) Partners in nursing:

a mentoring initiative to enhance nurse retention. *Nursing Education Perspectives 32* (4), 250–255.

de Bruijn, G., Wiedemann, A. and Rhodes, R. E. (2014). An investigation into the relevance of action planning, theory of planned behaviour concepts, and automaticity for fruit intake action control. *British Journal of Health Psychology, 19*(3), 652–669. doi:10.1111/bjhp.12067

Franciscan Visiting Nurse Service. 2016. Journey to Excellence Score Card. Unpublished internal document.

Gupta, M. (2015). A study on employees perception towards employee engagement. *Globsyn Management Journal, 9*(1/2), 45–51.

Hairr, D. C., Salisbury, H., Johannsson, M., & Redfern-Vance, N. (2014). Nurse staffing and the relationship to job satisfaction and retention. *Nursing Economic$, 32*(3), 142–147.

International Council of Nurses (2006) The global nursing shortage: Priority areas for intervention. Geneva:International Council of Nurses/Florence Nightingale International Foundation.

Jones, J. (2015). Effective leadership in the 21st Century. *Radiology Management, 37*(6), 16–19.

Lather, A. S., & Jain, V. K. (2015). Ten C's leadership practices impacting employee engagement: A study of hotel and tourism industry. *Vilakshan: The XIMB Journal of Management, 12*(2), 59–74.

Lesaux, N. K., Marietta, S. H., & Galloway, E. P. (2014). Learning to be a change agent: System leaders master skills to encourage buy-in for reforms. *Journal of Staff Development, 35*(5), 40–45.

Michaelidou, N. and Hassan, L. (2014). New advances in attitude and behavioural decision-making models. *Journal of Marketing Management, 30*(5/6), 519–528. doi:1 0.1080/0267257X.2014.884368

Mone, E., Eisinger, C., Guggenheim, K., Price, B., & Stine, C. (2011). Performance management at the wheel: Driving employee engagement in organizations. *Journal of Business & Psychology, 26*(2), 205–212.

Moran, G. (2011). The hidden costs of employee turnover. Entrepreneur. Retrieved from http://www.entrepreneur.com/article/220254

Nurse Reinvestment Act Background. (n.d.). Retrieved from http://www.nursingworld. org/MainMenuCategories/Policy-Advocacy/Federal/NurseReinvestmentAct.html

Nursing Solutions, Inc. 2015. 2015 National healthcare retention & RN staffing report. Retrieved from: www.nsinursingsolution.com

Pooreh, S., & Hosseini Nodeh, Z. (2015). Impact of education based on theory of planned gehavior: An investigation into hypertension-preventive self-care behaviors in Iranian girl adolescent. *Iranian Journal of Public Health, 44*(6), 839–847.

Salanova, M., Lorente, L., Chambel, M. J. and Martínez, I. M. (2011). Linking transformational leadership to nurses' extra-role performance: the mediating role of self-efficacy and work engagement. *Journal of Advanced Nursing, 67*(10), 2256–2266 11p. doi:10.1111/j.1365-2648.2011.05652.x

Set, communicate, and achieve buy-in to expectations. (2014). *Medical Staff Briefing, 24*(1), 3–6.

Shuck, B., Reio, T. G. and Rocco, T. S. (2011). Employee engagement: an examination of antecedent and outcome variables. *Human Resource Development International, 14*(4), 427–445. doi:10.1080/13678868.2011.601587

Tips to tackle the employee engagement crisis. (2016). *Health Care Registration: The Newsletter for Health Care Registration Professionals, 25*(6), 3-5.

Toller, C. (2016). If you're happy and you know it. Canadian Business, 89(1), 36-40.

Walsh, C. (2012). Employee Engagement and the role of leadership: Creating alignment, synergy and balance.

Zafar, D. F., Nasir, H. M., & Abbas, A. F. (2014). Four factors to influence organization & employee commitment to change within Pakistan. *IOSR Journal of Business and Management, 16*(1), 43–53. doi:10.9790/487x-16144353

Zhang, T., Avery, G.C., Bergsteiner, H. and More, E. (2014). The relationship between leadership paradigms and employee engagement. *Journal of Global Responsibility* 01/2014; 5(1). DOI: 10.1108/JGR-02-2014-0006

CHAPTER 15

Enhancing Cultural Competence Among the Psychiatric Population

GERLYN CAMPBELL, DNP, APRN, PMHNP

INTRODUCTION

The excitement of entering a Doctor of Nursing Practice (DNP) program is often very intriguing and indulging for most. Often times, students find that their program expectations incite numerous challenges, especially during the initial phase of a DNP project. The purpose of the DNP degree is to enable nurses to practice at a terminal degree level, incorporating their many years of expertise and knowledge to help influence healthcare outcomes. Since most DNP programs require projects with specific concentrations, candidates can expect to direct their attention towards project initiatives in alignment with their programs focus. The focus of my DNP program was to initiate leadership objectives that could help to improve healthcare outcomes. Like most readers, it was very challenging to find a clinical exemplar that was primarily leadership based, yet not educational or interventional. In addition, I had to ensure that the basis of my project was not attempting to institute any types of research activities or manipulation of variables. Having a passion for psychiatry, I quickly zoomed into ideas that could better improve the health and outcomes of that population. Although there were many avenues that could be addressed with that population, I chose initiatives that felt more feasible, yet fulfilling and gratifying, for both the facility and patient population. This was also the option that involved the least cost to implement.

One will find that any feasible project outcome first requires a review of data already posted. A primary struggle I experienced during this phase was ensuring that my project initiatives were geared toward data already published versus ones of unknown outcomes. After completing an exhaustive and inclusive search of several databases, such as EB-SCOhost, PubMed, CINHAL, Medline, and professional organizational websites, I made the decision to pursue a project initiative that included methods which enhanced cultural competence among the mental health population. This population was chosen because of the many complexities that are usually involved in their care, ranging from a lack of access to equitable services due to limited resources, lack in health insurance, stigma of mental illnesses, and general underrepresentation in the healthcare arena. Use of key terms and proper identification of peer-reviewed articles were also invaluable to this search.

Objectives

Clear objectives are a necessity when establishing any project guideline. These objectives not only help to provide a stronger basis for initiatives, but also help to set a clear understanding and standard, especially when seeking stakeholder support. I understood that the timeline of the project would be limited to a very short time span, which resulted in choosing objectives that could be tested and measured within a 30-day period. As the project progressed, I also realized that this time frame helped to boost participant enthusiasm and eagerness to fulfill the project initiatives.

PICO

Once I understood the nature of my project question, I then implemented a PICO format that would better outline my objectives. This PICO format was a lifesaver, as it helped to provide clearer outlines, especially during the process of gaining faculty approval. As the project progressed, I also discovered that the format assisted to better identify my objectives.

Selecting a Project Mentor and Content Expert

Once the above steps were achieved, the next steps involved pairing with a Project Mentor (PM) and Content Expert (CE). Some programs require both, whereas others allow freedom of choice in regard to the content expert. Both the PM and CE should be individuals who hold doctorate degrees in one's field and who have significant experience with DNP projects. The PM is also that person who can help to facilitate a project along, especially those in which there are various data analyses that you might not have experience applying and evaluating. Once everything has been set in place, all candidates including the PM and CE, can collaborate on the project objectives, making sure that you've adequately addressed roject guidelines as initially anticipated.

Stakeholder

Stakeholder support was a necessary yet arduous process during the initial project phase. The project was targeted to review interdepartmental policies and procedures, as they related to cultural services the targeted facility provided to the psychiatric patient population. Many of the potential stakeholders were willing to support the project, yet funding remained a primary factor. At the time of the project, the policies already in place were aimed at providing comprehensive mental health services through cultural screening, yet there continued to be a problem in their referral rates and patient satisfaction. Their most recent Press Ganey results yielded an 80% satisfaction rate among staff and patients, which showed that they had not met their interdepartmental benchmark of 90% as previously envisioned. Several key stakeholders recognized my project initiatives as a quality improvement intervention and were all in full support of its implementation.

During the initial phase of the clinic, a cultural tool was implemented, but it was not well adopted by all staff personnel, which resulted in lower success rates. As a result, most of the stakeholders were eager to implement cost-effective strategies such the ones I suggested to help boost patient satisfaction. In addition, timing, budgeting, and compliance were all primary considering factors. Several meetings and presentations of the project objectives were required to gain full stakeholder support. Once this phase was agreed upon, it was then approved to fully implement the project.

Clinical Problem

A thorough and exhaustive literature review is first needed before any DNP project can be successful. This includes not only knowing one's topic, but also understanding various treatment modalities and approaches. Oftentimes, DNP candidates might find that literature review may or may not fully support their interventions, which can be painstaking for most. During my literature review, I discovered not only the importance of culture as it related to psychiatric practices, but also a component leading to misdiagnoses, which often presents when an individual appears disorganized largely due to cultural norms, mores, and practices. Core beliefs can often be misinterpreted in psychiatric settings, where standard beliefs and practices may appear ambiguous. Gaining further insight into my problem, I was able to identify that mandatory use of cultural tools, especially during patient admission, had the ability to decrease mortality and morbidity. In addition, these tools were not only shown to improve standards of care, but also helped to improve the stance of the therapeutic client-provider relationship. The research further showed an overwhelming necessity for these types of practices, especially in the United States, where a migrant population has significantly increased during the recent decades (United States Census Bureau [USCB], 2015; Multicultural Mental Healthcare [MMH], 2017). I then completed exhaustive research on types of cultural tools and questionnaires that could provide clear and reliable outcomes. Because gaining approval for tool utilization is usually a necessary process, I then wrote the owners of the selected tools and questionnaires, in hopes for full written approval to use in this project. One should note that full approval of tools and questionnaires can take considerable time to complete and should request for permission of selected tools, as early as the tool has been decided upon.

Framework

Frameworks provide a basis for care delivery and are useful components of a successful DNP project. In undergoing this phase, I utilized the Theory of Transcultural Care, modeled by Madeline's Leininger. This Transcultural Nursing Theory (TNT) is also referred to as Culture Care Theory (CCT). The CCT was developed to assist researchers in studying transcultural human care phenomena and establish the knowledge required by nurses to deliver care in a multicultural world (Betancourt, 2015). According to McFarland and Alamah (2015), the theory was developed after integrating nursing care with cultural anthropology to address the varying patterns of caring among cultures. The rise in globalization of many different cultures also made the need for the services I was proposing, a necessity to providing equitable access to healthcare.

As a fellow psychiatric nurse and doctoral candidate, I had identified a lack in cultural sensitivity when working with the psychiatric population. Although culture has largely been stressed as a paramount basis of care in the United States, it appeared that this lack often resulted due to the many crisis, debilitation, population growth, and lower economic status that existed among many of that population. Because of these instances, the data showed that many patients tend to experience delays in having their cultural needs fully understood and included in their care. In addition, it was shown that numerous patients felt that a number of needs were not fully met, which often lead to non-adherence and dissatisfaction in the delivery of care. Issues such as socio-economic backgrounds, racial disparities, stigma, a lack of ethnic and linguistic services, and health insurance were shown as contributory factors affecting the standards of care (United States Department of Health and Human Services [UDHHS], 2016; Crowley and Kirschner, 2009). The presentation and manifestation of mental illnesses was shown not only to increase the likelihood of nonadherence among patients, but also to potentially increase the incidence of recidivism. The American Psychiatric Association (APA, 2016) also mentioned that cultural barriers and a lack of access to culturally competent care continued to affect the levels of care currently received by the psychiatric population. Based on these criteria, the demand for cultural awareness and competence remained in high demand and required high recognition of such by all healthcare organizations. In a position statement by the National Institutes of Health (2016), it was reiterated that cultural and linguistic competency are paramount to effective healthcare delivery and should be the cornerstone care delivery. The provision of competent care does not suffice for complete cultural knowledge of specific backgrounds but provides a basis for which standards of care can be established and adopted. By the improvement of cultural competency among the psychiatric population, standards of care are increased, helping to eliminate health disparities—a direct initiative of Healthy People 2020 (Healthypeople.gov, 2016). In the TNT framework, the focus of cultural mores, norms, beliefs, and practices were largely compounded as a basis for effective care, which had the potential to increase standards of care for the mental health population. The TNT also provided further insight into a person's upbringing, values, and beliefs, which might affect their acceptance toward care. Understanding the challenges and perplexities involved in providing holistic psychiatric care to individuals with mental illnesses also abetted to providing more specific accommodation and cultural preservation. Since the research showed that barriers to adequate cultural services were a crucial factor when providing care to the psychiatric population, the benefits of implementing the proposed interventions far outweighed traditional approaches employed by the targeted facility. Given that my project was focused on integrating cultural practices and preferences into care, the theory further assisted in defining, aligning, and manipulating the project outcomes.

Tools/Instrumentation

Approval of the selected tool was fully authorized by each owner prior to the initialization of the project. The selected tool was also very broad and could be utilized in a variety of settings to enhance cultural services. The tool has an inter-rater reliability of 0.73 and $p > 0.059$. In addition, the tool was implemented for use in psychiatric settings and had been broadly adapted in mental health settings. Because the tool was already evaluated for its efficacy in addressing the needs of individuals affected by psychiatric illnesses, it was considered a reliable tool in working to identify the specified data needed.

Description of Project Design

A quantitative project design was utilized to enhance the necessary required project initiatives. Their outpatient clinic has been operating for the last four years and is a relatively new department, added to broaden mental health services. The organization has been striving to utilize a uniformed cultural assessment tool, to help serve the large population of immigrants and various ethnicities in the community. The department aims to incorporate the use of a cultural tool to help enhance their delivery of culturally sensitive care and commitment to values among their patients. According to Ziebland and Hunt (2014), this design was appropriate to help validate the pre and post test data collection process, which is invaluable in the formulation of quality improvement measures at an organizational level. A pre and post test design was applied to gather pertinent data about the delivery of cultural services within the organization. The pre test was administered prior to live and online presentation on the need for the enhancement of cultural services within the organization. Participants additionally had the chance to ask questions and include feedback. Post test results were gathered after a 30-day trial period of the tool, through interdepartmental surveys and feedback.

Recruitment Methods

After carefully selecting my project question, stakeholder support, and identifying my tools, the next phase of recruiting was then initiated. This process involved presenting to nursing and auxiliary staff and elaborating the basis for the project objectives, methods, and expected outcomes. The project was approved as a quality improvement project and, therefore, the organization did not require any articulation agreements to facilitate its implementation. The initial steps taken to initiate the strategies mentioned above were included in full written approval from the doctoral committee and permission from the owners of the tools to incorporate it as part of anticipated project. Secondly, a presentation to staff detailing current and expected practices on cultural awareness was initiated. Prior to implementation of the tool, staff who volunteered to utilize the tool completed an online training module, which was approved by the facility. Implementation of the tool and how it would be used was also discussed. Staff was provided with the opportunity to ask detailed questions about the tool. A survey was also given with pre-and post-feedback of the tool. Key stakeholders then were to review staff feedback, referral rates, and efficacy of the tool, and to decide on approval. Once fully approved by stakeholders, after the 30-day departmental trial period, the Information technology (IT) department was then expected to take on further duties to upload the questionnaire in the admissions checklist for electronic use. To initiate execution of the project, approval was first needed by the school, in addition to signed agreements from stakeholders of their support for the identified initiatives. Once these were completed, participants were then required to sign agreement forms stipulating their willingness to complete the project within the allotted time frames. A total of 30 volunteers were initially expected to participate in the process, of which only 27 completed.

Timeline

My project was completed in a 30-day period after written approval was received from faculty, Institutional Review Board (IRB) approval was granted, stakeholder support was granted and articulation agreements were initiated, and approval of the selected tools were granted. During the first weeks of the project phase, an orientation to participating staff, including an online training module designed to refresh them on cultural competence, was conducted. During this period, the pre-questionnaire tool was also administered. The participants completed the pre questionnaire evaluation as a component of the online orientation module. During the second and third week, the staff completed at least 25 referrals in the community, as anticipated. Referrals made for culturally based psychiatric services were based on the needs identified by selected cultural tools. Routine use of the tool was used to help clinicians identify the unique needs and preferences of their patient's needs, by understanding an individual within his or her cultural context. The efficacy of the tool was evaluated based on the results of the post test. At the final week, the results were analyzed with the findings documented accordingly. Key stakeholders were then invited to disseminate the results.

Ethics and Human Subjects Protection

The DNP project focused on quality improvement measures and was intended to generate knowledge and quality care supplied by the organization. The primary purpose of institutional review of research is to protect human subjects and ensure proper scientific conduct (Grady, 2015). This project did not include exposure of human participants to any types of clinical interventions, and their identities were not involved. Application of the survey tool used was for the sole purpose of supplying organizational data rather than human health data. The employee participants included in the project were volunteers who decided to complete the pre- and post-questionnaire, for the sole purpose of improving care across the organization. Baker (2012) stated that the nature of confidentiality presents complex ethical questions and should be addressed at all points of contact involving research. Confidentiality and protection of the data obtained from employee participants was placed in a locked storage cabinet on the nursing unit, which was accessible to only the project leader. This project was intended to serve as a quality improvement project for the sole purpose of improving services within the organization. Patients were not directly enrolled in this project, negating the use of access to medical records or their permission to participate.

Data Collection Procedures

Data were collected from employee participants within various disciplines in the organization. This included up to 30 volunteer employees who provided feedback. Individuals completing the pre and post questionnaire included nurses, psychiatrists, social workers, and nurse practitioners. To recruit the volunteers, individuals had the opportunity to sign up both at a workshop given about the tool and after completing the 45-minute online module, which was required prior to the initiation of the tool. Full written approval of all selected tools was granted by their owners. These tools were utilized to administer both the pre and post questionnaire. This questionnaire aimed to assess employee feedback within the healthcare organization, based on their knowledge of cultural services needed within community settings and the types of referrals that are made based on cultural services identified. A pre and post program comparative analysis of the outcome measures was conducted to determine the effectiveness of the tool's implementation.

Data Analysis

A refresher course in biostatistics is necessary to help interpret data during this phase. Candidates who have not completed a statistics class within the past 5 years might want to consider hiring a statistician to help review and interpret the data. For the purpose of this project, use of the Statistical Package for the Social Sciences (SPSS) 17.0 statistical software for analysis was invaluable. A quantitative analysis was conducted in relation to the pre- and post-test scores of the selected cultural tools. Data were collected from participant questionnaires and entered into SPSS 17.0 for analysis. Pre- and post-analyses of the collected data were carried out via the use of paired sample t-tests to establish if the incorporation of culturally influenced policies enhanced culturally competent care. My PM suggested the use of the t-test to examine the data, because it was considered the best to explain the pre and post analysis. Also, there was not equal representation between the units, which required massaging the data for a more accurate analysis.

The statistical significance was held at $p \leq 0.05$. Given the nature of my project, all analyses were exploratory and did not represent the power required to adequately interpret statistical significance. A pre and post comparative analysis of the outcome measures of the intervention was carried out to establish the effectiveness of the selected tool's implementation in promoting cultural competency awareness. Significant changes in the feedback were noted in the pre and post intervention results in regard to the participants' knowledge of cultural services required within community settings and the kinds of referrals made.

For the descriptive statistics related to the participants, the survey data were tabulated and analyzed data were associated with demographic characteristics. To undertake an assessment for the change in the level of competency achieved, data collected via the selected tool were pooled and compared. The comparisons were closely assessed based on participant responses during both the pre and post tests. These comparisons were necessary because they helped to determine the efficacy of the tool by establishing if the policy resulted to a statistically significant change in cultural competency levels among the participant population. After the analysis was completed, the findings were presented in the form of Microsoft Excel tables and graphs.

Limitations

Limitations associated with this project were connected to the timeframe of the project's measurement. Because of the limited time associated with this project, a more systematic follow-up with all participants was not achievable. This means that all of the findings were confined to a one-month period. Accordingly, it was impossible to undertake follow-ups to establish the levels of competency of participants and the efficacy of the cultural competency policy. Additionally, the DNP project did not include any qualitative data, such as the description of cultural situations experienced by the participants working in the mental health facility. Subsequently, the latter limitation can be used as a likely area for future research.

In addition, a small participant size of 30 individuals was used for the project, of which only 27 completed the entire process. The participants did not only focus on mere psychiatric specialists (such as psychiatrist, psychiatric nurse practitioners, and psychologists), but also included nurses, psychiatrists, social workers, and nurse practitioners who did not have mental health as the focus of their practices. As of such, the project's findings were based on multi-disciplinary professionals, rather than a particular group of mental health professionals. Nonetheless, this inclusion of a diverse population did not negatively impact the reliability of the intervention findings because, in most cases, mental health facilities make use of an interprofessional team to meet the patient's mental health needs.

Needs and Significance

As expected, the integration of cultural competency in primary care settings was shown to be an imperative component in improving patient-based care. According to Khanna *et al.* (2009), improving knowledge and skills associated with culturally competent care among administrators and providers is necessary for quality improvement. Cultural competency in psychiatric care is of paramount importance and can be implemented via policy change and awareness creation among healthcare professionals. The need for cultural competency is directly associated with the increase in diversity in the national population that requires patient-specific-care based on specific needs. Cultural barriers and a limited access to culturally competent care affect the levels of nursing care received currently by the psychiatric population. The purpose of the quality improvement project was to increase the levels of cultural competency awareness among primary care facilities serving the psychiatric population. The suggested way to increase the level of cultural competency at a local primary outpatient clinic is to develop a policy that requires the integration of cultural screening during all intake assessments. Findings from this project indicated enhanced professional understanding of the healthcare experiences of patients with diverse backgrounds. This improvement supported an effective outcome when cross cultural understanding was required.

The increasing diversity experienced in the United States (U.S) presents challenges and opportunities for healthcare providers, policy makers, and the healthcare system, especially in the creation and delivery of culturally competent services. The field of psychiatry has patients and psychiatric professionals from different cultural, racial, and ethnic backgrounds. Thus, a competent healthcare system is required to assist in improving quality of psychiatric care and health outcomes and to eliminate racial and ethnic health disparities (Aggarwal *et al.,* 2016). The adoptions of culturally competent strategies that are inclusive to all are necessary, because they would move professionals and the organizational culture toward the realization of a healthcare system that focuses on cultural competence. The primary purpose of this quality improvement project was to help increase the awareness of cultural competency among healthcare organizations serving the psychiatric population. The pre and post findings revealed that participants experienced a significant increase in cultural competency following the implementation of a cultural policy. The pre and post survey findings are an indication that during patient evaluations at a local outpatient center, the cultural questionnaire that was implemented led to a significant increase in the cultural awareness by 30% among the professionals participating in this intervention project.

The increased competency levels are associated with improved knowledge and skills relating to the provision of culturally competent healthcare to patients in a primary care clinic. This increase in knowledge was based on the pre and post testing participant scoring. Thus, cultural competency is a core requirement for mental health professionals providing healthcare services to culturally diverse patient groups. Better understanding of race, culture, and ethnicity allowed easier comprehension by these professional participants as to the meanings and the applicability of the diversity in mental nursing (Khanna, Cheyney, and Engle, 2009). Generally, mental illness nursing care is focused on individualized needs. Thus, the consideration of patients' views is important because it allows mental health providers to better understand the specific needs for a culturally diverse perspective. The project findings lead to support the development or revision of policies at local and state levels that mandate the integration of a cultural screening tool during all intake assessments. Subsequently, culturally competent care among the mentally ill population assists psychiatric health providers to improve patient outcomes, safety, and satisfaction (Aggarwal *et al.,* 2016). To nursing practice, especially psychiatry, the project plays a significant role in quality care, by showing how the development of culturally specific policies and implementation in primary outpatient clinics could promote cultural competence (Truong, Paradies, and Priest, 2014). Subsequently, the culturally influenced policy could be used to improve the standards of care, increase cultural awareness, and improve the quality of psychiatric care. Embracing culturally competent care is a core component for any organization providing care to the psychiatric population. Hence, use of cultural tools are indispensable in helping to continuously boost organizational productivity and patient satisfaction in future years.

To implement a policy, it is necessary to perform cultural competency training to improve the quality of psychiatric and mental healthcare for diverse groups. The implementation of cultural competency strategy at the organizational level is encouraged, because it promotes skills development and ongoing awareness among staff on issues concerning diverse cultures.

Cultural competency is composed of a set of congruent skills, policies, and communication strategies that are implemented to facilitate effective delivery of services in healthcare across different cultural backgrounds. Calzada and Suarez-Balcazar (2014) noted that past research has emphasized the need for the role of cultural competency improvement to improve knowledge and skills of healthcare providers in mental care to enable them to work in cross-cultural situations in an effective manner. The incorporation of culturally influenced policies in the healthcare arena can help to enhance culturally competent care especially among the diverse psychiatric population. An increase in cultural awareness can result to improvements in providers' self-reported skills and knowledge as a result of cultural competency training (Truong, Parodies, and Priest, 2014). Subsequently, the local primary care facility will have improved delivery of culturally sensitive care followed by better health outcomes. As noted in this project, cultural competency training can also improve experiences of patients from diverse backgrounds, because the staff members not only work effectively in cross-cultural situations, but also provide high quality patient-centered care.

The findings of this project support the hypothesis that the development and implementation of practical cultural competency policies and framework by healthcare organizations could result in health promotion. The policy that entails assessment and screening of staff during intake could be promoted by diversifying the workforce, integrating cross-cultural training for providers, and providing interpreter services to promote healthcare that meets the needs of a diverse patient population. Almutairi *et al.* (2015) contended that when patients are provided with culturally sensitive care, they are more likely to be satisfied and show an increased level of adherence toward medical advice and treatment.

Cultural competency in psychiatric care is of paramount importance and can be implemented via policy change and awareness creation among healthcare professionals. The need for cultural competency is directly associated with an increase in diversity in the national population that requires patient-specific care based on specific needs. Cultural barriers and a limited access to culturally competent care affect the levels of nursing care received currently by the psychiatric population.

Implications for Nursing

Nurses are the forefront of healthcare and are enabled with increased opportunities to enhance patient care delivery. Because of diversity in the workplace, nurses work with patients from various backgrounds and disciplines. Nurses are the primary advocates of patients and are the main liaisons between patients and the healthcare system (Manesh *et al.*, 2012). These dynamics require the application of quality improvement measures that work to eliminate barriers to optimal care. Nurses are the forefront of healthcare and interact with patients affected by psychiatric disorders on a daily basis (McKeown, Ridley, and Fleischmann, 2015). Embracing culturally competent care helps the nurse to serve as a patient liaison and advocate. The ability to identify and understand quality measures that contribute to the enhancement of culturally competent care among the psychiatric population, not only are paramount to effective healthcare practices, but also contribute to optimal patient outcomes.

Dissemination of the Findings

Once the data have been collected and analyzed, the next phase is the dissemination process. A meaningful dissemination of one's analytic results can be carried out in two ways. The first is to ensure that data and findings are made available to all interested researchers and healthcare professionals. The second approach to meaningful dissemination of the findings involves publications. The publications could be made available to different stakeholders through poster presentations; refereed journals; and proceedings of seminars or conferences; and annual reports of institutions. Posters can also be used to disseminate the evidence-based findings and data to the involved stakeholders including nurses, researchers, policy makers, and other health and community care professionals. In comparison to publications, poster presentations are beneficial because they allow the presenter to distribute the findings in a relaxed, informal, interactive, and ocial manner (Ranse and Hayes, 2013). Additionally, posters, compared to manuscript publications in a peer-reviewed journal, are easy to publish and disseminate to the audience.

Doctoral candidates are also encouraged to publish their findings in peer-reviewed journals in efforts to disseminate and appeal to different stakeholders. Publication is based on the acceptance of an article topic, which will be later pursued at a later date. Publication is an appropriate approach to findings dissemination, because it promotes sharing with different stakeholders, including patients, nurses, physicians, and other healthcare professionals (Ranse and Hayes, 2013). The available publication opportunities include book reviews, electronic journals, evidence-based guidelines, and policy briefs.

Seminars and conference presentations are also invaluable in cases in which the DNP candidate has the ability to present their project outcomes orally to various stakeholders within the healthcare arena (Brownson, Colditz, and Proctor, 2012; Ranse and Hayes, 2013). Presentations in conference and seminars are also effective means of disseminating findings to impart knowledge and awareness to others. Moreover, these types of settings allow for immediate feedback and critique from peers prior to presentations of final manuscripts and publications.

Post Project Thoughts

DNP prepared nurses are constantly faced with several challenges within the healthcare arena. Their ability to identify, appraise, implement, and evaluate system changes are the one of the most useful assets they possess. A solid basis of the DNP project and program outcomes are insurmountably invaluable to any DNP candidate. Understanding one's initiatives and project flows additionally brightens the path for a stellar project. Proper time management; early initiation of project initiatives, including stakeholder support; permission of applicable tools; and faculty approval are invaluable to a successful project. In addition, working in close alignment with one's project mentor and content expert enhances the smoothness and stance of a project. The DNP degree empowers nurses to practice at the highest standards of the nursing profession. In this capacity, nurses assume leadership roles, which empower not only their areas of expertise, but also that of clinical practice and research settings. The DNP possesses several qualities that enhance nursing practice, serving as a base for theoretical practices and research utilization. As DNP scholars, advocates, and leaders, nurses have the ability to work from behind the scenes, holding positions in faculty and healthcare settings to help students and staff challenge everyday demands while applying knowledge at the highest levels to critically think and improve standards of care. Given the autonomous role of the DNP, nurses should strive at developing expert DNP projects that continually influence healthcare policies, enhancing nursing care and enriching healthcare delivery initiatives.

REFERENCES

American Psychiatric Association. (2013). *Diagnostic and statistical manual of mental disorders*: DSM-5. (pp. 749–759). Washington, D.C: American Psychiatric Association

Aggarwal, N. K., Cedeño, K., Guarnaccia, P., Kleinman, A., & Lewis-Fernández, R. (2016). The meanings of cultural competence in mental health: An exploratory focus group study with patients, clinicians, and administrators. *SpringerPlus, 5*, 384. doi:10.1186/s40064-016-2037-4.

Almutairi, A. F., Dahinten, V.S. and Rodney, P. (2015). Almutairi's Critical Cultural Competence model for a multicultural healthcare environment. *Nursing Inquiry, 22*(4), 317–325. doi:10.1111/nin.12099

Baker, T. D. (2012). Confidentiality and electronic surveys: How IRBs address ethical and technical issues. *IRB: Ethics & Human Research, 34*(5), 8–15.

Betancourt, D. A. (2015). Madeleine Leininger and the Transcultural Theory of Nursing. *The Downtown Review, 2*(1). 1-6. Retrieved from http://engagedscholarship. csuohio.edu/cgi/viewcontent.cgi?article=1020&context=tdr

Brownson, R. C., Colditz, G. A. and Proctor, E. K. (2018). *Dissemination and implementation research in health: Translating science to practice*. Oxford, UK: Oxford University Press.

Calzada, E. and Suarez-Balcazar, Y. (2014). *Enhancing cultural competence in social service agencies: A promising approach to serving diverse children and families.* Washington, DC: Office of Planning, Research and Evaluation, Administration for Children and Families, U.S. Department of Health and Human Services.

Crowley, R. A. and Kirschner, N. (2015). The integration of care for mental health, substance abuse, and other behavioral health conditions into primary care: executive summary of an American College of Physicians position paper. *Annals of Internal Medicine, 163*(4), 298–299. https://doi-org.proxy.library.maryville.edu/10.7326/M15-0510

Grady, C. (2015). Institutional review boards: Purpose and challenges. *Chest*, (5), 1148. https://doi-org.proxy.library.maryville.edu/10.1378/chest.15-0706.

Khanna, S. K., Cheyney, M., & Engle, M. (2009). Cultural competency in health care: Evaluating the outcomes of cultural competency training among health care professionals. *Journal of the National Medical Association, 101*(9), 886–892. Retrieved from http://www.journalnma.org/article/S0027-9684(15)31035-X/pdf.

Manesh, H., Tafreshi, Z., Ashktorab, T. and Majd, A. (2012). The comparison among perspective of doctors, nurses and patients towards nursing advocacy role. *Journal of Nursing & Midwifery, 22*(76), 10p.

McFarland, M. R. and Wehbe-Alamah, H. B. (2015). *Leininger's Culture Care Diversity and Universality* (Vol. Third edition). Burlington, MA: Jones & Bartlett Learning. Retrieved from http://proxy.library.maryville.edu/login?url=https://search.ebscohost.com/login.aspx?direct=true&db=nlebk&AN=666051&site=eds-live&scope=site

McKeown, M., Ridley, J. and Fleischmann, P. (2015). Doing the right thing: Mental health nursing support for independent advocacy. *Mental Health Nursing, 35*(3), 10–12.

Multicultural Mental Healthcare. (2017). Responding to cultural diversity in mental health. Retrieved from: http://www.multiculturalmentalhealth.ca/clinical-tools/cultural-formulation/

National Institutes of Health. (2016). Cultural respect. Retrieved from: https://www.nih.gov/institutes-nih/nih-office-director/office-communications-public-liaison/clear-communication

Office of Disease Prevention and Health Promotion (2016). *Healthy people 2020.* Retrieved from https://www.healthypeople.gov/2020/topics-objectives/topic/Access-to-Health-Services

Ranse, J. and Hayes, C. (2013). A novice' s guide to preparing and presenting an oral presentation at a Scientific Conference. *Australian Journal of Paramedicine, 7*(1), 1–9. Retrieved from http://ro.ecu.edu.au/cgi/viewcontent.cgi?article=1314&context=jephc

Truong, M., Paradies, Y. and Priest, N. (2014). Interventions to improve cultural competency in health care: A systematic review of reviews. *Biomed Central Health Research Services, 14* (99), 1–17.

United States Census Bureau. (2015). Demographic analysis 2010: Estimates of coverage of the foreign-born population in the American community survey. Retrieved from: https://www.census.gov/content/dam/Census/library/working-papers/2015/demo/POP-twps0103.pdf

United States Department of Health and Human Services (2016). Cultural competency. Retrieved from: http://minorityhealth.hhs.gov/

Ziebland, S. and Hunt, K. (2014). Using secondary analysis of qualitative data of patient experiences of health care to inform health services research and policy. *Journal of Health Services Research & Policy, 19*(3), 177–182. doi:10.1177/1355819614524187

Interprofessional Collaboration to Improve Postnatal Care Transitions by Revising an Innovative Application

SHAWANA BURNETTE, DNP, RN, NE-BC, RN-C

INTRODUCTION

The phenomenon of innovation and informatics in healthcare once seemed foreign to nursing practice. Healthcare is evolving, and the delivery of care must keep up. Healthcare leaders must think outside of the healthcare arena and engage the expertise of other professions. Nursing leaders have the capacity to be the pioneers who build the bridge to integrate innovation with the delivery of high-quality care outcomes. Innovative nursing leaders are vital for the sustainability of high-quality care processes. Engaging the expertise of other successful professions can enhance the efforts to meet the demands of an ever-changing society and demanding market for accessibility.

Over the years, scholarship has evolved into more than just knowledge. Scholarship is now valued as a level of credibility and standard of professionalism (McMillin, 2004). The role of a Doctor of Nursing Practice (DNP) prepared nurse is to apply evidence-based knowledge and clinical expertise to develop nursing practices and policies aimed at assisting nursing professionals in providing safe and efficient care. Ideally, the DNP nurse works as a clinical engineer. Engineers rely on the detailed accuracy of architects to research and draw the blueprints for development. Then the engineer studies the design, gathers the resources, and develops a plan for implementing the architect's ideas into physical form. PhD prepared nurses are like the architect. They provide the blueprints in the form of research and the DNP prepared nurse evaluates the evidence, develops a plan, gathers resources, and implements the research into practice. DNP nurses investigate and decipher complicated processes. They integrate evidence-based practices

295

into healthcare systems to ensure the care delivered in the organization meets standards based on research recommendations for positive outcomes (Conrad, 2014).

Conquering the world alone is impossible, making interprofessional collaboration a necessity for being a successful leader in today's healthcare environment. Having the ability to connect multiple disciplines of healthcare directly impacts the improvement of population health. By producing a scholarly project that validates the impact of interprofessional collaboration to integrate a care transition app into nursing practice, others can be inspired to think outside of the clinical setting to come up with creative ways to approach clinical concerns. Being able to see the possibilities, in similar situations, is fundamental in leading collaborative efforts to improve practice. Through scientific underpinning, the DNP prepared nursing leader is trained to evaluate scholarly works to improve practice. The DNP program has a high regard for innovative and evidence-based practices that reflects the application of information found in research (Conrad, 2014).

Facilitating interprofessional collaborations that improve patient and population health outcomes is an untapped skill that DNP prepared nurses possess. Because the healthcare environment is multifaceted, enlisting the knowledge and skills of other professional experts is vital to creating synergetic practices, policies, and processes. Essential VI of the *Essentials of Doctoral Education for Advanced Nursing Practice* elicits the DNP nurse to lead interprofessional teams through effective communications and a collaboration of skills to develop, implement, analyze, and evaluate professional practices and standards (AACN, 2006). An article in the *Journal of Interprofessional Care* describes the advanced practice nursing profession's training in nursing theory and practice as a key factor that "engenders trust," aiding in the ability to build connections across professions. Education and trust support a DNP nursing leader's ability to facilitate diverse collaborations within complex systems (Perkin, 2011).

Healthcare is being engulfed by technology. This project depicts an opportunity for nursing to lead the way in integrating alternative platforms for providing care. The childbearing population is at the forefront of technology so meeting the patients where they are most comfortable is imperative for successful interactions. Essential IV of the *Essentials of Doctoral Education for Advanced Nursing Practice* empowers the DNP leader to master skills related to information technology systems and patient care technology for the improvement and transformation of healthcare (AACN, 2006). By using system thinking to positively impact healthcare processes, ideas can be transformed to enhance outcomes. Innovation sounds compelling on the surface, but it can pose some resistance from the executive stakeholders due to risk and uncertainty for sustainability. Dixon-Woods *et al.* (2010) says that limited evidence exists to support innovative methods and products that create a risk and gamble for the technology executives to buy-in to ideas (Dixon-Woods *et al.*, 2010).

BACKGROUND

One issue piercing perinatal services is an increased push to decrease length of stay (LOS) for postnatal patients and improve satisfaction related to care experience. In the past 25 years, hospital LOS for the postnatal patient has progressively decreased, transforming the way nurses deliver care. In 1992, the American Academy of Pediatrics (AAP) and the American College of Obstetricians and Gynecologist (AGOC) jointly published *Guidelines for Perinatal Care* that recommended 48 hours LOS for vaginal deliveries and up to 96 hours LOS for Cesarean deliveries (Eaton, 2001). With the current changes in healthcare, for some women, the inpatient birth experience is their first hospitalization. The transition from frequent monitoring and healthcare support in the prenatal period to the postpartum period with less frequent healthcare interactions can be a challenge for new mothers (Pai, 2013).

A current focus for hospitals is to decrease the LOS for maternal patients to create capacity for the increasing volume. Because of the multi-layered care and education being compiled in the postnatal stay for the mother and baby, nurses struggle to properly prepare mothers for this transition. Federal agencies and organizations such as The Joint Commission on Accreditation of Hospital Organizations (JCAHO) have challenged healthcare to improve care quality, especially regarding handoff communication and transitions of care (The Joint Commission, 2012). Research suggests that the increased focus on early discharge of maternity patients after delivery leads to the need to improve discharge processes. The push for decreased hospital stays coupled with a lack of structured support for women has been tagged as a major factor in making this transition difficult for the postpartum population (Barimani & Vikstrom, 2015). Mobile health is infiltrating the healthcare domain at a rapid speed; therefore, to continue providing affordable high-quality care, healthcare systems must find cost-effective ways, such as technology integration, to improve the way care is delivered (Williams, 2012).

Applications (apps) have been identified as patient-centered ways consumers are receiving health information. Reports show that in January 2014, nineteen percent of smartphone users have at least one health application on their phone (Houdek *et al.*, 2015). Per a business intelligence article by Meola (2016), wearable health tracker devices and mobile health app usage have increased by 50% since 2014. The survey referenced in the article spanned over seven countries with over 8,000 people included. In a similar 2014 survey cited in the same article, 16% of respondents were said to use mobile health apps, whereas 33% responded as users of mobile health apps in 2016 (Meola, 2016).

The idea for this project to develop and implement an app was relevant, yet the complexity of app development and implementation realistically superseded the timeframe allowed. Thus, collaboration with an app company to improve and enhance a current product became the focus of this project, aimed at improving postpartum transitions. An app company named Baby Scripts was established in 2014, with the vision to use technology to advance healthcare. The company's foundational team is made up of engineers, designers, marketers, doctors, and scientists who all have a common passion for improving the status quo of pregnancy care delivery. Over the years, Baby Scripts has collaborated with major healthcare systems to create a product that improves patient outcomes for the maternity population, improves patient satisfaction, and creates additional office visits for obstetrical (OB) offices (1EQ Incorporated, 2016). With fundamental success of the app, a collaboration with this company to enhance the existing product became the best tactic for this scholarly work. Through idea sharing and structural consultations, a team approach was taken to gain support to collaborate with and engage new stakeholders.

PROBLEM STATEMENT

Based on the background information given, the problem identified is related to the propulsion to decrease LOS after delivery, which limits the time available to adequately educate and provide postnatal patients with the support needed to make the transition. There is a need for more innovative interventions to help better prepare maternity patients for care transitions in the postnatal period, and there are opportunities to connect with maternity patients using technology. Technology is invading health-care, and there are opportunities to leverage mobile health approaches to improve care practices for this population across the continuum.

There are some gaps in the literature for current clinical recommenda-tions that show impacts in LOS for the postnatal patient. There were lim-ited quantitative case studies to provide stronger levels of evidence. One of the challenges with innovate project implementation is that the data to support the project are not plain and easily deciphered. Creative inquiry is necessary to integrate the evidence-based literature to produce innova-tive practices with the necessary literature support. Many of the articles reviewed made suggestions for further research related to this topic.

This scholarly project will help contribute evidence supporting the value of interprofessional collaboration when innovative ideas attempt to blur the lines between healthcare and technology. There is limited re-search that provides high level evidence on the use of technology, such as mobile apps in healthcare. Most studies are more descriptive and lack statistical validity. Because of the increased access to technology, more research is in development that is designed to produce a higher level of evidence. This scholarly project will serve as the foundation of knowledge to continue to build premises for future research implemen-tation to help contribute to this up and coming knowledge base.

Purpose/Objective

The development of an enhanced postnatal care transition app was identified as an intervention that would give maternity patients access to multimedia methods to receive educational information, resources, and support after delivery. The app allows providers to prescribe educa-tion earlier, gives reminders, has ways to monitor remotely, and allows patients to access their discharge information through the app. The use of apps has been identified as a patient-centered way consumer are re-ceiving health information and, as of January 2014, 19% of smartphone users have at least one health app on their phones (Houdek *et al.*, 2015).

There is value in establishing diverse professional groups to leverage each professional's expertise when developing and implementing proj-ects. Mitchell and Boyle (2015) imply that the problem with innovation is that its value is based mainly on perception. On the other hand, hav-ing multiple perspectives can enhance innovation. Being able to trans-late a common vision into action and engage multiple professions to better healthcare is a necessary skill for a DNP leader. Many use the creation of diverse teams to address complex problems and issues. High open-mindedness has been linked to the production of highly innovative ideas (Mitchell and Boyle, 2015).

The short-term objectives of this scholarly project were to use clinical scholarship and scientific underpinnings to evaluate evidence-based practices that support the need to incorporate innovative technology into the care processes for maternity patients. Also, to translate scholarly information to facilitate a diverse interprofessional collaboration with an established application company to enhance a postnatal mobile app that to improve care transitions for postnatal patients. The third objective was to gain interdisciplinary support and approval from a complex healthcare system, using Roger's Diffusion of Innovation Theory, the Interprofessional Competency Frameworks, and Jean Watson's Caring Science, to incorporate the app into maternal care processes through system thinking.

Implementing new practices into a multi-facility healthcare system is a complex undertaking that starts with collaboration and a common goal to improve outcomes. The multiprofessional relationships formed because of this project provide the foundation for ongoing work that will continue to be facilitated among the diverse interprofessional collaborative group. The long-term goals of the scholarly project focused on defining an implementation plan to pilot use of the app in a maternity office setting, evaluating the effectiveness of the app usage related to the impact on maternal outcomes after the postpartum period and dissemination of the finding into the body of scholarly works led by a DNP nursing leader.

A strength, weakness, opportunity, and threat (SWOT) analysis was complete to identify the feasibility of the project. This analysis identified the strengths of supporting the development of an app, the weaknesses to getting revisions implemented, opportunities created from use of the app, and threats to using the app in practice. The findings of the analysis helped identify ways to approach the app company and organization to convey the need for collaboration to develop enhancements and use of the app. Findings were also used to entice hospital and nursing executives to get project buy-in.

CLINICAL QUESTION

The PICOT question for this project is, in a complex healthcare system, does the interprofessional collaboration with a DNP prepared nursing leader help increase innovative care technology resources for postnatal patients and providers to improve care transitions during the business interaction period with a software company?

Data show that women are 200% more likely than men to use health apps and young adults aged 25 to 34 years old use health and fitness apps twice as much as other age groups on average (Pai, 2013). Women are noted as being the primary healthcare decision makers for their families. Studies by Kaiser Family Foundation in Research show that 80% of healthcare choices are made by women. It states that 85% decide which pediatrician to use, 84% are the ones taking family members to appointments, and 79% are responsible for ensuring their families get recommended care (Salganicoff, Ranji and Wyn, 2005). This makes the childbearing population ideal for compliance with healthcare app utilization.

Pregnancy app usage is on the rise. A software company by the name of Citrix did a study on the use of pregnancy apps using mobile data usage information. In the study, they report that, on average, of those that use one or more mobile health apps, 47% of the total subscribers also used a pregnancy related app. Pregnancy apps were identified as not using as much data traffic as fitness apps. Although pregnancy apps aren't downloaded as much as fitness apps, the usage of the pregnancy apps is said to have a larger user base (Dolan, 2013).

The DNP nurse is strategically prepared to evaluate populations and systems to innovatively blend new knowledge and research with high quality clinical practice to influence optimal outcomes for the communities they serve. Being able to identify key experts to collaborate with to ensure synergy in these processes is vital. To do this, the DNP nurse leader must be able to identify potential catalyst to bridge the practice of nursing with administrative expectations and goals. Knowledge, technology, and patient preference are taken into consideration to help translate the evidence into everyday patient care.

Interprofessional collaboration has been identified as a positive driver of patient outcomes. Each profession brings a different value to a collaboration that helps foster shared understanding of all entities. Having a professional practice environment fosters greater nurse control. Magnet designated facilities foster a culture of collaboration and promotes nursing leadership. A study published in 2016 stated that interprofessional collaboration is enhanced when the concepts of structural empowerment, authentic leadership, and a professional nursing practice

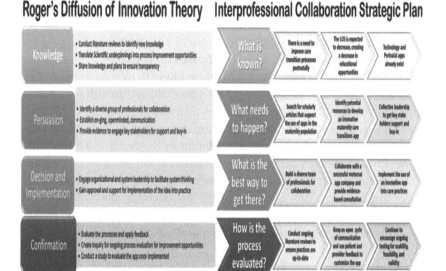

FIGURE 16.1. This diagram (self-created) shows the strategic plan as it correlates to Roger's Diffusion of Innovation Theory.

exists. A predictive non-experimental design was used to show the effectiveness of those concepts are present. Multiple regression analyses and descriptive statistics were used. Results showed that when those three concepts were present, the perception of interprofessional collaboration was also higher (Regan, Laschinger, and Wong, 2016).

PROJECT DESIGN

The project design of this scholarly project may differ greatly from traditional DNP projects. Most scholarly projects have an emphasis on implementation of evidence-based ideas with proven accomplishments through statistical data and outcomes. In this project, the approach is to translate evidence into practice. The literature has shown a need for interprofessional collaboration on the use of technology in practice and has supported the need to improve processes for care transition for the postnatal patient. This project has shown how establishing a diverse group of professionals to infiltrate the current practices of a complex healthcare system is attainable with the right evidence to support its impact. The efforts applied in this project help funnel evidence-based practice to the bedside, clinics, and healthcare providers and the populations they serve.

Methodology

This project targeted a specialty population, yet required a global approach to make the process possible. Figure 16.2 depicts the 12 groups of professionals who took part in this interprofessional collaboration to get the app approved for the pilot study. The ebbs and flows of the diagram show the momentum of the process as an additional group took stake in the collaboration. As shown, the initial process started with great momentum and, as involvement increased, the decision-making process grew slower.

SETTING

A large healthcare system that consists of over 900 locations with over 7,600 licensed beds and growing daily. The hospital is a 1,132 bed, quaternary care, level I trauma facility that serves as the referral center for many out-skirting facilities (Health Care, 2017). The maternity

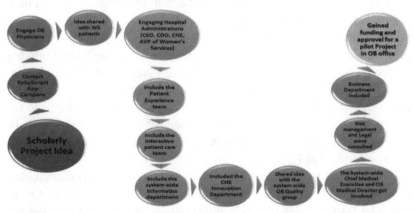

FIGURE 16.2. *Self-created diagram shows the accumulation professional groups as the project progressed.*

floor with 23 laboring suits experienced close to 7,000 births in 2016. The current practice at the facility encourages discharge at 36 hours for vaginal deliveries and 72 hours for cesarean section deliveries, creating a greater need to improve the care transition for new mothers and their families.

TOOLS/MEASUREMENTS

The DNP Residency/Scholarly Project Log will serve as the tracking tool used to document clinical interactions that contribute to the work related to this scholarly project. Hours will be documented and categorized by the DNP essential that the activity applies. A description of the scholarly activity will be recorded as it relates to the identified objectives to be complete for the scholarly project. All interactions documented are related to the collection, analysis, dissemination, or evaluation of knowledge and expertise possessed by the DNP nursing student.

The success of this scholarly project was measured by the ability of the DNP nursing student to interprofessional collaborate with others to implement an innovative app. The initial plan for implementation was not achieved in the given timeframe and, therefore, the focus was limited to the dissemination of knowledge and expertise to provide evidence-based consultation and collaboration with an app company and a complex healthcare system. Because it is impossible to statistically validate collaborations, the interaction process was tracked.

A survey was generated through the Survey Monkey application. This brief five question survey was used to evaluate the interactions with the DNP nursing student and the *Baby Scripts* app company to help provide constructive feedback for the benefits of having a DNP nursing leader involved. The survey used two questions based on a five-point Likert scale. Two questions were multiple choice, and one required a response in the form of a comment. The informal results were used for constructive develop for the DNP nursing leader only. It was distributed to Bryan King, Sales Executive of *Baby Scripts*; Anish Sebastian, Co-Founder/Chief Executive Officer (CEO) of *Baby Scripts*; and Juan Pablo Segura, Co-Founder/CEO of *Baby Scripts*. It was also distributed to hospital administration, nursing administration, the Chief of OB at involved hospital, the facility's information specialist responsible for app development, and representatives from the patient experience team.

The ultimate measure of the achievement of deliverables is the formal contract established between the complex healthcare system and the *Baby Scripts* application company. This proves that the interprofessional collaborative efforts were effective and contributed to the building of a professional relationship between two different industries to produce an innovative process that will benefit the perinatal population. In February 2017, a business agreement was secured and approval was received to pilot the basic *Baby Scripts* product in an outpatient OB gynecological (Gyn) office within the hospital system.

Feedback from the brief survey taken by the app company helps validate the desire to continue the interprofessional collaboration with a DNP nursing student to continue the efforts to create innovative ways to approach perinatal care. This business collaborative will lead to further research and process improvements that will inspire additional innovative practices in healthcare as evidence by decreased LOS, greater patient satisfaction in the maternal population related to the discharge process and transitions of care, and work flow efficiencies.

DATA COLLECTION

Interactions were documented on the clinical log to show how each effort supported the DNP essentials. An interaction was defined as an occurrence or activity completed in one session. Examples of interactions include emails, text message conversations, telephone conversations, and but not limited to face to face interactions. Interactions were tracked based on the DNP essential, as well as its relationship to the app company, the healthcare system, and assimilation/integration of knowledge. The categories were logged by interaction and hours spent engaging in the activity. The hours and interactions logged by the DNP essential overlapped in the fact that some activities comprised efforts that supported more than one category. Interactions were tracked through electronic email documentations, text message logs, telephone logs, and Microsoft Office electronic calendar.

The three categories for grouping the interactions were *Baby Scripts* interactions, hospital administrative interactions, and interactions that consisted of assimilation and integration of knowledge. Interactions placed in the *Baby Scripts* category were defined as any interaction with the *Baby Scripts* company or concerning the *Baby Scripts* app. Hospital administrative interactions included any interaction with a hospital professional in which the idea of the *Baby Scripts* app was discussed or mentioned as a possible solution to a problem. The last category included any activity that the DNP student gathered, evaluated, or integrated scholarly knowledge or evidence-based practice related to a concern that the app idea could address.

INTERVENTIONS

An exemplary approach will be taken to describe the process. Details of how the idea was derived and the steps taking to form the collaboration and engage stake holders will be described. A chronological timeline of events was created to show the progress of the collaboration over the year. Examples of products produced from the dissemination of knowledge and expertise are included in the appendices.

Interventions for this DNP project are also nontraditional and expand the potential for impact from the DNP nursing student. This project involved the DNP nursing student evaluating the literature and practice setting to identify a problem. Once identified, further research took place to find innovative evidence-based practices to support the idea of developing a postnatal care transition app that would meet the needs of the targeted population and healthcare system. The app idea was shared with patients and staff involved with the hospital women's services patient experience group. Brainstorming then began to plan the specifications of the app and identify opportunities for impacting outcomes. It was decided that the originating of an app would take longer than time allowed and, therefore, a search was done to collaborate with an existing app company that would benefit from the ideas for improvement the DNP student assimilated from the evidence and experience.

The *Baby Scripts* app company was identified as it aligned with the vision of the DNP student. The ideas and need for assistance with the DNP project were shared with the company. An instant connection was built based on the shared thrill for innovation and opportunities to impact the perinatal population. Coincidentally, the company had already tried to engage the outpatient OB offices at the complex healthcare system. The sales executive of the app company invited the DNP student to join the initial business meeting with the Chief of OB at the facility, in which the overview of services of the app was reviewed and the product was demonstrated. From that point, the app company included the DNP student in all additional meetings and email discussion to help translate visions, processes, and ideas to other healthcare professionals. The added perception of a nurse helped engage the inpatient administration, also sparking the attention of other system-wide leaders.

Multiple interactions took place that allowed the DNP student to combine knowledge and expertise to share ideas for new paradigms and insight on additional opportunities to improve the current app and create additional versions of the app. Translating evidence into practice was a major component of most interactions. The student shared current practice changes as they related to new The American College of Obstetricians and Gynecologists (ACOG) guidelines regarding conservative management of hypertensive disorders in pregnancy and identified opportunities for incorporation in a future high-risk postnatal app. Input was given to help the company develop a Memorandum of Understanding (MOU) that proposed collaboration with the complex healthcare system to co-develop an initiative using technology to help providers better manage postpartum patients.

Evaluation of the current app's information was completed, and evidence-supported feedback was provided for the app's postpartum education component. New practice recommendations were researched for improving morbidity of the postpartum patient. A postpartum discharge education initiative was identified through the Associations of Women's Health, Obstetrics, and Neonatal Nursing (AWOHNN) related to POST BIRTH warning signs that are recommended to be integrated into postnatal care and teaching. This information was translated and shared with the app company for future collaboration in the development of the postpartum component of the app.

Another key role that the DNP student served was a resource for the app company to understand the culture of the organization. The student informed the company about the many levels of leadership and connected them to key stakeholders to engage their support. Help was also provided to coordinate meetings. Advice was given concerning the best approaches to appeal to key stakeholders and information to have proactively prepared for meetings.

Additional interventions included the following:

- Evaluation of case review to provide additional evidence for stakeholder buy-in
- Translated current practices to support the need for an innovative intervention

- Evaluated current policy and practice to identify opportunities and ensure suggestions meet regulatory expectations
- Provided a nursing perspective for pilot study implementation

On a facility level, the DNP student engaged a diverse group of professionals representing different aspects of healthcare that would be impacted by using the innovative app. OB physician, nursing leadership, and the patients were most supportive and adopted the idea early. Nonpatient care departments such as marketing, information services, legal, finance, and business departments were brought into the collaboration to offer unique perspectives based on their expertise. Other groups that are not responsible for direct patient care yet focus on patient care concerns were also a part of the team. These groups consisted of professionals from hospital executives, the patient experience, interactive patient care, and risk management departments. It was interesting to hear each group's perspectives, apprehensions, and acceptance of the ideas. It was also interesting to see others express interest in the process once they saw the potential impact of the idea.

PROJECT FINDINGS/RESULTS

Overall, a total of 253 interactions were related to this interprofessional collaboration. Assimilation and integration of knowledge and expertise made up 40% of those interactions. Figure 16.3 shows that 22% of the interactions were with the *Baby Scripts* app company, and the other 38% involved hospital professionals and administration. The greatest portion of the DNP student's time was spent searching for, translating, and disseminating evidence-based information to share with the organization and the app company.

When the interactions were divided by semester, it was evident that the knowledge and concepts learned were applied to practice in the clinical setting. Clinical residency II was the period when the collaboration began, and it is interesting to see that was the semester in which the greatest number of interactions occurred. The initial process was very productive and exciting. As the semesters progressed and more professionals got involved, the progress of the project slowed, as shown, with less overall interactions in clinical residencies III and IV. By clinical residency III, the project had been almost completely consumed on a system-wide level, in which the DNP student had less opportunity to impact.

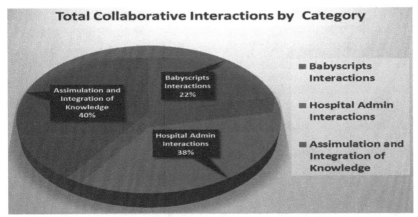

FIGURE 16.3. Graph showing the total distribution of interactions grouped by collaborative category.

A primary focus of this DNP project was to ensure the DNP essentials were integrated into the project. It was fascinating to identify that the most hours spent assimilating and integrating scholarly knowledge and expertise was during clinical residencies I and II, in which the objectives were more related to the learning expectations. As the DNP student learned new concepts, clinical residencies II and III showed the greatest number of hours spent in activities related to interprofessional collaboration, which these two semesters focused on more. Relating

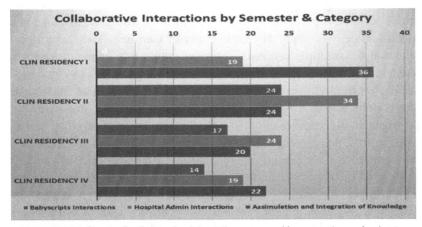

FIGURE 16.4. Graph of collaborative interactions grouped by semester and category.

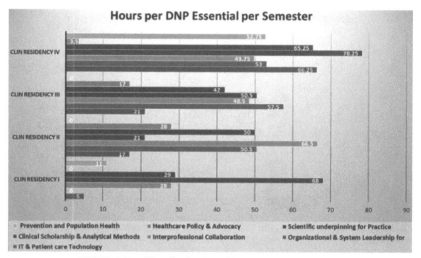

FIGURE 16.5. The distribution of hours by DNP essential.

the DNP essentials to the hours spent helps validate the mastery of skill obtained through the DNP educational program. The progression of this scholarly project shows how the objectives of the DNP program align with the needs for nursing leaders in the clinical setting. The data show that having a DNP nurse collaboratively lead interprofessional teams is an appropriate role to assume based on the preparation of the DNP program.

Project implementation in a large healthcare system is very complicated. Knowing the culture and customs helps to navigate the people, yet it doesn't prepare one for the layers of infrastructure and processes that must be overcome. The complexity of Carolinas Healthcare System and the multiple layers of approval required to change processes created huge delays in the project. By introducing the idea to key stakeholders early and mentioning the potential for the idea of the app in conversations with the different levels of administration, the hope was to create an eagerness to adopt the idea for implementation when paired with topics such as length of stay (LOS) and patient satisfaction. Although the hospital executives were eager to implement the idea, many system level groups waved multiple flags of caution regarding current opportunities for improvement. Because the system already had an app platform, it was thought that the addition of the postnatal care transition component should be easily received.

Strengths

Because of clinical practice recommendations for early discharge in the postnatal period, some strengths of forming a collaboration with the app company to develop a postnatal care transition component of the app will be to provide multiple methods of education and ease of access for referencing the information early and on an ongoing basis. It will create an interactive way for the nurse to make teaching personal and meet individual needs of the patient through on-demand communication creating connectivity, so the patient still feels he or she has access to healthcare advice after discharge. This connection could help increase patient loyalty for the healthcare facility.

Another strength of this scholarly project is that the interprofessional team was diverse and crossed a spectrum of professions. Categorization of professional identity can cause complications when forming an interprofessional collaboration. Professional identity encompasses professional insight into the practices and expertise of each professional group. Innovation is said to occur when multiple vessels of knowledge intersect. Knowledge sharing across professional boundaries is seen to paramount to multi-professional collaboration effectiveness. Engaging all perceptions of practice is a valuable attribute to have in an organization. Being able to overcome and understand the boundaries of each profession can contribute to opportunities to produce innovative solutions (Mitchell, R., 2010).

Based on the survey results of the Interprofessional Collaboration Survey that the DNP student sent to key members of the collaboration, 100% of those that responded to the survey said that it was very helpful having a DNP nursing leader to collaborate with for relationship building. It was agreed upon 100% that it was very helpful having someone within the organization to collaborate with. There was 100% of responses that said they would use a DNP prepared nurse to help with evidence-based practice in the future. Respondents included three representatives from the Baby Scriptts company, the President of the facility, the Chief of OB for the facility, the Assistant Vice President of Women's Service at the facility, the Clinical Expert for the DNP project, and a patient experience representative.

OBSTACLES

Throughout the process, as more and more professionals and groups became involved, the project expanded beyond the DNP students' control. The ideas were shared with the patient experience and interactive patient team for support and additional collaboration. To recruit additional support, the interactive patient care representative reached out to the director of informatics for the healthcare system, which created a huge obstacle.

Because the system already has an app, the issue of territoriality arose. The information technology (IT) department became very defensive related to the idea of using an outside company's product. The implementation was held up for several months because of the systematic debate as to whether the organization should create their own version of the app or use *Baby Scripts*. There were several meetings to state the case for using the existing app, which had proven results and consumer credibility. Collaborative leadership of the efforts was taken over by executives of the *Baby Scripts* company, and they presented supportive information as to why, from a business aspect, it made better sense to go with the app that had already been developed. After long deliberation, the idea was accepted.

The system-wide OB chair also got involved, attempting to assume leadership of the process and use the app to impact a different quality matrix. The app company continued to include the DNP student in the conversations, allowing the student to provide input from a nursing process perspective. Eventually it was decided the app was appropriate for implementation and it was advanced through several levels of system wide approval.

Roger's Diffusion of Innovation Theory suggests that it takes time for change to become routine. Time is often a barrier for implementing ideas. The complexity of the system created a delay in the implementation of the pilot study, which needed to take place before further collaboration could occur to develop the additional components of the new app idea.

SIGNIFICANCE OF IMPLICATIONS

During the collaborative efforts, being a mediator for conflict resolution was vital. Establishing a trusting relationship with the app company and the organizational leaders proved to be effective. Knowing that the DNP student shared the same vision and purpose helped others to be involved and more transparent with their opinions concerning the collaboration. Keeping an open line of communication with the multiple groups involved helped the DNP remain neutral and represent all perspectives. Respecting the expertise of each profession was consistently maintained, and constructive feedback was shared freely. As the DNP student, it was imperative to stay informed and constantly review the literature for opportunities to share.

By showing fewer interactions as the project reached more system wide levels, it is evident that having more DNP nursing leaders on a system level could help facilitate and translate ground level concepts to the higher-level executives. DNP students are trained in facilitating efforts to improve outcomes. Trusting the global perspective of DNP leaders would benefit larger facilities and organizations because of the intricate training to be system thinkers through organizational and system leadership.

Lack of understanding of the process could also be a barrier, yet in this case it helped gain early support from the hospital executives. Technology is a challenge for different generations, creating a hesitance to adopt ideas that are technology based. Because the organization was a magnet designated facility, there was an environment of professional practice and an open-mindedness for innovation. This level of acceptance was not present on a system level. Because the primary contact was confined to the obstetrical specialty, when the idea reached the system Medical Director, the sense of urgency to adopt the innovative ideas dwindled. It was very difficult to get the idea on the system level agenda for final approval despite constant communication with the facility level executives.

LIMITATIONS

There are a few limitations that exist in this project. The lack of statistical data weakens to level of evidence and representation of scholarly practice. Because the quantitative data of the interactions was compared to the qualitative data in the categories, there could have been some recoding of information to show more statistical validity to the assumptions and correlations. Also, the data represented in the budget model included general information that would be uncontrollable altered by populations and volume. This would make the information less transferable to smaller populations with lower acuity. The sample size of the feedback received was small and represented only those on a facility level. More efforts could have been made to elicit feedback from system-wide administration and the IT department. It would have been interesting to see a comparison to a collaboration that did not include a DNP student to quality and timing of the process and outcomes.

ADVICE TO THE DNP STUDENT

Ensuring the project implementation is within the individual's scope of practice is important. My greatest lesson learned was regarding the potential magnitude on innovative ideas. Ensuring the work is realistic and able to be completed in the timeframe is crucial. Understanding the entire extent of all layers of approval and formalizations prior to project planning could help present delays and allow DNP students to map out the implementation plan more accurately. The span of control in some organizations crossed several layers of administration and domains. Knowing the complexity of a system can help overcome these barriers. Finally, remember that innovation requires the ability to embark one's vision on a platform that multiple groups understand, support, and embrace. Stay diligent, do not give up, and utilize the expertise of surrounding professionals.

APPENDIX A: CLINICAL HOURS CHARTED AND GRAPHED BY CATEGORY OF INTERACTION

The information below shows the breakdown of clinical hours by category of interaction. This information was collected from the WCU clinical residency hours' log. These charts and graphs show the changes in focus that occurred each semester as they relate to the DNP essential.

Course	Babyscripts Hours	Hospital Admin Hours	Assimulation and Integration of Knowledge	Total Hours
Clin Residency I	0	34.5	106.5	141
Clin Residency II	33	53.5	60	146.5
Clin Residency III	37	55.5	50	142.5
Clin Residency IV	15.75	47.5	84.75	148
Total	85.75	191	301.25	578

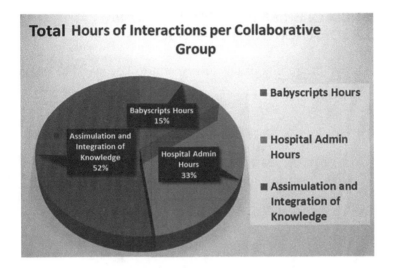

APPENDIX B: CLINICAL INTERACTIONS GRAPHED BY DNP ESSENTIAL BY SEMESTER

The information below shows the breakdown of interactions by DNP essential. This information was collected from the WCU clinical residency hours' log. These charts and graphs show the changes in focus that occurred each semester as they relate to the DNP essential.

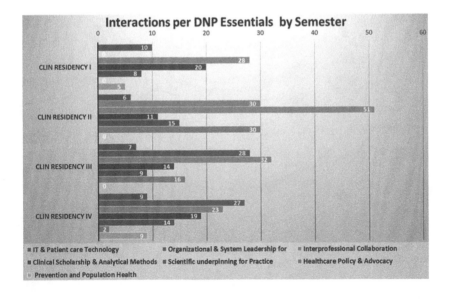

APPENDIX C: BRIEF INTERPROFESSIONAL COLLABORATION SURVEY RESULTS

These are the results of the survey sent to key stakeholders in the project.

Was it helpful to have a DNP prepared nursing leader to collaborate with in order to build a relationship with the Healthcare System?

Answered: 8   Skipped: 0

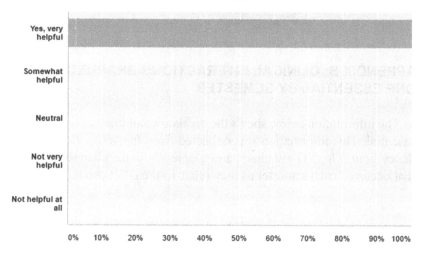

Answer Choices		Responses	
Yes, very helpful		100.00%	8
Somewhat helpful		0.00%	0
Neutral		0.00%	0
Not very helpful		0.00%	0
Not helpful at all		0.00%	0
Total			8

What is the average number of times that you have to interact with an organization when establishing a business partnership?

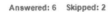

Answered: 6   Skipped: 2

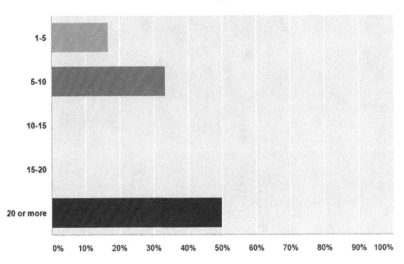

Answer Choices	Responses	
▼ 1-5	16.67%	1
▼ 5-10	33.33%	2
▼ 10-15	0.00%	0
▼ 15-20	0.00%	0
▼ 20 or more	50.00%	3
Total		6

On a scale of 1 to 5 how helpful is it to have someone within the organization to collaborate with?

Answered: 8   Skipped: 0

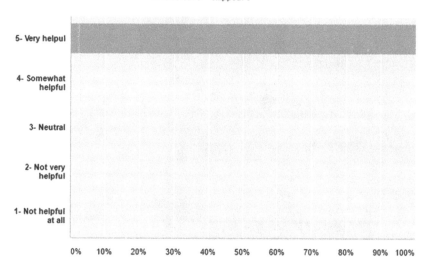

Answer Choices	Responses	
5- Very helpul	100.00%	8
4- Somewhat helpful	0.00%	0
3- Neutral	0.00%	0
2- Not very helpful	0.00%	0
1- Not helpful at all	0.00%	0
Total		8

Would you use a DNP prepared nurse to help your company with future evidence based practice?

Answered: 8   Skipped: 0

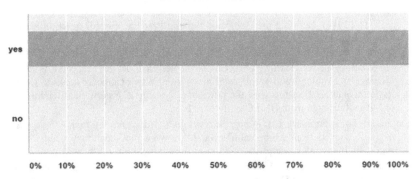

Answer Choices	Responses	
yes	100.00%	8
no	0.00%	0
Total		8

How else could you use nursing to benefit your company?

Answered: 4   Skipped: 4

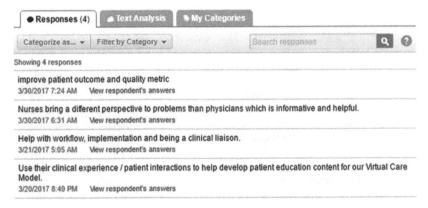

● Responses (4)   ▲ Text Analysis   ● My Categories

Categorize as... ▾   Filter by Category ▾   Search responses

Showing 4 responses

improve patient outcome and quality metric
3/30/2017 7:24 AM   View respondent's answers

Nurses bring a different perspective to problems than physicians which is informative and helpful.
3/30/2017 6:31 AM   View respondent's answers

Help with workflow, implementation and being a clinical liaison.
3/21/2017 5:05 AM   View respondent's answers

Use their clinical experience / patient interactions to help develop patient education content for our Virtual Care Model.
3/20/2017 8:49 PM   View respondent's answers

REFERENCES

AACN. (2006). *Essentials of doctoral education for advanced nursing practice*. Retrieved from Americal Association of Colleges of Nursing: http://www.aacn.nche.edu/publications/position/DNPEssentials.pdf

Barimani, M. and Vikstrom, A. (2015). Successful early postpatum support linked to mangement, informatinal, and relational continuity. *Midwifery*, 811–817.

Conrad, D. (2014). Defining the Doctor of Nursing Practice: current trend. In K. Moran, R. Burson and D. Conrad, *The Doctor of Nursing Practice Scholarly Project: A Framework for Success* (pp. 33–51). Burlington, MA: Jones & Bartlett Learning.

Dixon-Woods, M., Amalberti, R., Goodman, S., Bergman, B. and Glasziou, P. (2010, October 9). Problems and promises of innovation: Why healthcare needs to rethink its love//hate relationship with the new. *BMJ Quality & Safety*, Suppl 1(Suppl_1 i47–i51. Retrieved from BMJ Quality & Safety.

Dolan, B. (2013, February 13). *Report finds pregnancy apps more popular than fitness apps*. Retrieved from MobihealthNews: http://www.mobihealthnews.com/20333/report-finds-pregnancy-apps-more-popular-than-fitness-apps/

Houdek, L. A., Hypolite, K. A., Carrt, B. G., Shofer, F. S., Winston, F. K., Hanson, W. and Merhant, R. (2015). Use of mobil apps: A patient-cented approah. *Acedemic Emergency Medicine*, 765–768.

1EQ Incorporated. (2016). Our solutions. Retrieved from *Baby Scripts*: https://get Baby Scripts .com/solution.html

Journal of Interprofessional Care. (2011). Nurse practitioners and interprofessional collaboration. *Journal of Interprofessional Care*, 243–244.

McMillin, L. (2004, Spring). *Creating the "complete scholar": Academic professionalism in the 21st century*. Retrieved from Association of American Colleges & Universities: https://www.aacu.org/publications-research/periodicals/creating-complete-scholar-academic-professionalism-21st-century

Melnyk, B. and Fineout-Overhold, E. (2015). Creating a vision and motivating a change to evidence-based practice in individuals, teams, and organizations. In B. Melnyk and E. Fineout-Overhold, *Evidence-Based Practice in Nursing and Healthcare* (pp. 316–323). China: Wolters Kluwer Health.

Meola, A. (2016, May 7). *Business intellegence*. Retrieved from Business Insider: http://www.businessinsider.com/fitbit-mobile-health-app-adoption-doubles-in-two-years-2016-3

Mitchell, R. (2010, February). Toward realizing the potential of diversity in composition of interprofessional health care teams: An examination of the cognitive and psychosocial dynamics of interprofessional collaboration. *Medical Care Research and Review*, pp. 3–26.

Mitchell, R. and Boyle, B. (2015). Professional diversity, identity salience and team innovation: The moderating role of openmindedness norms. *Journal of organizational Behavior*, 873–894.

Pai, A. (2013, June 17). *Mobi health news*. Retrieved from http://mobihealthnews.com/23117/millennials-use-health-and-fitness-appsmore-than-other-age-groups/

Perkin, K. (2011). Nurse practitioners and interprofessional collaboration. *Journal of Interprofessional Care*, 243–244.

Regan, S., Laschinger, H. and Wong, C. (2016). The influence of empowerment, authentic leadership, and professional practice enviornments on nurses' perceived interprofessional collaboration. 24(1), *Journal of Nursing Management*, E54-E61.

Salganicoff, A., Ranji, U. and Wyn, R. (2005). *Women and healthcare: A national profile*. Kaiser Family Foundation.

The Joint Commission. (2012). Transitions of care: The need for a more effective approach to continuing patient care. *Hot Topics in Healthcare*, 1–8.

Williams, J. (2012). The Value of mobile apps in healthcare. Healthcare Financial Management, 96–101.

CHAPTER 17

DNP Contributions to the Future of Nursing Practice, Nursing Education, and Healthcare Policy Introduction

PATRICK LAROSE, DNP, MSN/ED, RN
JILL WALSH, DNP, 1RN, CEN, NEA-BC, CNE

INTRODUCTION

The Doctor of Nursing Practice (DNP) degree, also known as the practice doctorate, represents one of the highest or terminal levels of education in clinical nursing. Prior to the development of the DNP terminal degree, universities and institutions of higher learning had a number of terminal degree designations in nursing, most of which were focused on empirical or primary research. In 2004, the American Association of Colleges of Nursing (AACN) released a position statement on the need for and the support of a practice doctorate as a means of addressing the need for a terminal clinical degree in nursing (AACN, 2004). Since the release of this position statement by the AACN in 2004, 336 programs have been developed awarding the doctor of nursing degree designation, with an additional 121 in the planning stages (AACN, 2018). Some critics of the DNP degree asserted a practice doctorate would negatively affect enrollment into PhD programs, but this has not been the case. In fact, enrollment in both DNP programs and PhD programs have demonstrated significant increases, with PhD programs demonstrating a 43% increase in graduation rates between 2008 and 2017 (AACN, 2018b). For some DNP prepared nurses, enrollment in a PhD program after the completion of a DNP program is driven by the lack of recognition for the DNP degree by some universities as an acceptable teaching credential (Sebach and Chunta 2018). Although this has been an issue in the past, many universities today are beginning to recognize the important contributions DNP prepared nurses can make, in terms of clinical teaching/learning, grant funding, and practice scholarship.

323

A general misunderstanding of the purpose of the DNP degree is not uncommon and, in fact, is discussed in the literature quite often. However, as graduates of DNP programs begin to enter the workforce and demonstrate increased ability to improve patient outcomes and practice quality through translational science, it is simply a matter of time before the DNP degree is more clearly understood and accepted. Dunbar-Jacob *et al.* (2013) state, "DNP graduates bring to primary care an enhanced understanding of the health care system, policy issues, finance, and professional leadership" (Dunbar-Jacob, Nativio, and Khalil, 2013, 426). This understanding is certainly not lost on those that have a high degree of faith and belief in the practice doctorate. Today, many healthcare organizations are looking to employ nurses prepared at the DNP level to manage quality improvement departments, become Chief Nursing Officers, and in many organizations, the DNP prepared nurse is sought after to lead differing service lines. Nancy *et al.* (2018) suggest nurses prepared at the DNP level of education have already demonstrated the positive impact of this clinical doctorate through the contribution being made in healthcare leadership, clinical practice, and healthcare policy advocacy.

Despite some of the challenges DNP prepared nurses may face, the integration of nurses prepared at the practice doctorate level is an imperative if the discipline of nursing is to reach parity with other healthcare disciplines that already require a terminal degree for entry into the profession. Some examples of professions requiring a practice doctorate for entry level include medicine, physical therapy, audiology, pharmacology, and clinical psychology to name a few (Dunbar-Jacob, Nativio, and Khalil, 2013). Historically, nursing as a professional discipline has been slow to change in terms of developing a consensus on educational standards for each level of practice. While the battle for BSN entry into initial licensed practice continues, the same is happening with DNP education as a means of entry into practice for nurse practitioners (NPs). It is clear nurses struggle with the cost benefit of advancing to this level of education, as more recent studies have concluded that DNP-prepared nurses are focused on the use of evidence to frame practice. To this end, professional organizations such as the American Association of Nurse Anesthetists and the National Organization of Nurse Practitioner Faculty (NONPF) will require DNP education as an entry point to practice by 2025. Following suit, the National Organization of Clinical Nurse Specialist will require the DNP as a point of entry to practice by 2030 (Nancy *et al.*, 2018).

The controversy over DNP preparation is not at the heightened level that entry into initial licensed practice is, but the idea that a DNP degree may be the formal entry-level education for NP practice promises to have the same passion. In a recent Rand (2015) report, nursing programs across the country are beginning to shift educational focus with increased programmatic offerings of the bachelor of science in nursing (BSN) to DNP option, citing a survey they conducted from 400 schools of nursing, in which 57% are now offering BSN to DNP options for advanced practice nurses (APRNs). The master of science in nursing (MSN) degree remains the most popular avenue to entry into NP practice, but it appears the climate of NP education is beginning to shift. As the DNP degree continues to gain momentum, graduates from both the NP and non-NP options will be entering the workforce in larger numbers than in the past. It is expected DNP-prepared nurses will have a significant impact on health systems thinking, healthcare policy, clinical practice, and academia (Nancy *et al.*, 2018).

In 2010, the Institutes for Medicine (Institute for Medicine, 2011) released *The Future of Nursing: Leading Change, Advancing Health* as a call to action for nurses and healthcare leaders across the country. These recommendations were largely identified as a means to call attention to ways in which nurses could improve healthcare and impact care for populations and aggregates across the country. Since the release of this historic report, nursing and healthcare organizations began developing action committees to better define the role nursing can play in some of the healthcare challenges presented today and into the future. Of course, nurses prepared at the DNP level have a unique and exciting opportunity to influence change in healthcare with translational science and to reduce bench to bedside time as a primary means of bringing relevant and current research findings into practice much sooner.

A DNP prepared nurse is practicing at a very exciting time: (1) A time with major shifts and changes to healthcare; (2) A time in which the contribution of nurses is expected, valued, recognized and, more importantly, respected; and (3) A time when nurses can lead change as empowered professionals with autonomy, scientific knowledge, and the ability to make a difference in the lives of patients, families, communities, populations, and aggregates. This is the time in which nurses continue to influence positive and exciting changes in nursing practice and healthcare in general. For example, see Part 4, Chapter 16, "Interprofessional Collaboration to Improve Postnatal Care Transitions by

Revising an Innovative Application," which highlights empowering professionals.

Transitioning—The DNP-Prepared Nurse, Networking, Authorship, Establishing Practice Credibility, Credibility as a Writer, and Manuscript Submissions

Nurses completing the DNP degree education come from all lifestyles and nursing situations. Some have completed this education as a means of personal fulfillment, others as a requirement for a current position or a position they seek in the future. Yet others have completed this education with the notion that having a DNP degree will open new doors of opportunity. Despite the reasons for completion of this education, many nurses wonder how this new degree will affect or influence their careers and if the industry has enough understanding of the degree designation to assign value in the job market. Some nurses may even ask the question, "What do I do with this education and how can I influence and lead change within my nursing situation, with the care my patients receive or within my organization?"

To this end, DNP graduates, employers, universities, and professional organizations have come to realize the value and importance of this practice doctorate as a means to influence changes in the delivery of care, improvements in the development of healthcare policy, and the way nurses are educated. Nursing scholars now write about ways in which the DNP prepared nurse can help to change the shape of care or the delivery of care and clinical practice. Carter and Moore (2015) say, "In the future, [this] care will be required to be continuous across episodes, provide comprehensive services including new emphasis on health promotion and disease prevention, and be highly coordinated across the care continuum. To do less fails to provide the expected quality of care and places the patient in potential harm" (Carter and Moore, 2015, 16). Moreover, although the statement by Carter and Moore (2015) may be true, it will take time for DNP-prepared nurses to demonstrate the positive changes they bring to healthcare and the discipline of nursing. The DNP degree brings value to organizations, the community, healthcare, and nursing as a science driven discipline by enhancing the knowledge and actions of nurses in an effort to utilize best evidence for practice (Nancy *et al.*, 2018). The use of best evidence is most notably driven by the use of empirical research, as a means to improve patient outcomes, streamline care processes, and shape policy within care environments and through legislative pursuits. These competencies align with the DNP Essentials published by the American Association of Colleges of Nursing (AACN, 2006) and speak to the culminated learning expected from any DNP graduate.

As nurses prepared at the DNP level graduate and begin to transition, many have already begun to demonstrate their value and worth through scholarship; improvements in systems thinking; and helping to shape and influence healthcare policy at the organizational, local, and national levels and are influencing the care provided to patients across the country every day (Carter and Moore, 2015; Nancy *et al.,* 2018). Role transition is largely dependent upon the individual and the goals and outcomes associated with returning to school and completing this important education. Role transition, at the very least, is about how the nurse prepared at the DNP level of education sees himself or herself, the discipline of nursing, and how each individual can lead change that promotes the best possible outcomes for patients and practice in healthcare overall.

Conducting Real World Projects as a DNP Prepared Nurse

The culmination of any accredited DNP program results in the completion of a significant body of work by the DNP student, reflecting a practice change that is informed by a needs assessment at the site where the DNP student plans to conduct the project. This culminating body of work provides the DNP student with the experience to design, implement, and provide final analysis of a project that brings meaning to the overall educational experience and demonstrates competency for project management at the doctoral level (AACN, 2004). The expectation at the conclusion of the DNP program is that graduates will continue to demonstrate practice scholarship in the real world of nursing practice. Practice doctorate graduates are now working in all aspects of the nursing discipline across the country and have the opportunity and some would say obligation to lead change within the respective environment.

DNP graduates work in academia; some may be primary care providers and function as nurse practitioners or perhaps clinical nurse specialists. Some graduates may be leading teams as directors of nursing service lines, and some may even be in the role of chief executive officers or chief nursing officers. Regardless of what role the nurse may play, a DNP graduate is prepared with a unique and qualified skill set to assess, conceptualize, design, implement, and manage a practice change within his or her specific nursing situation with translational science. Publishing the results of these practice changes provides evidence of the contributions many DNP-prepared nurses are making to improving healthcare. (Examples in Part 4, Chapters 13 and 14.)

In a study conducted by Redman *et al.* (2015), the authors determine the majority of publications produced by DNP graduates alone or in collaboration with PhD colleagues largely focused on clinical practice issues or nursing education. Not surprising, the study demonstrated the primary topics of interest centered on patient safety across all spectrums. In addition, the study showed greater than 50% of the DNP authored articles were written by DNPs employed within a university system. The lowest percentage of DNP authored articles was 7.3%; these articles were from those employed in primary care. This might indicate DNP-prepared nurses in primary care are not publishing at the rate of their university colleagues. Whatever the case may be, DNP graduates must begin to publish their work as a means for the discipline to provide true evaluation of the effect of the DNP degree on bench to bedside timeframes. Redman *et al.* (2015) say "Whether DNP graduates are able to speed up the translation of new knowledge into practice will be of primary importance in improving healthcare. The leadership activities of DNP graduates and the evolving impact of their role enactment will need to be evaluated" (Redman *et al.*, 2015, 128).

Although evaluating the published works of DNPs may be of primary importance, there is convincing evidence today that DNP-prepared nurses are making a difference. Nancy *et al.* (2018) assert the contribution of DNP prepared nurses is far reaching and is influencing change in healthcare systems, clinical practice, education/academia, and healthcare policy. Most notable is the idea that DNP-prepared nurses are also influencing change in areas not previously reported. Nancy *et al.* (2018) state "The DNP nurse impacts other areas of healthcare including health economics, health insurance, administration, and information technology" (Nancy *et al.*, 2018, 7). The important work being done by DNP prepared nurses will only continue to evolve as graduates begin to assume roles that foster and embrace the translation of science into reasonable and needed practice change. These changes will not only be the impetus for improved quality outcomes, but also will be the discerning factor in how we, collectively, as a profession go about helping to improve healthcare for individuals, families, communities, populations, and aggregates.

Identification of Problems, Problem-Solver, Translational Science and the Important Role the DNP-Prepared Nurse May Play in Healthcare Today

Identification of Problems

Healthcare is becoming more complex, and healthcare systems and processes continue to evolve rapidly. DNP-prepared nurses are in a unique position to identify health systems problems and practice gaps and to address the almost endless amount of problems in the real world of practice. DNP-prepared nurses possess the knowledge and skills to address problems using best available evidence to improve healthcare systems and care delivery and to improve safety, quality of care, and patient outcomes. These individuals are well positioned to meet the Institute of Medicine's (2010) "Future of Nursing Report" mandate that nurses act as full partners with their interprofessional colleagues and provide their unique perspectives to improve healthcare and lead healthcare reform.

Translation Science

Translation science is a rapidly growing field of research (Titler, 2018). Although research evidence is being generated at an increasing rate, applying research evidence to clinical practice has lagged behind. A gap therefore exists between the availability of evidence based practice (EBP) recommendations and application in care delivery that contributes to poor health outcomes.

As an emerging area of science, translation science offers an empirical base for guiding the selection of strategies to promote adoption and use of evidence-based interventions in the real world of practice. According to Titler (2014), the focus of the field of translation science is "testing implementation interventions to improve uptake and use of evidence to improve patient outcomes and population health, and to explicate what implementation strategies work for whom, in what settings, and why" (p. 270). Titler (2018) further explained that although translation science and EBP are related, these terms are distinct and not interchangeable. Translation science is research focused, whereas EBP refers to application of proven interventions.

There are many theories and models in translation science. Nilsen (2015) identified five categories of theoretical approaches used in translation science. Process models are utilized to describe and/or guide the research-to-practice process. Determinant frameworks, classic theories, and implementation theories aim to understand and/or explain what influences implementation outcomes. Evaluation frameworks provide a structure to evaluate implementation efforts.

Process models are often referred to as action models of EBP. These models identify the steps for promoting the use of research evidence in practice. One commonly used process model that originated from the nursing discipline is the "Iowa Model of Evidence-Based Practice to Promote Quality Care" (Iowa Model Collaborative, 2017). The Iowa Model is a very practical model for the systematic implementation of EBP. This process model is applicable in diverse settings, including academic settings and healthcare institutions, and is intended for nurses and other clinicians at the point of care. The Iowa Model consists of a flowchart to guide decision-making that includes problem solving steps and feedback loops to guide the change process.

The DNP practice scholar has an important role to play in translating best research evidence to clinical practice to improve healthcare outcomes. It is this ability to translate evidence to improve outcomes that sets the DNP practice scholar apart from the PhD scholar. DNP-prepared nurses possess the skillset and knowledge to apply evidence to address patient care problems and improve outcomes. Additionally, DNP prepared nurses have the capacity to generate new knowledge through application and evaluation of (1) practice innovations, (2) translation of evidence, and (3) implementation of quality improvement initiatives to improve outcomes (AACN, 2015).

Bench to Beside to Bench—Relationships With the PhD Prepared Nurse, Important Collaborative Relationships Between PhD Prepared Nurse and the DNP Prepared Nurse

Nurse scientists engage in research to inform EBPs to improve healthcare systems and patient outcomes. Collaboration between PhD and DNP prepared nurses is important for establishing an efficient repeating loop from bench to bedside to bench. Melnyk (2013) emphasized the importance of PhD and DNP prepared nurses working collaboratively to "rapidly and effectively translate evidence-based interventions supported by research into clinical settings for the ultimate purpose of improving healthcare quality and patient outcomes (Melynk 2013, 443). The results of collaboration between nurse scientists and advanced practice leaders ensure that current nursing practice remains relevant to meet changing patient needs (Trautman *et al.,* 2018).

DNP-prepared nurses are expert practitioners who have the knowledge and ability to apply and translate evidence into practice (AACN, 2004). They are well-equipped to bridge the gap from bench science (i.e., knowledge produced through research) to use of evidence at the bedside. DNP-prepared nurses have the knowledge and skills to ensure that best evidence is effectively implemented at the bedside and in healthcare systems to improve outcomes.

DNP-prepared nurses as systems thinkers play an important role in problem identification and analysis of current practice. Through collaboration with the PhD nurse scientist, clinically relevant questions can move from the bedside to the laboratory. Following testing and completion of bench research, the PhD nurse scientist transfers the updated current best evidence back to the DNP-prepared nurse for incorporation in patient care and healthcare delivery systems.

Identifying the Contributions DNP Prepared Nurses Have Made to Nursing Practice (Section Heading, Clinical inquiry, findings, what did they do, and what was the outcome—dissemination)

As leaders and change agents in a complex and ever evolving healthcare delivery system, DNP-prepared nurses are educationally prepared to translate best available evidence to improve patient and health systems outcomes. As the number of DNP graduates continues to increase, there is a growing body of knowledge to demonstrate DNP contributions to nursing practice.

A review of current literature and published DNP students' scholarly projects found that DNP-prepared nurses and DNP students have implemented projects to improve outcomes across settings. In this section, examples of evidence-based projects implemented in nursing practice to improve patient and healthcare delivery system outcomes will be described.

Russell *et al.* (2018) identified a practice problem in their academic medical center on the adult cardiovascular thoracic step-down unit; the catheter associated urinary tract infection (CAUTI) rate had increased higher than the target rate. Using a problem-solving approach, this team of two DNP-prepared nurses and one PhD-prepared nurse first reviewed the literature for best available evidence for decreasing the risk of CAUTIs. They found that use of evidence-based nurse-driven algorithms to prevent CAUTIs successfully decreased CAUTIs in similar settings. For this quality improvement project, they used the Plan-Do-Study-Act (PDSA) model for implementing the practice change. In addition to meeting the objective to decrease the CAUTI rate, the team noted that because of participation in this project, the nurses on this unit felt a new sense of empowerment and enthusiasm to improve patient outcomes that are nursing sensitive.

LiVolsi (2018) implemented her DNP scholarly project in the Maternal-Child clinical practice setting in a community hospital. The purpose of her project was to implement a delayed infant bathing program based on current best evidence recommendations that have been shown to improve outcomes for neonates when the first bath is delayed for 12 to 24 hours after birth. Results of this project included an increase in in-hospital breast-feeding rates, a decrease in formula supplementation, a decrease in the frequency of hypoglycemia, and a decrease in the incidence of hypothermia in low-risk infants. Additionally, the project ignited the spirit of inquiry and heightened the nurses' awareness of implementing evidence based best practice to improve quality and safety.

An outpatient healthcare clinic was the setting Bentum (2018) used for his DNP scholarly project. The purpose of his project was to determine whether promoting diabetes knowledge and self-efficacy would improve self-care behavior and glycemic control in a sample of middle-aged persons with Type 2 diabetes mellitus. Bentum used the American Association of Diabetes Educators (AADE) AADE7 Self-Care Behaviors program to educate the participants about patient centered diabetes self-management and care. The project used a pre test/post test design in which hemoglobin A1c (HbA1c) values and confidence scores in managing patients' diseases were compared pre and post intervention. The Stanford Diabetes Self-Efficacy Scale was used for quantitative evaluation of participant confidence before and after the teaching intervention. Results of this 12-week intervention showed a moderate reduction in HbA1c percentage and a substantial improvement in self-efficacy scores. Findings showed a positive correlation of higher self-efficacy on self-care behaviors and positive health outcomes.

For his DNP scholarly project, Linthicum (2018) implemented the patient Admissions Predictor Tool (APT) in the triage area of a busy emergency department (ED) to improve ED throughput of admitted patients. This quality improvement project included a two-step process: (1) utilize the APT tool at triage to identify patients with a high probability of admission and (2) expedite the admissions process by initiating a bed request after triage (BERT). Linthicum used the PDSA quality improvement design for this project. ED throughput is a complex issue and during this two-month pilot project, Linthicum was not able to meet the goal of improving patient throughput. Further evaluation of the APT tool may be indicated. Based on findings of this pilot implementation, Linthicum plans to share suggestions for future ways to improve the tool.

Heart failure is one of the most costly diagnoses for Medicare. Literature shows that the transition from hospital to home is a critical time when patients are prone to exacerbations and at risk for readmission to the hospital. DNP-prepared nurse Whitaker-Brown and her multidisciplinary team implemented a 4-week multidisciplinary, transition-to-care program following hospitalization to determine the feasibility of the program and the impact on quality of life for heart failure patients (Whitaker-Brown *et al.,* 2016). The pre- and post-test study design was used for this study. The Minnesota Living with Heart Failure Questionnaire (MLHFQ) was used to measure participants' quality of life before and after participation in the program. Results showed a significant improvement in quality of life. Additionally, only 2 of the 36 participants were readmitted to the hospital within 30 days and with non-heart failure related causes. Findings from this study demonstrated support for a 4-week multidisciplinary, transition- to-care program to enhance quality of life and decrease the 30-day readmission rate for persons with heart failure.

Identifying the Contributions DNP Prepared Nurses Have Made to Nursing Education (Section Heading, Clinical inquiry, findings, what did they do, and what was the outcome—dissemination)

Over the past two decades, faculty have increasingly integrated simulation into undergraduate nursing curricula. There is an abundance of literature on simulation and a growing body of research evidence to demonstrate effectiveness of simulation-based education (Aebersold, 2018). Although many think of simulation as the use of high-fidelity simulators, a variety of simulation methods are available. Simulation today includes role-play, standardized patients, computerized manne-quins, and virtual simulation.

A review of current literature and published DNP students' scholarly projects found that DNP-prepared nursing faculty and DNP students have implemented projects in undergraduate and graduate level nursing programs that explore the effect of simulation and debriefing interventions on the knowledge, skills, and confidence of nursing students. In this section, examples of evidence-based projects implemented in nursing education will be described. These projects focused on communication skills, caring competencies, self-awareness, use of simulation to replace traditional clinical hours, and debriefing.

Millwater (2015) studied the effects of high-fidelity human patient (mannequin) simulation on the quality of hand-off communication skills among undergraduate nursing students for her DNP scholarly project. Millwater used a mixed methods research design that used post-test only analysis for her study. Thirty-eight students participated in the study with the experimental group and the control group, each comprised of 19 students. Findings of this study support use of human patient simulation as a method for teaching communication skills in undergraduate nursing curricula. Results from this study suggest a need for more human patient simulation experiences in undergraduate nursing curricula for improving the quality and safety outcomes for patients.

The purpose of Threatt's (2017) DNP scholarly project was to determine if after incorporating caring competencies in didactic lectures and two simulation-based experiences with debriefing would there be an increase in students' perceived level of caring. This project was implemented in a Fundamentals of Nursing course in an Associate Degree in Nursing (ADN) program. A convenience sample of 32 students participated in this project. The Caring Efficacy Scale (CES) was used to evaluate the effectiveness of the project post implementation. The results showed a slight increase in students' perceived level of caring ability. Qualitative data showed a heightened awareness of the importance of caring competencies. Results suggest that there is a need to incorporate caring competencies throughout the didactic, clinical, and simulation curriculum.

Poverty is one of the major social determinants of health in the United States (U.S.). The purpose of Ehmke's (2018) DNP scholarly project was to determine if the addition of a poverty simulation for nursing students would positively affect their self-awareness and individual-level beliefs and attitudes towards poverty. Ehmke implemented an evidence-based poverty simulation practice into the Bachelor of Science in Nursing (BSN)/DNP curriculum. The participants in this simulation project included 45 BSN and 29 DNP students. The Attitude Toward Poverty Scale—Short (ATPS) form was administered pre-simulation and post-simulation. Significant findings were present in both groups; however, more were found for the DNP student cohort. Results showed nursing students benefitted from the addition of a poverty simulation experience. The simulation experience positively affected their self-awareness and individual-level beliefs and attitudes towards poverty.

For her DNP scholarly project, McCoy (2018) created an eight-hour maternal-newborn high-fidelity simulation to replace a portion of traditional clinical hours necessary to meet undergraduate nursing clinical requirements. The participants in this project were second-level nursing maternal-newborn faculty in an ADN program. Pre-simulation and post-simulation surveys were administered to the participants. Results showed an increase in participants' familiarity and comfort with simulation and its use in the course, as well as participants indicating that they would be more likely to use simulation in the course in the future.

DNP-prepared nurse educator Gordon (2017) implemented WebEx, an online conferencing platform to conduct synchronous online debriefing sessions following virtual simulation in an asynchronous virtual learning environment with family practice nurse practitioner students in an online graduate program. Results of this pilot program showed that use of the online Web conferencing tool "provided an environment conducive for learning and supported confidentiality, trust, open communication, self-analysis, feedback, and reflection" (Gordon, 2017, 671).

Identifying the Contributions DNP Prepared Nurses Have Made to Healthcare Policy (Section Heading, Clinical inquiry, findings, what did they do, and what was the outcome—dissemination)

The contributions being made today by DNP-prepared nurses are helping to shape healthcare policy at the organizational, local, and national levels (Nancy *et al.*, 2018). Armed with the understanding of translation science and front-line experience, DNP-prepared nurses are providing insight and understanding into complex healthcare issues and are serving as valuable resource to policy makers. Although this is a new area of practice and specialization for many nurses, the ability of nurses to network and be trusted as knowledgeable partners by legislative colleagues makes the emergence of nurses into the political environment a welcome addition. Arabi *et al.* (2014) state "Nurses have individual views on healthcare issues and influence healthcare policies in different ways." (Arabi *et al.,* 2014, 315). This influence is largely informed by the nurse's own practice experience and the understanding of what is needed within a community to promote improved health outcomes. Nurses are healthcare experts and need to utilize the knowledge they have to collaborate with elected officials as a means to address important issues for constituents. In addition, a nurse's influence is also impacted by power, knowledge, and networking within the legislative body. Nurses who have experience and are well respected often serve as a battle tested allies when advocating for healthcare issues that may be considered contentious or not entirely popular (Arabi *et al.,* 2014).

Central to the success of any nurse hoping to gain political influence is the idea and notion that the nurse needs to have a broad knowledge of many different healthcare issues. Leveraging knowledge, education, and experience allows the nurse to provide advocacy for legislative change that provides positive outcomes to patients, communities, and populations (Salmond and Echevarria, 2017). DNP-prepared nurses are uniquely qualified through education to lead change like this and to partner with elected officials to design, advocate, or support legislation that meets the needs of the community. There is a limited, but slowly emerging, body of evidence that DNP-prepared nurses are leading change, advocating for patients and communities, and making a tangible difference on the organizational, local, and national level through healthcare policy advocacy.

To illustrate this point—we need to look no further than the EBP change (student project) completed by Dr. Holly Ortega (2018). Dr. Ortega recognized a disparate health issue among Hispanic women within her community and postulated a change in care regimen would help to influence positive outcomes within her community and with the participants of her project. Dr. Ortega focused her project on obesity in woman, more specially from a disadvantaged socioeconomic perspective (those receiving benefits from the Women, Infant, and Children—WIC program). She provided the foundation for her project based on the literature and the clear practice gap, which existed for her intended population. Dr. Ortega believed women from disadvantaged socioeconomic circumstances in her community would benefit from Bandura's self-efficacy theory as a means of improving healthcare outcomes through improved self-care behaviors. The premise to her project was to engage participants in activities that would enhance self-esteem and provide motivational, decisional, and emotional support as a means to meet the overall objective for the project (Ortega, 2018). Use of support strategies coupled with exercise modification, diet changes, and motivational support were the primary interventions to this practice change. Dr. Ortega's DNP project demonstrated a strong foundation of literature and evidence to frame the work she proposed to do with participants. Her goal as a change leader was to provide preventative care strategies designed to improve overall patient outcomes within her community.

Change in any fashion is often uncomfortable for those in the path of change. DNP prepared nurses recognize the importance of change management and can be a powerful influence on designing programs of advocacy based on the evidence, with a focus on change management. Inherent to this management is the understanding that DNP-prepared nurses have the skills to focus healthcare policy change within organizations, the community, or local government or on the national level as a colleague with an elected official. The role of a political advocate requires a period of self-reflection to determine the skills that are needed for success.

Nurses prepared at the DNP level need to assess political competency as a means of addressing a self-development plan that can lead to advocacy roles with elected officials if this is an area of interest. Although DNP-prepared nurses may possess rudimentary skills with political advocacy, there is value in the recognition that an advising role with a policy-maker requires time and exposure for competency development. Salmond (as cited in Salmond and Echevarria, 2017) asserts nurses must take the lead in advancing healthcare. She says nurses can no longer take a "back seat" (Salmond and Echevarria, 2017, 23) and must begin to lead the change. Leading change as a political advocate takes strength, courage, and a desire to make a difference within the community or area of interest.

THE IMPACT OF THE DNP PREPARED NURSE

Since the release of the Institute of Medicine (IOM) report *To Err is Human: Building a Safer Health System* (Kohn, Corrigan, and Donaldson, 2000), healthcare systems leaders have been required to pay greater attention to quality and process improvement, with an increased emphasis on the use of EBPs to improve outcomes. The recommendations put forth in the IOM report required greater skill and knowledge from nurses than master's education could support.

The DNP degree programs were first introduced in 2004. This new practice doctorate degree programs' curricula were developed to build upon master's programs by providing education in systems leadership, EBP, quality improvement, and other key areas (AACN, 2018).

Anecdotal reports of DNP graduates using their skills and expertise to solve important practice problems, increase quality, decrease costs, and increase patient satisfaction are becoming more prevalent (Waldrop, 2017). Furthermore, many reports about DNP scholarly projects are being published or presented as podium or poster presentations at professional meetings. Broome *et al.* (2013) analyzed the publication practices of DNP prepared nurses. One hundred seventy-five articles published between 2005 and 2012 met inclusion criteria. They found that studies evaluating the effectiveness of an intervention with nurses or patients were the most frequent, with studies of self-report surveys of nurses or patients the second most frequent type of study. Kleinpell (2017) reports, however, that there is limited evidence in the literature regarding the impact of DNP-prepared nurses. Kleinpell cautions that until robust research studies are conducted to evaluate their impact on patient and healthcare system outcomes, the ultimate impact of the DNP-prepared nurse will not be known.

SUMMARY

This chapter addresses the important and valuable work being done by DNP-prepared nurses across the entire healthcare spectrum. The primary focus centers on role transition and the overall perception of the DNP degree from many stakeholders, including the graduate discipline of nursing, other healthcare professionals, and healthcare in general. Upon graduation, DNP-prepared nurses need to determine the future course of career goals and to consider taking on a new role, publishing, or advancing in the role currently held.

The contribution of DNP-prepared nurses is well documented and continues to evolve as graduates of this education enter the work force and begin to lead change in differing clinical situations. DNP-prepared nurses must publish the important work being done as a way for programs offering DNP education to measure and evaluate effectiveness of the degree and the programmatic offerings. This is an area in which graduates need to be consistent and take credit for the work being done within healthcare. Overall contributions of the DNP-prepared nurse can be felt in nursing education/academia, clinical/nursing practice, and within healthcare policy. Again, publishing the work being done is stressed as a way to highlight the impact of DNP graduate overall.

Tool Kit

The Iowa Model Revised: Evidence-Based Practice to Promote Excellence in Health Care© (Iowa Model Collaborative, 2017) is a widely used, very practical model for the systematic implementation of EBP. The Iowa Model is applicable in diverse settings, including academic settings and healthcare institutions, and is intended for nurses and other clinicians at the point of care. The model consists of a flowchart to guide decision-making that includes problem solving steps and feedback loops to guide the change process.

The Iowa Model Revised: Evidence-Based Practice to Promote Excellence in Health Care figure

Citation: Iowa Model Collaborative. "Iowa Model of Evidence-Based Practice: Revisions and Validation." Worldviews on Evidence-Based Nursing 14, no. 3 (2017): 175 182. doi:10.1111/wvn.12223

In written material, please add the following statement:

Used/reprinted with permission from the University of Iowa Hospitals and Clinics, copyright 2015.

DNP Project Final Paper—Sample Table of Contents for a Practice-Change DNP Project

The DNP course of study culminates in the completion of the DNP Project. The DNP Project is a scholarly experience that provides evidence of the DNP student's ability to critically think, demonstrate leadership, and use best available evidence to improve outcomes. DNP projects include problem identification, planning, implementation, and evaluation phases. The completed DNP Project final paper should provide a detailed account of all phases of the completed DNP Project.

Sample Table of Contents for a Practice-Change DNP Project

Dedication

Acknowledgements

Executive Summary

CHAPTER 1: INTRODUCTION

Problem Statement
Objectives and Aims
Significance of the Practice Problem
Synthesis of the Literature
Practice Recommendations
Evidence-based Practice: Verification of Chosen Option

CHAPTER 2: THEORETICAL FRAMEWORK

Theoretical Framework
Change Model

CHAPTER 3: PROJECT DESIGN AND METHODS

Organizational Need
Organizational Support
Project Stakeholders
SWOT Analysis
Strengths
Weaknesses
Opportunities
Threats
Barriers and Facilitators
Project Schedule
Resources Needed
Project Manager Role
Plans for Sustainability
Project Vision, Mission, and Objectives
PICOT Question
Population
Intervention
Comparison
Outcome
Time Frame
Feasibility
Sample and setting
Implementation Plan/Procedures
Data Collection Procedures
Recruitment and Selection
Data Analysis Plan
Instrumentation
Instrument Reliability and Validity
Ethics and Human Subjects Protection

CHAPTER 4: RESULTS AND DISCUSSION OF DNP PROJECT

Summary of Methods and Procedures
Summary of Sample and Setting Characteristics
Major Findings

CHAPTER 5: IMPLICATIONS IN PRACTICE AND CONCLUSIONS

Implications for Nursing Practice
Recommendations
Discussion
Plans for Dissemination
Conclusions and Contributions to the Profession of Nursing
References

Appendix A

REFERENCES

Aebersold, M., (April 3, 2018). Simulation-based learning: No longer a novelty in undergraduate education. *OJIN: The Online Journal of Issues in Nursing, 23*(2).

American Association of Colleges of Nursing. (2004). *AACN position statement on the practice doctorate in nursing*. Washington, DC: Author. Retrieved from http://www.aacn.nche.edu/publications/position/DNPpositionstatement.pdf

American Association of Colleges of Nursing. (2006). The essentials of doctoral education for advanced nursing practice. Washington, D.C.: author.

American Association of Colleges of Nursing. (2018a). DNP factsheet. Retrieved from https://www.aacnnursing.org/News-Information/Fact-Sheets/DNP-Fact-Sheet

American Association of Colleges of Nursing. (2018b). PhD in nursing. Retrieved from https://www.aacnnursing.org/News-Information/Research-Data-Center/PhD

American Association of Colleges of Nursing. (2015). The Doctor of Nursing Practice: Current issues and clarifying recommendations: Report from the task force on the implementation of the DNP. Retrieved from https://www.aacnnursing.org/Portals/42/DNP/DNP-Implementation.pdf

Arabi A, Rafii F, Cheraghi MA, and Ghiyasvandian S. Nurses' policy influence: A concept analysis. *Iran Journal Nurse Midwifery Res. 2014; 19*(3):315-22.

Auerbach, D. I., Martsolf, G. R., Pearson, M. L., Taylor, E. A., Zaydman, M., Muchow, A. N., Spetz, J., and Lee, Y. (2015). The DNP by 2015: A study of the institutional, political, and professional issues that facilitate or impede establishing a post-baccalaureate doctor of nursing practice program. *Rand Health Quarterly, 5*(1), 3.

Bentum, E. 2018. Promoting diabetes self-efficacy to improve glycemic control (Order No. 10978169). Available from ProQuest Dissertations & Theses Global (2136286098).

Carter, M. A and Moore, P. J. (2015). The necessity of the doctor of nursing practice in comprehensive care for future health care. *Clinical Scholars Review, 8*(1), 13-17. Retrieved from https://chamberlainuniversity.idm.oclc.org/login?url=https://search-proquest-com.chamberlainuniversity.idm.oclc.org/docview/1676823515?accountid=147674

Dunbar-Jacob, J., Nativio, Donna G. and Khalil, H. (2013). Impact of doctor of nursing practice education in shaping health care systems for the future. *Journal of Nursing Education, 52*(8), 423–427. doi:http://dx.doi.org.chamberlainuniversity.idm.oclc.org/10.3928/01484834-20130719-03

Edwards, N. E., Coddington, J., Erler, C. and Kirkpatrick, J. (2018). The impact of the role of doctor of nursing practice nurses on healthcare and leadership. *Edwards Medical Research Archives, 6*(4). Available from: https://doi.org/10.18103/mra.v6i4.1734

Ehmke, M. (2018). *Implementing a CAPS simulation to increase nursing education practice students' self-awareness of attitudes and beliefs about poverty* (Order No. 10843007). Available from ProQuest Dissertations & Theses Global. (2102483711).

Gordon, R. M. (2017, December). Debriefing virtual simulation using an online conferencing platform: Lessons learned. *Clinical Simulation in Nursing, 13*(12), 668-674. http://dx.doi.org/10.1016/j.ecns.2017.08.003.

Institute of Medicine (US) Committee on the Robert Wood Johnson Foundation Initiative on the Future of Nursing, at the Institute of Medicine. The Future of Nursing: Leading Change, Advancing Health. Washington (DC): National Academies Press

(US); 2011. Available from: https://www.ncbi.nlm.nih.gov/books/NBK209880/ doi: 10.17226/12956

Iowa Model Collaborative. (2017) Iowa model of evidence-based practice: Revisions and validation. *Worldviews Evid Based Nurs. 14*(3):175–182. doi:10.1111/wvn.12223

Kleinpell, R. M. 2017. *Outcome Assessment in Advanced Practice Nursing, Fourth Edition* (Vol. Fourth edition). New York, NY: Springer Publishing Company.

Kohn, L. T., Corrigan, J. and Donaldson, M. S. (2000). To err is human: Building a safer health system. Washington, D. C.: National Academy Press.

Linthicum, B. O. (2018). Improving emergency department throughput by adoption of an admissions predictor tool at triage (Order No. 10786495). Available from ProQuest Dissertations & Theses Global. (2058749769).

LiVolsi, K. (2018). Improving neonatal outcomes through the implementation of a delayed bathing program (Order No. 10823295). Available from ProQuest Dissertations & Theses Global. (2046938441).

McCoy, T. L. (2018). *Implementing high-fidelity simulation to meet undergraduate clinical requirements* (Order No. 10814662). Available from ProQuest Dissertations & Theses Global. (2124443522).

Melnyk, B. M. (2013). Distinguishing the preparation and roles of doctor of philosophy and doctor of nursing practice graduates: National implications for academic curricula and health care systems. *Journal of Nursing Education, 52*(8), 442e448.

Millwater, T. L. (2015). *Effects of human patient simulation on communication skills among nursing students* (Order No. 3707300). Available from ProQuest Dissertations & Theses Global. (1696055111).

Ortega, H. E. (2018). *Female obesity an evidence-based program for wic participants.* Available through the Doctor of Nursing Practice Project Repository. https://www.doctorsofnursingpractice.org/project-repository-details/?postid=196

National League for Nursing. (2016). Accreditation standards for nursing education programs. Retrieved from: http://www.nln.org/docs/default-source/accreditation-services/cnea-standards-final-february-201613f2bf5c78366c709642ff00005f0421.pdf?sfvrsn=12

National Research Council (US) Committee for Monitoring the Nation's Changing Needs for Biomedical, Behavioral, and Clinical Personnel. (2005). *Advancing the nation's health needs: NIH research training programs.* Washington, DC: National Academies Press. Retrieved from http://www.ncbi.nlm.nih.gov/books/NBK22631/

Nilsen, P., Making sense of implementation theories, models, and frameworks. *Implement Sci.* 2015; Apr 21:10:53. doi: 10.1186/s13012-015-0242-0

Redman, R. W., Pressler, S. J., Furspan, P. and Potempa, K. (2015). Nurses in the United States with a practice doctorate: Implications for leading in the current context of health care. *Nursing Outlook, 63*(2), 124–129. https://doi-org.chamberlainuniversity.idm.oclc.org/10.1016/j.outlook.2014.08.003

Russell, J. A., Lemming-Lee, S. and Watters, R. (in press). Implementation of a nurse-driven CAUTI prevention algorithm. *Nurs Clin N Am.* (2018). https://doi.org/10.1016/j.cnur.2018.11.001

Salmond, S. W. and Echevarria, M. (2017). Healthcare transformation and changing roles for nursing. *Orthopedic Nursing, 36*(1), 12–25. https://doi-org.chamberlainuniversity.idm.oclc.org/10.1097/NOR.0000000000000308

Sebach, A. and Chunta, K. (2018). Exploring the experiences of dnp-prepared nurses enrolled in a dnp-to-phd pathway program. *Nursing Education Perspectives, 39*(5):302–304.

Threatt, R. M. C. (2017). *Incorporating caring competencies in the academic setting through simulation* (Order No. 10258377). Available from ProQuest Dissertations & Theses Global. (1914681570).

Titler, M. G. (2018). Translation research in practice: An introduction. *OJIN: The Online Journal of Issues in Nursing, 23*(2), Manuscript 1.

Titler, M.G. (2014). Overview of evidence-based practice and translation science. *Nursing Clinics of North America, 49*(3), 269–274. doi:10.1016/j.cnur.2014.05.001

Trautman, D. E., Idzik, S., Hammersla, M. and Rosseter, R. (2018). Advancing scholarship through translational research: The Role of PhD and DNP prepared nurses. *Online Journal of Issues in Nursing, 23*(2), 1. https://doi-org.chamberlainuniversity.idm.oclc.org/10.3912/OJIN.Vol23No02Man02

Waldrop, J. (2017). Are nurse practitioners with a doctor of nursing practice degree making a difference in health care? *Journal for Nurse Practitioners, 13*(4), 13.

Whitaker-Brown, C. D., Woods, S. J., Cornelius, J. B., Southard, E. and Gulati, S. K. (2016). Improving quality of life and decreasing readmissions in heart failure patients in a multidisciplinary transition-to-care clinic. *Heart & Lung, 46*, 79–84.

CHAPTER 18

Words of Wisdom (Comments to Support the Students)

MARY BEMKER, PhD, RN, CNE

NICHOLAS GREEN, DNP, RN, Alumnus CCRN

Having overseen and taught in a Doctor of Nursing Practice (DNP) program for a number of years, students have repeatedly stated they wish they knew in the beginning what they had discovered by the end of the project. Therefore, this chapter will include a general overview of key requests for clarity regarding the DNP project. In addition, words of wisdom from successful DNP learners are offered as a first-hand perspective of what these DNP prepared nurses wished they had known prior to starting their DNP project.

The first piece of information often requested is what exactly is a DNP project and how do I successfully complete one? The DNP project is an overarching term that offers a student the ability to demonstrate her or his skills in the key areas of DNP education. Typically, it is focused on a problem or topic area within the student's advanced nursing specialty. As described in Chapter 1 of this book, specialty areas focus upon a specific clinical area (neonatology, emergency department/acute care). In addition, earners can obtain a DNP with a specialization in education or leadership.

Within each of these areas, the project may translate evidence into practice, focus on a quality improvement initiative, evaluation of a new practice model, or a consultation project. Regardless of what an individual chooses as an advanced focus area or type of project actualized, the DNP project synthesizes evidence from the DNP educational experience (didactic and experiential) and utilizes this knowledge toward investigating a practice (education, leadership, or clinical focused) based problem within nursing or healthcare. As indicated previously in this

345

text, it is imperative that students are able to justify the topic is relevant to nursing/healthcare, has a wealth of research that provides a solid underpinning for the project, and has the potential to have a positive impact on nursing practice.

The true experts in relation to the DNP project are those who have successfully completed and mastered the skillset needed to be a DNP. It is as much the overall process that makes one have a paradigm shift regarding nursing and healthcare as any one experience or knowledge gleaned. If this were not the case, students could be given a set of texts and articles, told to read them, and then be assigned a DNP degree. Therefore, to assist the student with the overall project experience, the following "words of wisdom" are offered by nurses who successfully navigate the DNP waters and are practicing at an advanced level within nursing.

As a student working towards their Doctor of Nursing Practice (DNP), it is important to allow yourself time to grow and develop as a student. The journey you have chosen to embark on will have its share of stressful moments. However, the path you have chosen to pursue is one which will open numerous doors in your ability to not only affect current practice but also mold the future of healthcare.

As you transition through your courses required and work on your deliverable project to successfully complete the terminal degree it is important to remember the difference in pursuing a DNP versus those who choose to pursue a Ph.D. As a DNP student, your objective is to focus on a project which will implement change through evidenced-based practice. In short, the person who has obtained their Ph.D. establishes scholarly work through the development and execution of quantitative or qualitative research. The role of the DNP prepared nurse is to take the findings of the Ph.D. prepared individual and disseminate those findings into the clinical arena. It is important to remember this distinction as numerous DNP students find themselves falling into the research trap due to not having a clear understanding of the differences between the two terminal degrees.

You must now take the time to fully understand the steps provided to you during your education. It is best to keep open communication with the faculty as they are the individuals who are assisting you in developing a conceptual idea into something deliverable. What may seem like obvious tips have been found to sideline many students as they find themselves struggling to keep up with the demands of a DNP program.

Lastly, it is important to remember the road traveled does lead to a final destination. When it seems as though the task at hand seems overwhelming, remember you have chosen to take the step in touching the profession through understanding, knowledge, and selfless acts which comprise the core essence of what it means to be a nurse.

GERLYN CAMPBELL, DNP, APRN, PMHNP, RN

The role of a DNP defines not only the students' academic accomplishments, but also the nursing profession. As a past doctoral candidate, there are many tools which can help to make the arduous accomplishment of a doctorate more inviting. Some of these include the student's willingness to connect with fellow students and professors, entering the program with a project focus in mind, and having a passion for their assigned topic of interest, as well as being well versed in conducting research and appraising evidence. The essence of the DNP degree not only encapsulates the true enigma of nursing education, but also promotes a basis for higher standards of care.

Upon entering the program, students can expect to commit between 25 and 40 hours of weekly effort to ensure successful project completion. Working closely with one's academic adviser and project mentor is also invaluable. Students who shy away from asking questions might find themselves struggling in this area, especially as the topic and approaches of the DNP project require advanced knowledge for successful coordination and academic aptitude. A review of statistical measures is also invaluable throughout most phases of the project, to help ensure proper testing and credible analysis of one's data. All of these elements are critical to building a strong infrastructure for project success. Lastly, many students tend to struggle in the areas of balancing family life and school, which calls for the need for proper time management and dedication. Appropriate time management and prioritization skills are also optimal in meeting project guidelines. Once the student embraces a spirit of academic wellness, the factors mentioned above will assist in making the project phase eagerly meaningful and rewarding. Apart from the blossoming of one's profession, successful candidates also become more recognized in their mission toward helping to improve the human phenomena of care.

OBED ASIF, DNP, RN

My student journey during the DNP Leadership Program began soon after registering in the summer term of 2017. The DNP program at the university where I attended is a unique school, because it is based on Judaic values. This was important to me, as one of my needs was for flexibility in my school schedule with the observance of the Sabbath, which begins Fridays at sunset and goes through Saturday at sunset. As the DNP program started, I failed to notice the fast pace we were expected to follow. Being accepted into the program close to the start date of courses meant I didn't have enough time to explore the program syllabus in a timely fashion. This meant that I was lacking in knowledge related to the program's expectations and course timelines.

During the first week of school, there was a lot of study material to review. I spent many hours trying to learn and understand various functions of Blackboard navigation, use of the semester calendars, review of course and program objectives, and overall acclimation to various other required components linked to the program. Even though portal features were well organized, it appeared I needed more time to learn the usual functions within the portal that were specific to this program. It took me awhile to steer through all of the available content and to understand the timelines for course requirements. Later, toward the end of the program, I learned some of the other classmates faced similar types of portal navigation challenges. I wished I had attended the orientation before the start of this program. A mandatory orientation via phone/zoom collaboration between a potential DNP student and project course professor, prior to starting the DNP program, would definitely help the student. This type of orientation could prepare the student for immediate timelines and expectations, especially with portal log-in and course templates (Hande, Beuscher, and Phillippi, 2017).

The program syllabus is designed to identify and describe the DNP courses, as well as the DNP Scholarly Project. This program overview reflects the progression and required courses over the entire length of the program (American Nurses Association, 2014). Before the courses started, I felt as though I would be fine, but within the first two weeks I began to feel unaccomplished and exhausted. Every new course had something to be submitted "yesterday." Understanding the rubrics was a nightmare. With the pressure of timelines and fear of losing points, my level of frustration and disappointment raised quickly. I wished if I could ask someone, "What are they asking us to do for these particular assignments?" In the agonizing hours, I felt as though I was disorganized. I feared I had fallen behind on assignments and the submission timelines. The time constraints with reading assignments were too hasty. I was continuing to get less organized, and my performance outcome was becoming unproductive.

Through these frustrating moments, I wished for additional help and guidance, but from where? Various questions arose dashing through my mind in late hours of the night. "What should I do? "Maybe I should send an email to the professor? My concern was that it would, and what if the course professor thinks I am so dull that I can't understand simple instructions?" In my hesitation, I didn't reach out but tried to satisfy my concerns. Until this time, I always thought people joked around when referring to busy individuals as multitaskers. I quickly found out that was not true, as I found myself multitasking between assignments.

Through many sleepless hours, a slew of unusual physical symptoms accompanied this insomnia. I noted that I was anxious, experienced racing heartbeat, and projected shallow breathing. I felt a lot of frustration and felt mild pressure on the left side of my chest. I began losing weight without dieting. I got nervous about these physical symptoms, and I made an appointment with my Primary Care Physician. They ran tests and an EKG, upon my request, which all turned out to be clear. I began treatment for my lack of sleep by taking over the counter relaxants, but they would stop working after a few doses, then sleepless hours again began to pile up as I thought about my weekly assignments. As a daily routine, I would plan for two to three-course submissions and meet requirements to fulfillment assignment timelines.

Often, I wished I could talk to someone who was going through similar experience as to what I was going through. I noticed I had access to other students' email addresses, but I didn't know if my program allowed direct communication with them. During my second week into the program, I had bad feedback on one of my assignments. It was not good; all night I was awake worried, thinking this program is hard. I came to a conclusion this program was not meant for me, and I decided I was going to drop the program. I briefly discussed my decision with my family as they saw me going through a rough start. They advised me that I should first discuss this decision with my professor; they also recommended that I email my classmates to see if anyone want to connect and help each other out. With that in mind, I sent an email to my professor and some classmates. I heard back from one classmate right away. Fortunately, the student lived in the same state yet at a fair amount of distance. Although this student was not assigned in the same group as I was, the student was very positive and supportive. We exchanged our contact information and later three more students connected with me. During the program, we tried to encourage and support each other. It was a tremendous help to me, and things began to shift toward success.

Weekly Virtual Meetings with my Professor

As I made a final decision to drop the program right away, I still prayed and sent an email to my first-semester professor Dr. MB. We discussed my situation based on my assignment results, and my physical symptoms, and then I shared my final decision of dropping the DNP program. The professor began with sharing personal experiences as well and what coping strategies were helpful for her and other students. The professor encouraged me to try each strategy and broke it down to what I should do and when I should do it. Since I had been out of school for a while, my worst nightmare was grammar and sentence structure. The professor provided me with tools and resources, and the support especially from the student support department at the university became my number one resource in dealing with these issues. I learned to work ahead on my assignments and summit them for editing, proofing, etc., before final submission to the course.

I made sure that I spoke to my professors every week, because the help was real and essential to succeed in the DNP program. I Zoomed my professor every week and experienced gradual progress in my overall success. Each time I spoke to the professor, I gained additional knowledge, ideas, and information, which led me toward academic success. I began to use various strategies that helped to calm my nerves, such as relaxing music at bedtime. Student professor collaboration once a week was a key tool in my success.

What Did I Learn at the Completion of the DNP Program?

The American Association Colleges of Nursing (AACN) Position Statement on the Practice Doctorate in Nursing (AACN, 2004) transformed the course of nursing education by advocating that advanced nursing practice education is progressed to the doctoral level (AACN, 2006). The national dialogue about the DNP has strengthened the need to clarify and restate how advanced nursing practice is defined. Advanced nursing practice is any form of nursing intervention that influences healthcare outcomes for individuals or populations, including the provision of direct care or organization of care for individual patients or management of care populations, and the provision of indirect care such as nursing administration, executive leadership, health policy, informatics, and population health. Also, it is important to remember that the DNP is an academic degree, not a role (AACN, 2004).

The DNP leadership program where I attended is an outstanding program. As a graduate of this program, I plan to continue working at my current position but participate effectively in the current health organization with policy updates and quality improvement processes. The key to success during the DNP program is to develop frequent communication with the course professors. As a student, one must know and learn about the available resources and tools and helpful hints and ideas. During group immersion assignments, I was able to pursue a successful outcome in this academic arena. A DNP student may seek peer interaction to enhance learning through activities such as collaborating and synthesizing evidence, discussing issues regarding project implementation, team communication, access to or gathering data, and outcome evaluation methods (Commission on Collegiate Nursing Education, 2013). It is also important to develop a DNP student toolkit with information regarding such topics as requirements, available resources, timelines, scholarly writing, and publishing guidelines.

JAYANTHI HENRY, DNP, MSNCH, MSNIPC, GNEd, RN-BC, CIC

I consider this question an important one. I am a foreign educated graduate. I have completed my basic Bachelor of Science in Nursing (BSN) in India in 1979 and a Master of Nursing in Community Health in 2004. I migrated to the United States (U.S.) in 2006 with my family. I had to start all over on the medical surgical floor. In 2009, I did the credential evaluation, and my Master of Science in Nursing (MSN) credentials showed that I had a 4.0 GPA, then I started clinical and lab for the PN and ADN students. I had a plan to do a doctorate in nursing and wanted to experience the online education system. In India, it was a traditional education program combined with clinical practice, and most of the classroom seminars were led by the MSN students as part of the MSN program. I earned an online post masters nursing education certificate in 2012 at Kaplan University and an online Master of Nursing in Infection Control in 2015 at the American Sentinel University.

When I started the application for the DNP program at Touro University, the response was quick. But the credentials to be submitted before the start of the program. As a foreign educated student, I wanted at least six to eight weeks' time to get the credentials from India; when I requested it was granted. As a DNP student, I wished I had known the sequence of all the classes, and I realize that there was very clear information about all the semesters and the classes were opened early for the students to plan effectively.

I had a very good peer group who were supportive of each other and all the online discussions went on with great learning. I wanted to know about the off days and the time to submit the assignments. The information that I wished to know was announced earlier so that I could start the Institutional Review Board (IRB) requirements earlier before the start of the third semester. I got kudos from my professor that "You were the first one to come out of the crack pot." That helped me to start the data collection on time. I had a group of ED registered nurses and a group of ED physicians to interview, but everything went on well within the given time frame. I want to say, I got an answer for all my questions when I went through the program.

COLLEEN CROSBY, DNP, MSN, RN BC-NE

Returning to college to pursue my DNP degree was a big decision for me. I had completed my master's degree in the 1990s. It is a very different world now. Reflecting on my doctoral program, I would say I had supportive instructors who helped guide me when I didn't understand an assignment. I had a variety of nursing experiences, extending back 35 years, that I was able to utilize to complete assignments and respond to my classmates and instructors in a knowledgeable manner on Blackboard. I utilized many resources from the university where I obtained my DNP degree, including instructors, the library, other students in my class, former DNP students, and colleagues for support and guidance in completing assignments. Early on, I hired an editor to review my papers; this was the best thing I did. I also hired a statistician to help me determine what data to collect, what tests to use, how best to utilize SPSS software, and how to interpret SPSS analysis. This was invaluable, and I would recommend all DNP students strongly consider this.

I encountered many obstacles along the way while completing my DNP degree program. First, my computer skills were lacking. I had never heard of Blackboard, let alone used it. I hadn't used American Psychological Association (APA) formatting for 17 years and the Mac computer I had was not working properly and had to be replaced. I had to learn how to use the online university library and related resources. Generally, my instructors were patient, helping me deal with obstacles. I had a prolonged and gradual learning curve. One of my biggest frustrations this past year was a PowerPoint presentation I completed and had to redo, because the instructor felt it did not meet all necessary requirements. I learned a valuable lesson: ask for instructor clarification if you have uncertainty about expectations for an assignment. Also, I did not initially understand how a rubric works; however, once I did, I unswervingly kept a printed copy next to me when doing an assignment or writing a paper.

Finally, instructors could alleviate somewhat the inherent stress felt by future DNP students if they acknowledged that not all the students are at the same level of computer literacy. I really struggled, especially the first few months, with a variety of computer issues. I lacked experience with a lot of the computer software: Word, Excel, PowerPoint, Blackboard, SPSS, and CINAL raised a variety of challenges I did not anticipate. That was stressful, especially when instructions seemed unclear, inconsistent, or inaccurate. Occasionally, instructions stated one thing in one place, but something unexpectedly different in another; more attention to consistency across the platform would be helpful to students balancing busy professional lives and a rigorous academic program. That instructor attention would likely also result in fewer subsequent student requests for interpretation.

Also, group assignments can be tricky, working with classmates in different time zones and with different schedules. Students need to set clear expectations for one another, especially regarding individual responsibility and timelines. Inherent differences in work ethic or desire to excel among students can cause frustration for everybody in a group. Group assignments are necessary on the one hand because they build collaborative skills, a core competency of the profession, but on the other hand they give rise to a host of interpersonal frustrations. Finally, instructors need to foreground open communication with students and respond to communications promptly when students seek clarification.

Most students are juggling full-time employment, family obligations, and academic work. When students are in possession of the information they need to complete assignments properly earlier, rather than later, they find it easier to maintain that balance without altering work schedules or frustrating family members who have their own needs. All of this makes for better student retention, less stress for students, and greater esteem for the program.

STACI HARRISON, DNP, RN

Beginning a DNP educational journey can be a daunting and overwhelming experience. There are many things to consider. All universities have criteria that require a certain number of hours for degree completion. Where will you obtain those hours? Many students assume their respective place of employment will suffice; however, this assumption may not always work in your favor. Prior to starting your terminal degree, you should investigate if your workplace and university have a relationship that would allow you to obtain the hours. It is also important to identify who you will have as your mentor(s); it is critical to make connections early and communicate frequently with your designated mentor(s). Most importantly, take your terminal degree one step at a time, and don't forget to breathe.

SELENA A. GILLES, DNP, ANP-BC, CNEcl, CCRN

In reflecting on my own journey, I often think about the things that I wish I knew as a DNP student. I knew that embarking on a doctoral degree was not going to be easy; however, I didn't anticipate the mental stamina that it would take. In fact, it was the toughest academic experience I have ever had. I underestimated how truly intense the program would be. Prior to embarking on my journey, I didn't know anyone who had previously completed a DNP program and was not really sure what to expect. I wish someone would have instilled in me the importance of having an external mentor who could guide and support me. I was confident that I had the will to succeed, but there were several points through my program that I was unsure if I would make it. I think having someone in my corner who had experienced being in a DNP program would have helped me feel more prepared and equipped to handle the intensity. I wish I would have been better at managing my time and that someone would have told me to prioritize my self care. I would get so caught up in my work schedule and work so hard to do well in school that I would forget to take moments to breathe and decompress. Despite it all, I learned a lot along the way and I'm a better and stronger person, nurse, and educator because of it.

AUDREY SUTTON, DNP, RN

First, being accepted into a DNP program is an exciting time for one wishing to obtain a DNP degree. In my personal journey, it was difficult being an older student and working full time while I returned to a university for this advanced degree. It was easy to articulate my thoughts, but putting them in perfect APA format was a challenge. An APA refresher course would have been a great support if taken just prior to starting this program.

Secondly, it would be helpful to have a student mentor early in the program. Someone who can assist the student with narrowing down the DNP project, talking through pros and cons of topic areas, and sharing their experiences with the new DNP student could offset additional work and repel any anxiety a student might have about this. One of the complaints I heard from fellow students was, "I wish someone would have told me my project idea would be difficult to implement." That is something important to consider when selecting your project. Personally, the biggest challenge for me was finding a practicum site that was affiliated with the university where I attended for my DNP degree. Furthermore, spending months working on getting my clinical practicum approved only, to have my project rejected due to my work title was a major setback. Make sure you have a "Plan B" and even a "Plan C" in case something comes along to alter.

In my case, I contacted a women's health clinic and inquired about their Code Blue and team builder training. It was a surprise to learn the staff did not routinely practice Code Blue training or team building exercises. The clinic owners were very excited to have someone come in and provide education/training to the staff. The opportunity left a lasting impression on my journey to become a DNP prepared nurse. The opportunity to educate the staff on why Code Blue training and team building exercises are so important when considering improving patient care. Team building exercises create a positive and conducive work environment and can assist with staff retention and support overall quality patient care.

Consider meeting early with your academic advisor and/or student mentor. A weekly connection via phone conversation or video chat can do much to keep a student on track when developing, implementing, and evaluating the DNP project. The rationale for this action is to receive continuous feedback regarding his or her progress and/or to discuss any issues that are presenting themselves.

It has been my experience that many older students returning to college or university feel embarrassed about asking for help. Therefore, many drop out of the program early due to feeling overwhelmed. A good example of this is many DNP cohorts will start out with a group of 20 students, but by graduation there may be 10 left that completed. If this happens to you, reach out as soon as you are aware of these feelings. Almost everyone has these feelings at some point in the process, and your faculty do not think less of you for asking questions and staying on top of things.

REFERENCES

American Association of Colleges of Nursing. 2004. *AACN position statement on the practice doctorate in nursing.* Washington, DC: American Association of Colleges of Nursing.

American Association of Colleges of Nursing. 2006. *The essentials of doctoral education for advanced nursing practice.* Washington, DC: American Association of Colleges of Nursing. http://www.aacn.nche.edu/publications/position/DNPEssentials.pdf

American Nurses Association. (2014). *Nursing informatics: Scope and standards of practice* (2nd ed.). Washington, DC: Author.

Commission on Collegiate Nursing Education, (2013) *Standards for accreditation of baccalaureate and graduate nursing programs.* Retrieved from http://www.aacn.nche.edu/ccne-accreditation/Standards-Amended-2013.pdf

Hande, K. Karen. a. hande@vanderbilt. ed., Beuscher, L., Allison, T., & Phillippi, J. (2017). Navigating DNP student needs: Faculty advising competencies and effective strategies for development and support. *Nurse Educator, 42*(3), 147–150. https://doi.org/10.1097/NNE.0000000000000332

Understanding the Collaboration Between the Professor and Student for Successful DNP Project Completion

LINA NAJIB KAWAR, PhD, RN, CNS

STACI HARRISON, DNP, RN

INTRODUCTION

One of the most important aspects of the Doctor of Nursing Practice (DNP) project is finding and collaborating with a mentor. The mentor is the individual who will guide, direct, and support the DNP student's clinical experiences. Without the connections, insights, and support of a professional where the student is conducting the DNP project, the student could have a more difficult time in obtaining the right experiences and completing the DNP project in a timely manner.

CHOOSING YOUR MENTOR

Many choose their mentor based on convenience or because the potential mentor is likable. Although those are reputable considerations, others also need to be addressed. Is the mentor, for example, someone with the education and experience needed to support the DNP student in receiving the needed experiences to be an expert in the area of his or her DNP project?

Some have chosen mentors because of the mentors' professional reputation, only to find that the individual was not a good fit for them. Unrealistic requests, inability to communicate effectively, and lack of time are but a few of the reasons identified that can extend a DNP student's completion of his or her project.

Beside the mentor's knowledge, experience, and competences, the DNP candidate has to ponder the mentor qualities, such as effective communication/good listening skills, patience, advocacy, patience,

357

constructive criticism/feedback, enthusiasm, respect, and empowerment.

An important issue worth mentioning is if the mentor is a PhD prepared individual, the mentor has to consider the DNP project and advise the student accordingly. It is easy to take a detour and guide the DNP student based on the familiar research process. Separation between mentoring PhD candidates is different than DNP candidates. The research study rules do not apply to DNP projects. To consider what one might want to consider when selecting a mentor, the following looks at the DNP project experience from the mentee and mentor perspectives. Much can be determined from considering this experience from the "eyes" of those who successfully navigated these roles.

SCHOOL SELECTION

When considering schools for a DNP program, it is essential to also look for a mentor. According to Merriam-Webster's collegiate dictionary, the definition of a mentor is "an experienced and trusted adviser" (Merriam-Webster Dictionary, n.d.). A mentor is also one who promotes independence and growth by creating an environment that fosters creativity and confidence. Thus, mentorship is a complex and vibrant relationship between two individuals in which the more experienced, skilled, or knowledgeable individual helps to guide the less experienced, skilled, or knowledgeable individual. Age is not a factor in determining this relationship. Mentors may be older or younger than the person being mentored; however, mentors are specialists in an area of expertise that supports the mentees in their academic or professional progression. The relationship is learning based and a development partnership between the individual who exhibits the extensive experience and someone who desires to grow in the specialty. The collaboration and partnership between the two parties is necessary to equip the mentee with the specific filed competencies.

According to Wiemer (2019), this relationship should occur naturally and should not be forced. One may want to think about the following: What are the potential mentors' interests outside of their professional world? What types of things do they enjoy? Are these similar to yours? To your project interests? Also, you will want to be open and transparent in sharing some personal things with your mentor. The goal is to make a personal and professional connection with your mentor. This relationship may last a lifetime.

MENTORING

Mentoring is an active developmental collaboration involving two individuals. The two parties usually share the same background or have something common between them. The main goal of this relationship is to help the mentee grow professionally. On the other hand, the mentor is the expert who desires to provide guidance, insights, and provision with the intention to help the mentee grow both professionally and personally.

Mentorship purposes vary. Mainly mentoring is used to develop the mentee professionally; however, this dynamic can be used to help mentees learn an organization, institution, or company roles and practices. Also, a mentor can help the mentee build lifelong professional relationships with colleagues and other specialists. Sometimes, the relationship could develop with well-known colleagues in the profession. Following is related to a DNP student mentorship.

The mentorship relationship starts upon the mentee requests to be mentored by the designated preceptor followed by both the mentor mentee agreement. The agreement could be written or verbal. Typically, the relationship is formal and highly specified when a DNP project is involved. Often times, not only do the mentor and mentee enter into a written agreement with each other and the university, but also the hosting organization may request an agreement with the mentee and the university.

Regardless of the format, commitment is guaranteed when a mentor and mentee agree to a relationship. It is always best for one to have the freedom to select his or her own mentor. Choosing the mentor is beneficial and usually leads to favorable outcomes.

This reciprocated relationship is time limited and can be summarized into three structured phases (Guidelines to the Stages of the Mentoring Relationship), including the following:

1. Selection phase
2. Engagement phase
3. Closure phase

What is the Mentor?

A mentor is a content expert who is an experienced and trusted counselor. Other terms to describe a mentor are used interchangeably with mentor are preceptor (Walker *et al.,* 2012); counselor or guide (Glynn *et al.,* 2017); or lead, tutor, and/or coach. Some of those expressions are context related; e.g., preceptor could be more to helping the mentee build skills. On the other hand, couch might align more with physical activity training and tend to focus upon a one to one relationship that does not involve organizational input or collaboration.

A mentor is also one who promotes independence and growth by creating an environment that fosters creativity and confidence. Why is this important? One may recall having mentors who have guided one through his or her career, but what is the importance of a mentor who will guide the student through a terminal degree program? Mentors in general have special characteristics that qualify them to take on this role. Those qualities are pivotal to thriving interaction, such as calmness, patience, approachable, listener, passionate, compassionate, and motivated (Gidman *et al.*, 2011; McIntosh, Gidman, and Smith, 2014) and supportive, confident, and available. Also, mentors are experts in the content area and exhibit a holistic perspective on the subject. Part of their responsibilities are to facilitate the learning process and maturation of the mentee. The above-mentioned qualities are inviting and vital to a successful mentoring relationship. According to Smith (2018), mentors usually have a similar set of experiences, and they help guide the mentee through life, a system, or organization. The mentee and mentor must build a relationship, not just a professional relationship, but also a personal one, which would be helpful on this journey.

Mentors act as advisers and advocates who work to guide mentees in the appropriate direction. In response to the set goals, the mentor keeps redirecting and keeps the mentee in line to achieve the desired goals. Mentors are usually more visionary; they support the mentee throughout a program or project. They share their knowledge and expertise to advise and recommend modalities and modifications to strengthen the project. Mentors use the appropriate opportunity to tutor on topics related to the discussed subject. Also, they provide feedback to advance and progress a specific project. Mentors offer advice on behavioral issues that aim at mentees' professional growth and progress.

Choosing a Mentor (Choosing the Team)

Choosing a mentor is part of the selection phase and a critical as well as delicate process. After the DNP student decides on the topic, the student can start a list of possible mentors' names. The list gathers names of experts in the area who are qualified to lead the student in the right direction. The mentor could be a person who the student knows, from before he or she begins the DNP program, through work or school. Also, a possible mentor could be a specialist's name garnered from reading specialty articles or an expert recommended to the student by fellow colleagues. If one is not familiar with the experts in the field, solicit advice from leaders and clinicians in the area.

Next meet the individual to learn if he or she is willing to work with you and support your goals. Additionally, it is important to think critically if this individual is good fit for you and if you can work with him or her. Ask yourself if the relationship is going to be productive. Is it what you were looking for? If you have any hesitation, approach the next person on the list. Mentors should not be forced on you. However, keep in mind that you are the novice at this level and will be feeling out of your comfort zone working with any preceptor.

Committee Member Selection

As you secure the preceptor, think of the other committee members. For your success and progress of your project, it is very important to have committee members that work together well. Consider and investigate if the potential committee members have friendly collegial relationships and that there is no friction in the relationships among them. Cohesiveness between the committee members helps your progress. If you are not sure of how well the mentor works with the other potential members, then ask the mentor. Harmony among the different members helps avoid delays in moving forward. Keep in mind that the mentor can suggest other colleagues with whom the mentor has good relationship.

Responsibilities of the Mentor and Committee

The mentor is committed to help the mentee to advance professionally. Therefore, the preceptor needs to familiarize himself or herself and understand the requirements of the DNP project being undertaken. If the mentor has experience with projects or dissertations, he or she will need to familiarize himself or herself with the DNP project and how it differs from these other means of evaluating competence for graduate nurses. It is a priority to read and discuss with the mentor the instructions provided by the syllabus and address the details necessary for consideration. The mentor keeps the student focused and refers the mentee to the syllabus to help in meeting the DNP project requirements.

The mentor keeps the mentee focused, especially when a subtopic looks attractive to divert the mentee attention. Time is limited and critical in this relationship. Mentors should be aware and respectful of the timeline; therefore, the mentor is responsible to keep the mentee concentrating, especially if the mentee goes on a tangent. A vital responsibility is to maintain the quality of work that adds to the nursing science and practice. Quality is not determined by the quantity, such as length of the product or time spent on the project; it is related to using precise understandable language to communicate the findings.

Mentors are role models that mentees try to mimic professionally. They are not teachers, therapists, or personal coaches. The time the mentor and mentee spend together should be used efficiently. It is not time to ventilate or complain about other factors, such as individuals, requirements, or the work environment. Mentors should avoid dominating the conversation; both need to be involved and engaged. Mentors have to provide safe environments and allow time for questions and answers. Also, they need to maintain confidentiality. A positive mentoring experience can affect the student's decisions and might contribute to creating a new successful mentor.

Mentorship Strategies

Mentors adapt different approaches during this profitable interaction, engagement phase. The main strategy is to create a respectful trustworthy relationship. Although the student is a novice at this point, respecting the student's feelings and what he or she offers is crucial. Students are emerging colleagues and professionalism should be the essence of this relationship (Jokelainen *et al.,* 2011). Professional relationships are civil interactions based on setting boundaries. However, leave room for personal visitation, for some time if needed. It is important to build caring supportive association (McIntosh, Gidman, and Smith, 2014).

Appropriate communication crowns every flourishing interaction. Use clear open communication throughout the engagement (Flott and Linden, 2016). Mentors need to provide specific direct instructions. This includes constructive feedback that helps advance the project and collaborations. Be sensitive to the student's needs and goals. Also consider the student's learning style. Mentors must be respectful and sensitive to the fact that people's comprehensions vary. Mentees' readiness differs; some individuals might need longer times to process the materials or instructions.

Make appointments for structured regular in person meetings with set agendas. In collaboration with the mentee, concentrate on the short-term goals that correspond with the respective agenda. This time is geared toward goal-oriented mentoring. Do your homework in advance and come prepared to lead a reflective dialog on the subject during the meeting. Meetings should reflect quality time of cogent debates (Hilli *et al.*, 2014). This is the time to problem solve and negotiate changes and revise.

Other tactics that might serve you well include taking notes. Notes keeps you tuned and help you assist in producing the agenda. Although it is the student's responsibility to prepare the agenda and find the place and time of meeting, notes act as a reference to the task at hand. Reflection during mentoring is necessary and can help both sides evaluate self and the interactions (Tuomikoski *et al.*, 2018). Encouragement goes a long way and reflects on the student experience positively. Always find something the mentee did that you can praise. Start your feedback positively, than deliver critiques or requests.

Moreover, keep humor as part of your interactions. Humor tends to reduce stress and provides a pleasant feeling. It changes the mood and helps ease frustrations. Transparency and sharing own experiences could be valuable in showing the mentee that you are human and you had some struggles; however, you achieved the desired goals. Your experiences can help the student learn new skills and apply them in real life. It helps the student realize that working hard pays off and leads to satisfaction.

Accountability is expected from both sides. Mentors are responsible to assist mentees in identifying their own needs and to compose corresponding SMART goals. Also, mentors observe and guide the mentees' progress in reaching their proposed learning outcomes. On the other hand, mentees need to understand that they have to work hard through their programs to attain their personal goals. To have conducive outcomes, both parties have to stay objective and leave their feelings out. The mentors have to recognize these are not personal projects and to stay focused on the mentees' goals. The mentees have to understand that DNP projects are just learning exercises, not life-long projects. Maturity of the mentees is expected, especially when the reviews are back; it is the students who fail or pass, not the faculty.

At the end of the mentorship, a final meeting needs to happen. During this time, a closure phase, evaluation, and reflection on the progress may take place. Reflections on how the experience was, what was learned, and the adjustments that could have been made to make this interaction better. Both parties need to ask each other for feedback (peer to peer feedback) to enhance future mentorship relations. Consider what worked, what did not work, and what worked well in the process to achieve the expected outcomes.

Evaluate and rate the set goals. Ponder if goals were met, unmet, or partially met. Are there new goals that evolved as a result of this interaction? Is there a need for further mentorship? If future mentoring is needed, then the cycle will start over. Upon mutual decision to continue the interaction, a new agreement is required. If goals are met, the mentorship could grow to a friendship or becomes a lifelong collegial relationship. After all, the mentor had invested in your success.

Our Story

Before selecting my mentor, I pondered a series of questions to ask my prospective mentor. I also thought about what I had to offer a mentor and what I would need from a mentor. There was a checklist of what I needed in a mentor: published author and speaker, organized, approachable, altruistic, and well respected in the profession. Being a published author and international speaker would let me know the person was well rounded and had determination and persistence. Having a mentor who had been published or was an international speaker was important to me, because these were things to which I aspired. A transformational leader with organizational skills allowed me to know this person would pay attention to my goals and guide me in areas in which I needed to develop. There are other characteristics that you may want to consider when looking for a mentor, such as empathy, communication skills, emotional intelligence, accessibility, and dependability and whether the mentor is an expert in his or her area. It is important to have a mentor who encourages the use of critical thinking skills to enhance personal and/or professional growth.

Pursuing an advanced degree and working can be an emotional rollercoaster. When you want to jump off the ride, your mentor will assist in guiding you in the right direction, encouraging you to stay focused, while assisting you with rebuilding confidence. A mentor can envision the big picture of the mentee's terminal degree and set expectations for the mentee. A mentor who is respectful and honest falls in line with transformational leadership. A good mentor listens without trying to solve problems. It is important for your mentor to help you discover your strengths and use those strengths to make difficult choices or decisions. Your mentor should help you discover who you are and what you want and help you identify options to reach your desired goals. A good mentor provides support for change and/or growth. Your educational journey is not your mentor's responsibility alone; you (the student) must take accountability for your own learning.

At the onset, it is imperative to establish good rapport and build a relationship. Be prepared for your mentor to challenge you to think through issues and approaches rather than solving your problems. Use your mentor as a source of wisdom when needed. Set regularly scheduled meetings with your mentor throughout your program. We all have busy work schedules, and life can get in the way. However, setting standing meetings with your mentor will keep you both on task. My mentor would read a chapter and question me on what direction I was trying to go with my writing or if my project was on time. As a mentee, it is essential to be flexible, adaptable, and open to constructive criticism. Being held accountable will help you keep on track, finish assignments, and complete your dissertation. Setting clear expectations for both parties should be outlined (Straus, Chatur, and Taylor, 2009). Have your mentor set clear expectations so there is understanding, and let your mentor know your expectations as a mentee.

Choose your mentor carefully. Consider not picking a close friend to be your mentor unless you can separate friendship from the mentee/mentor relationship; this can be a barrier to the relationship. Open communication and respect for one another must be maintained as well as confidentiality. As I was fortunate to find an outstanding mentor, I wish you the same. Do your homework when searching for a mentor as this experience will offer you life-changing benefits.

REFERENCES

Cowan, M. Mentorship. *Nursing Standard (through 2013)*, 26, no. 31 (2012): 59–60. Accessed December 11, 2018, https://search-proquest-com.contentproxy.phoenix.edu/docview/1000412077?accountid=134061

Dictionary by Merriam-Webster: America's most-trusted online dictionary. (n.d.). Accessed December 11, 2018, https://www.merriam-webster/

Flott, E., Linden, L. (2016). The clinical environment in nursing education: A concept analysis. *Journal of Advance Nursing, 72*(3), 301–313.

Guideline to the stages of the mentoring relationship. Retrieved December 11, 2018. https://womeninmanagement.info/wp-content/uploads/2011/07/Guidelines-to-the-Stages-of-the-Mentoring-Programme3.pdf

Glynn, D.M., Mcvey, C., Wendt, J. and Russel, B. (2017). Dedicated educational nursing Unit: Clinical instruction role perceptions and learning needs. *Journal of Professional Nursing, 33*(2), 108-112.

Hilli, Y., Melender, H., Salmuc, M., and Jonsend, E. (2014). Being a preceptor- a Nordic qualitative study. *Nursing Education Today, 34*(12), 1420–1424.

Jokelainen, M., Turunen, H., Tossavainen, K., Jamookeeah, D., and Coco, K. (2011). A systematic review of mentoring nursing students in clinical placement. *Journal of clinical Nurses, 20*(19–20), 2854–2867.

McIntosh, A., Gidman, J. and Smith, D. (2014). Mentors' perceptions and experiences of supporting students nurses in practice. *International Journal of Nursing Practice, 20*(4), 360–365.

Sattayarakas, T. and Boon-itt, S. (2018). The roles of CEO transformational leadership and organizational factors on product innovation performance. *European Journal of Innovation Management, 21*(2). 227–249. doi:10.1108/EJIM-06-2017-0077

Smith, L. S. (2018). A nurse educator's guide to cultural competence. *Nursing Management (Springhouse), 49*(2), 11–14. doi: 10.1097/01.NUMA.0000529933.83408.06

Straus, S. E., Chatur, F. and Taylor, M. (2009). Issues in the Mentor-Mentee Relationship in Academic Medicine: A Qualitative Study. *Academic Medicine, 84*(1), 135–139. doi:10.1097/ACM.0b013e31819301ab

Tuomikoski, A., Ruotsalainen, H., Mikkonen, K., Miettunen, J. and Maria, K. (2018). The competence of nurse mentors in mentoring students in clinical practice—A cross-sectional study. *Nursing Education today, 71*, 78–83.

Walker, S., Dwyer, T, Moxham, L. and Sander, T., (2012). Facilitator versus Preceptor: Which offers the best support to BN students? *Nurs Educator Today, 33*(5), 530–535.

Weimer, K. R. (2019). Maximizing Mentoring Relationships. *General Music Today, 32*(2), 12. https://doi-org.comtentproxy.phoenix.edu/10.1177/1048371318805226

Index

367